Mental Health

A person-centred approach

Mental Health: A person-centred approach aligns leading mental health research with the human connections that can and should be made in mental health care. It seeks to deepen readers' understanding of themselves, the work they do, and how this intersects with the lives and crises of people with mental health illness.

This book adopts a storytelling approach, which encourages engagement with the lives and needs of consumers and carers in mental health. It has a nursing focus but considers the broader health context and a range of practice settings.

Each chapter features learning objectives, reflective and critical thinking questions, extension activities and further reading. Chapters also include stories of those with direct experience recovering from mental illness, using mental health services or giving mental health support.

Mental Health: A person-centred approach is a comprehensive resource which utilises fresh thinking to support the development of safe, high-quality, person-centred care in both the Australian and New Zealand context.

Nicholas Procter is the University of South Australia's Inaugural Chair: Mental Health Nursing, and convener of the Mental Health and Substance Abuse Research Group, located within the Sansom Institute for Health Research.

Helen P. Hamer is a senior lecturer and nurse consultant in the School of Nursing and the Centre for Mental Health Research at the University of Auckland.

Denise McGarry is a lecturer in mental health in the School of Nursing, Midwifery and Indigenous Health at Charles Sturt University. She is a credentialled mental health nurse and a fellow of the Australian College of Mental Health Nurses.

Rhonda L. Wilson is a mental health nurse lecturer at the University of New England, in New South Wales. She is immediate-past Deputy Chair of the Research Committee for the Australian College of Mental Health Nurses.

Terry Froggatt teaches and coordinates undergraduate subjects and postgraduate courses at the University of Wollongong, in New South Wales. He is a credentialled mental health Nurse, a fellow and board member of the Australian College of Mental Health Nurses.

Mental Health

A person-centred approach

Edited by
Nicholas Procter, Helen P. Hamer, Denise McGarry,
Rhonda L. Wilson and Terry Froggatt

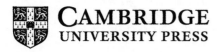

CAMBRIDGE
UNIVERSITY PRESS

477 Williamstown Road, Port Melbourne, VIC 3207, Australia

Published in the United States of America by Cambridge University Press, New York

Cambridge University Press is part of the University of Cambridge.

It furthers the University's mission by disseminating knowledge in the pursuit of education, learning, and research at the highest international levels of excellence.

www.cambridge.org
Information on this title: www.cambridge.org/9781107667723

© Cambridge University Press 2014

First published 2014

Cover designed by Jenny Cowan
Typeset by Integra Software Services Pvt Ltd
Printed in Singapore by C.O.S. Printers Pte Ltd

A catalogue record for this publication is available from the British Library

A Cataloguing-in-Publication entry is available from the catalogue of the National Library of Australia at www.nla.gov.au

ISBN 978-1-107-66772-3 Paperback

Additional resources for this publication at
www.cambridge.edu.au/academic/mentalhealth

Foreword: Carer

Earlier this year I was waiting to turn right at the traffic lights when I suddenly became aware of a young man standing at the pedestrian crossing on the opposite side of the road. I looked again at the handsome face. The blonde hair cut in a style I remember so well. He was wearing blue jeans and a denim jacket. My heart skipped a beat. Once again, the universe had found a way to bring him back to me for a few moments. My son, Nicholas. My son who, in November 2000, had died in the psychiatric ward of a public hospital in Adelaide. He was 26 years old.

I'd visited Nicholas in hospital shortly before he died. We went for a walk in the grounds of the hospital that day, and I noticed one of the other patients, an elderly woman, was following us. We sat down on a bench and the woman came and stood close by. After a while Nicholas got up and walked over to the woman. He put his hand on her arm very gently and in a quiet voice I heard him say, 'My mother and I are having some time together, would you mind very much moving further away?' The woman nodded and without speaking moved away a little. We started to talk but we were interrupted again; this time the woman had started to sing. Looking over at Nicholas she sang to him. The words of the song were: 'A certain smile, a certain place can lead an unsuspecting heart on a merry chase.' It was an unlikely serenade but he listened attentively to her until she finished singing, then he turned back to me, and we continued our conversation.

At that moment I knew that despite the illness, his essential kindness hadn't left him. That despite the illness, the essence of Nicholas had not changed. I knew, too, that he'd let her know that she mattered. Was valued. He did it by listening to her story. A story that she had sung to him with the words of an old love story.

In this book you will meet courageous men and women who live with mental illness, and also the people who love and care for them. You will come to know their experiences through reading their stories. It has taken trust for them to share their stories; a trust in you, that as you read them it will be with an open as well as an inquiring mind.

Are stories important? My children when they were little seemed to think so. 'Tell me a story,' was a favourite way for them to push back the night, to delay the lights being put out, or to chase away a bad dream with a happy-ever-after ending.

As a young wife and mother of newly born twins and a little one-year-old daughter, Sarah, one of my favourite times was when an invitation would come from my kindly neighbour, Vivian, to 'put the kettle on'. I'd bundle the children into the big old pram and set off to her house across the road.

Sarah had been born with a major heart abnormality and was often in need of urgent medical attention. I was often anxious in those days, and the chance to talk it over with my neighbour, to 'tell her my story' was a great release. 'Tell me about it,' Vivian would say and sitting in the sunny family room, drinking cups of tea, I'd tell her about the worries of the day.

Often, it concerned me not being able to coax Sarah to eat or even drink very much. The medication that was prescribed to help regulate her little heart also had the unfortunate side-effect of being an appetite suppressant.

'Is her colour too pale? Do her little fingers look blue to you?' I'd want to know. Sometimes, all I needed was simply reassurance that all was well. At other times we would decided that maybe it was best to call in the local doctor to have a look at Sarah. But always it was that listening ear – as well as wise counsel that my friend gave me – that was important to me.

The founders of Alcoholics Anonymous believed stories were important. The remarkable program of recovery from addiction devised by them includes the regular attendance of members at meetings, where they are encouraged to tell their stories and to listen to the stories of others. Along with the 12 steps or suggestions it is in the listening and in the telling of stories that Bill Wilson and Dr Bob believed a transformation could occur.

'Is it real or is it pretend?' my children would ask me sometimes as I'd start the bedtime story. The day that Nicholas arrived at my apartment and, looking wildly around, produced a notepad and pen and wrote 'Don't talk. We are being monitored by agents…' I knew that the pretend story he was writing was very real to him. I tried to reassure him that he was safe, but the words I wrote on the notepad that he gave me didn't help him. I knew that he was very ill, that something was terribly wrong. Eventually, I phoned a friend and together we managed to get Nicholas into my car and drive to the hospital. He was admitted immediately. A few hours later I was told that he'd been transferred to a psychiatric ward and that the diagnosis was drug-induced psychosis.

Nicholas was 22 years old when this first admission occurred. He'd been studying at university and had an ambition to become a writer. But after this time his life changed; there were more hospital admissions and he was diagnosed with mental illness and drug dependency – comorbidity.

Over the following four years there were some periods of relative well-being. Nicholas spent a number of times at a Buddhist retreat in New South Wales and learned the practice of meditation. He travelled to India and Nepal. He fell in love and told me that one day they would have an amazing child together. He tried to get back to studying again.

But drugs came back into his life, and this time the anti-psychotic medication he'd been prescribed was not effective. Nicholas rang me to tell me that he'd decided to go into hospital as a voluntary patient, to be introduced to a drug his doctor advised might help him. 'Clonazepam does have risks of major side-effects and would need to be carefully monitored', I was advised by his doctor. 'It's worth a try, Mum', he told me as I drove with him to the hospital. He was admitted and commenced the process of coming off one anti-psychotic medication and being introduced to another.

Some time later Nicholas rang me from the hospital. 'I've decided to quit drugs, Mum, and I'm going to start a methadone treatment tomorrow.' He went on to explain that it was all arranged. The hospital would organise a taxi to take him to the nearby clinic, and then after he'd been given the methadone a taxi would be called to return him back to the hospital. He'd decided to turn his life around. A new medication for the mental illness and a new treatment to come off heroin. He rang me the night before he died and we talked about the new treatments. We ended the call as we always did: 'I love you, Mum', he told me. 'And I love you too, Nicholas...'

Three days after starting the methadone treatment combination with Clonazepam Nicholas was found dead on the floor near his hospital bed. The autopsy result was death due to mixed drug toxicity. A coroner's report two years later resulted in a verdict of 'accidental death by drug toxicity', with strong recommendations of changes to procedures by hospital administration in relation to treatment of drug withdrawal combined with certain anti-psychotic drugs.

A week after Nicholas died I had a call from the hospital's social worker, who offered to deliver his possessions that were left at the hospital. They were given to me in a green plastic bin-liner. His doona with a large blood stain. Although I'd read in the autopsy report of the internal haemmorhage he'd had moments before he died, I had not understood that reality until I saw the blood-stained doona. His Doc Martens. Blue jeans. A denim jacket. A tee shirt with 'Champion' written across the front. A portable chess set. A transistor radio. A writing pad and biro. The book he'd been reading, with a piece of paper folded as a bookmark, Gore Vidal's *Judgement of Paris*. There was also a black wallet I'd given him a few years earlier. Neatly tucked into one of the folds was a receipt. It was dated two days before he died. It was a receipt for a layby; a $5 deposit on a black leather jacket at St Vincent de Paul's Opportunity Shop. The shop was near the clinic where Nicholas had gone to receive the methadone treatment.

In those last days he'd been creating a new life for himself –

A new medication to take away the psychosis
A way out of dependency on drugs
And a new-to-him black leather jacket to wear.

He'd been creating a happy-ever-after ending to his story.

To all the students reading this book, I wish you every success with your studies. It's my belief that mental illness is one of the great challenges of our time. To find a cure for schizophrenia. A medication without major side-effects. To care for people with mental illness in times of crisis with insight and compassion ... these are my hopes for you.

Margaret O'Donnell
Adelaide
June 2013

Foreword: Consumer

The best nurse I ever had walked beside me and never got in my way. She would appear unobtrusively by my side and gently encourage me to get off my bed and go for walks with her. She hardly said a thing to me, but I could feel her calmness and acceptance through all the static of my distress. Other nurses got in my way; they tore off my blankets, threatened me, berated me for being inappropriate or for not facing the world, or gave me strange looks when I expressed my pain.

In their training and professional development, nurses learn many things – much of it is irrelevant to the experience of the person using the service. I do not remember any of the nurses I encountered for their professional skills. But I do remember them for their human qualities. Above all, I remember the nurses who were kind and compassionate.

Compassion is hard to teach and impossible to enforce, but it is the single most important attribute any mental health professional needs to develop. Compassion means being able to stand in the shoes of the other and be with the person in her or his distress. It allows the helper to stand on the ledge between deflecting the other person's pain and losing herself or himself in it. Compassion takes a strong sense of self, patience and an acceptance of difference.

Unfortunately, compassion cannot thrive in services that control people and pathologise their experience. A recovery-based service promotes people's autonomy and respects their subjectivity; this is the best setting for compassion to grow. Wherever we work in the mental health system we have a responsibility to foster compassion, not only in our one-to-one relationships with the people who use the service and our colleagues, but in creating a service environment that encourages empowering and respectful relationships at all levels.

Mental Health: A person-centred approach is a recovery-based text for undergraduate nurses in Australia and New Zealand. This book is a compass on your journey to becoming a mental health nurse whose compassion service users will remember.

Mary O'Hagan

Contents

Foreword: Carer by Margaret O'Donnell   v
Foreword: Consumer by Mary O'Hagan   viii
About the authors   xvii
Acknowledgements   xxi

1 Introduction to mental health and mental illness: Human connectedness
   and the collaborative consumer narrative   1
   Nicholas Procter, Amy Baker, Kirsty Grocke and Monika Ferguson
   Introduction   2
   A narrative approach to mental health   3
   Defining mental health and mental illness   4
   Mental health nursing   13
   Mental state assessment   16
   Recovery   17
   Collaborative practice in mental health nursing   18
   Chapter summary   21
   Critical thinking/learning activities   21
   Learning extension   21
   Further reading   22
   References   22

2 Learning through human connectedness on clinical placement:
   Translation to practice   25
   Denise McGarry
   Introduction   26
   Mental health (nursing) education: An overview   26
   Attitudes, expectations and positive engagement within practice   28
   Application of interpersonal skills within the mental health practicum
   placement and other, non-mental health settings   31
   Power relations involved in the therapeutic relationship   31
   Development of emotional competence   34
   Reflective practice as a critical thinking process   34
   Clinical supervision for the beginning/novice nursing student within
   mental health nursing   35
   Developing objectives for clinical placements   38
   The process of self-assessment and personal problem solving   40
   Reflection, self, in-action and post-placement   40
   Ethical and political influences on care   41

And off to clinical placement: Pragmatic strategies for learning   42
Chapter summary   47
Critical thinking/learning activities   47
Learning extension   47
Further reading   48
References   48

3 The social and emotional well-being of Aboriginal Australians and the
   collaborative consumer narrative   51
   Debra Hocking
   Introduction   52
   Social and emotional well-being versus mental health   52
   Culture   53
   Colonisation   54
   Aboriginal worldviews   55
   Government policies   56
   The incidence of trauma   62
   The concept of healing   65
   Chapter summary   68
   Critical thinking/learning activities   68
   Learning extension   68
   Acknowledgement   69
   Further reading   69
   References   70

4 Māori mental health   72
   Jacquie Kidd, Kerri Butler and Reina Harris
   Introduction   73
   Kawa whakaruruhau (cultural safety)   75
   Whānau ora   77
   Hauora (health) and *oranga* (wellness)   78
   Engagement with *tangata whai i te ora*: The Ten Commitments   80
   Chapter summary   86
   Critical thinking/learning activities   86
   Learning extension   87
   Further reading   87
   References   87

5 Assessment of mental health and mental illness   89
Terry Froggatt and Susan Liersch-Sumskis
Introduction   90
The meaning of mental health and mental health conditions
within assessment   90
Therapeutic communication within the assessment process   92
The assessment process   95
Mental status examination   98
Strengths-based assessment   104
The Tidal Model   106
Aboriginal mental health assessment   107
Assessment in the context of forensic psychiatry   107
Diagnosis of mental illness   110
Chapter summary   113
Critical thinking/learning activities   113
Learning extension   114
Further reading   114
References   114

6 Legal and ethical aspects in mental health care   117
Helen P. Hamer, Anthony J. O'Brien and Debra Lampshire
Introduction   118
A legal and ethical framework for practice   118
Procedural justice and mental health nursing   126
Alternatives to compulsory treatment and the role of advance directives
and crisis plans   129
Mental health legislation in the year 2042   130
Chapter summary   133
Critical thinking/learning activities   133
Learning extension   133
Further reading   133
References   134

7 Mental health and substance use   137
Rhonda L. Wilson
Introduction   138
Harm minimisation   138
Overview of substance-use problems   139

An overview of drugs and the effects they have on people   140
Reasons people use drugs and alcohol   145
An holistic framework for understanding people who use drugs and those
who misuse drugs   146
Mental illness and substance-use problems in combination with each other   158
Mental health and drug and alcohol models of care   158
Chapter summary   162
Critical thinking/learning activities   162
Learning extension   162
Acknowledgement   162
Further reading   163
References   163

8   Nutrition, physical health and behavioural change   165
Denise McGarry
Introduction   166
Prevalence   167
Comorbidity   168
Common physical illnesses and conditions   174
Interventions   187
Chapter summary   191
Critical thinking/learning activities   191
Learning extension   191
Further reading   192
References   192

9   Mental health of people of immigrant and refugee backgrounds   197
Nicholas Procter, Asma Babakarkhil, Amy Baker and Monika Ferguson
Introduction   198
What is meant by the terms refugee, immigrant and asylum seeker?   200
Temporary Protection Visas   201
Mental health of people of immigrant and refugee background   202
Culture and explanatory models in mental health   204
Isolation   207
Engagement with mainstream mental health services   208
Traumatic stress   209
Access and engagement when in distress   211
Trust and human connectedness in mental health   211

Older people of immigrant background   212
Chapter summary   213
Critical thinking/learning activities   213
Learning extension   214
Further reading   215
References   215

10 Gender, sexuality and mental health   217
Helen P. Hamer, Joe MacDonald, Jane Barrington and Debra Lampshire
Introduction   218
Gender and health   223
Culturally competent human connectedness   224
Interpersonal abuse and psychological trauma   229
Interpersonal trauma and mental health   231
Trauma-informed care   233
Chapter summary   239
Critical thinking/learning activities   239
Learning extension   240
Further reading   240
References   240

11 Mental health of children and young people   244
Rhonda L. Wilson and Serena Riley
Introduction   245
Respect for young people   245
Developing a rapport with young people   246
Developmental stages   248
Reducing risk and vulnerability   249
Mental health promotion, prevention and early intervention for
young people   252
Common mental health conditions in young people   256
Chapter summary   258
Critical thinking /learning activities   258
Learning extension   258
Acknowledgement   259
Further reading   259
References   259

12 Mental health of older people   262
   Helen P. Hamer, Debra Lampshire and Sue Thomson
   Introduction   263
   Recovery   266
   Culture of older people   267
   Human connectedness   268
   When things go wrong: Common mental illnesses   271
   Cognitive decline, depression, delirium or dementia? Getting
   the diagnosis right   273
   An ethical framework to underpin practice   277
   The future of older people's mental health nursing   278
   Chapter summary   281
   Critical thinking/learning activities   281
   Learning extension   281
   Further reading   282
   References   282

13 Rural and regional mental health   287
   Rhonda L. Wilson
   Introduction   288
   What is *rural*?   288
   Overview of the rural and regional clinical context   291
   Prevalence of mental health problems in rural and regional communities   294
   Rural mental health promotion and prevention   297
   Travel implications for rural people with mental health care needs   303
   Natural disasters and rural implications   304
   Agriculture, mining and itinerant workforces   305
   Chapter summary   306
   Critical thinking/learning activities   306
   Learning extension   307
   Acknowledgement   307
   Further reading   307
   References   308

14 Mental health in the interprofessional context 311
Denise McGarry and Anne Storey
Introduction 312
Historical professional precedents 312
Arguments for an interprofessional mental health workforce 313
The composition of the mental health workforce: Preparation and
scope of practice 314
Regulation of the mental health workforce 321
Effectiveness of interprofessional workforces 323
Looking after yourself 326
Chapter summary 333
Critical thinking/learning activities 333
Learning extension 333
Further reading 333
References 334

15 Conclusions: Looking to practice 336
Nicholas Procter
Introduction 337
A message of leadership 337
The need to self-question 337
Clinical mentoring and empowerment 338
References 340

Index 341

About the authors

Editors

Nicholas Procter PhD MBA Grad Dip Adult Ed BA CertAdvClinNsg RN, CMHN. Nicholas is the University of South Australia's Inaugural Chair: Mental Health Nursing, and convener of the Mental Health and Substance Abuse Research Group, located within the Sansom Institute for Health Research. He is also convener of the University of South Australia's Human Rights and Security Research and Innovation Cluster, and adjunct professor at the University of Tasmania.

Helen P. Hamer is a senior lecturer and nurse consultant in the School of Nursing and the Centre for Mental Health Research at the University of Auckland.

Denise McGarry is a credentialled mental health nurse and a fellow of the Australian College of Mental Health Nurses. She teaches in the School of Nursing, Midwifery and Indigenous Health at Charles Sturt University, as a lecturer in mental health. In this capacity Denise enjoys working with nursing and paramedic students.

Rhonda L. Wilson RN BNSc MN(Hons). Rhonda is a mental health nurse lecturer at the University of New England, in New South Wales. She is immediate-past Deputy Chair of the Research Committee for the Australian College of Mental Health Nurses. Rhonda broadcasts a regular series, *Bush Remedies: You and your mental health*, on ABC Radio's New England North West.

Terry Froggatt PhD MSc BHA FAIM RN MHN FACMHN JP. Terry teaches and coordinates undergraduate subjects and postgraduate courses at the University of Wollongong, in New South Wales. He is a credentialled mental health Nurse, a fellow and board member of the Australian College of Mental Health Nurses and a coordinator of the Australian Government's Mental Health Professionals Network.

Contributors

Asma Babakarkhil BBus BA. Asma and her family emigrated from Afghanistan to Australia in the late 1980s. Asma has eight years of experience working as a professional interpreter in Pashto and Dari languages. In 2010 she worked in the Ministry of Women's Affairs in the Department of Statistics and Research, Kabul Afghanistan.

Amy Baker PhD BHSc(Hons)(OccTh) BAppSc(OccTh). Amy is a research fellow in the School of Nursing and Midwifery at the University of South Australia. She has undertaken research and projects in a diverse range of fields, including autism, palliative care, horticultural therapy and healing environments, community mental health care and environmental health of immigrants and refugees. Her interest in the field of mental health derives in part from providing support to a loved one who experiences mental illness. Amy's special interests include consumer and carer participation, innovative and creative approaches to engagement and human flourishing.

Jane Barrington is a registered nurse who works as a professional teaching fellow in the school of nursing at the University of Auckland. She coordinates a postgraduate program for nurses in their first year of mental health nursing practice.

Kerri Butler is *tangata whai ite ora* and has worked in the field of mental health in varying consumer and quality roles. She is from the Ngapuhi iwi in the Hokianga as well as having Ngati Porou affiliations from the east coast of New Zealand.

Monika Ferguson BPsych(Hons). Monika is a research assistant for the Mental Health and Substance Abuse Research Group, located within the Sansom Institute for Health Research at the University of South Australia.

Sandria C. Butler is Town Planner in Wagga Wagga, New South Wales.

Kirsty Grocke BN Grad Dip MHN. Kirsty is Lecturer and Course Coordinator in the Graduate Diploma in Mental Health at the University of South Australia. She is also a mental health nurse working in the acute and crisis mental health services in the Adelaide public mental health sector.

Reina Harris BA LLB. Reina has worked in various operational management and policy positions with a focus on indigenous development. She is employed as a consumer leader at Affinity Services, providing advice and leadership to the Auckland District Mental Health Board. Reina describes her consumer experience or pathway to wellness as *Te po ki te ao marama*, 'moving from darkness to light'.

Debra Hocking is a lecturer at the University of Wollongong in New South Wales, and coordinates postgraduate Indigenous health subjects. A Palawa (Tasmanian Aboriginal) who descends from the Mouheneenner people from south-east Tasmania, Debra is a Stolen Generations survivor.

Jacquie Kidd PhD MN RN. Jacquie is a mental health nurse of Māori (Nga Puhi) descent. She is a co-director of the Centre for Mental Health Research at the University of Auckland.

Debra Lampshire is a professional teaching fellow and an experience-based expert in the School of Nursing and the Centre for Mental Health Research at the University of Auckland. She is the chairperson of the New Zealand branch and executive board member of the International Organization Promoting Psychotherapy and Psychological (ISPS) treatments for persons with psychosis.

Susan Liersch-Sumskis RN MHN BN(Hons) PhD Churchill Fellow. Susan is a lecturer in mental health nursing at the University of Wollongong in New South Wales. She is also in private mental health nursing practice under the Medicare Nurse Incentive Program, and is actively involved in professional roles within the Australian College of Mental Health Nurses.

Joe MacDonald works in community development, mental health and social justice, as Rainbow Community Liaison and Trainer for Affinity Services in Auckland.

Anthony J. O'Brien RN BA MPhil(Hons) FNZCMHN. Anthony is a senior lecturer at the School of Nursing, University of Auckland and Nurse Specialist, Liaison Psychiatry, at Auckland District Health Board. He is also a researcher with the Centre for Mental Health Research, University of Auckland

Serena Riley is an undergraduate student in the Bachelor of Nursing program at the University of New England in Armidale, New South Wales. She is a young woman with personal experience of mental illness, and her experience as a consumer and in recovery have provided her with a lived experience background that enriches her understanding of the mental health needs of people in similar circumstances to her. Serena's road to recovery has been challenging but she has been able to reflect on her experiences and is now in a position to be able to share them for the purpose of helping others to learn about mental illness, and how to care sensitively for people with mental illness. Serena has travelled extensively, undertaking humanitarian work in many countries including India, South Africa, Uganda and Greece. She hopes to use her nursing education to continue to undertake humanitarian work in the future.

Anne Storey RN BHS (Nurs) MN. Anne completed her registered nursing course in Melbourne in 1982. After completing a hospital-based midwifery and mental health nursing course with Charles Sturt University in Sydney, she undertook the Master of Nursing program at the University of Technology, Sydney and is currently working towards a Master in Nursing (Nurse Practitioner). Anne works in a primary care role as a credentialled mental health nurse with asylum seekers

Sue Thomson works in planning, education and advisory services for Dementia Care for the Northern Region of New Zealand, and is based at the Northern Regional Alliance in Auckland.

Consumer contributors

Michael Barton PhD MEd (Counselling and Guidance) BEd. Michael is Director of Teaching and Learning at a New South Wales independent school.

Angie Bulic is a graduate intern paramedic in regional New South Wales.

Edwina Casey RN. Edwina completed her nursing degree at the University of New England in 2012. Throughout that time, she found her mental health placement one of the most eye-opening clinical placements she had been on. Not only did Edwina find mental health a completely different aspect of nursing, but she found it a demanding, yet a very rewarding area of nursing to be a part of – an area that many nurses and other health professionals underestimate. Edwina is in her new graduate year and is working in Hobart, Tasmania, in a cardiothoracic ward. Edwina encourages nursing students to make the most of their mental health unit and clinical placement, and to rise up to the challenge to promote a greater awareness of mental health in rural and remote areas in Australia.

Sally Drummond is a registered nurse and credentialled mental health nurse at Charles Sturt University, in New South Wales.

Kristen Ella is an Aboriginal woman whose family originated from the Yuin nation, in southern New South Wales. She is the Aboriginal Mental Health Clinician on the Aboriginal Infant Maternal Health Service team, based on the central coast of New South Wales.

James Robert Hindman MBA MBusMan BN. James is acting Clinical Nurse Consultant for Mental Health Emergency Care – Rural Access Program at Western NSW Local Health District. He also lectures to second-year paramedic students at Charles Sturt University.

Cindi McCormick is a Mental Health Drug and Alcohol Local Health District transitional support nurse educator.

Sandra Murphy is a Gadigal woman of the Eora nation.

Leigh Murray is co-Chair, National District Health Board, Family Whānau Advisors and Family Advisor for mental health services in Auckland District Health Board.

Barbara O'Neill is a Gadigal woman of the Eora Nation.

John C. Wade DipNurs GradDipEd. John is a registered nurse and also lectures and tutors at various New South Wales universities, and has facilitated nursing students on clinical placement. John is Secretary of Illawarra Local Aboriginal Land Council and has held positions on the board of the Illawarrra Aboriginal Medical Service, including as chairperson.

Stephanie Webster is a consumer educator who has delivered mental health education from a lived experience perspective since 2006.

Limor Weingarten is a registered nurse and clinical nurse educator working in a public residential and rehabilitation service for people experiencing serious mental illness in Sydney. Her passion is to enhance the status, knowledge and skills of nurses working in mental health, and to improve the quality of life of residents in the hospital environment.

Acknowledgements

The authors are extremely grateful to Nina Sharpe and other staff at Cambridge University Press for their thoughtful guidance and support, and to Renée Otmar of Otmar Miller Consultancy, for her patience during the development of the book. We thank Carmel Haggerty for her contribution to the book proposal. We also gratefully acknowledge the consumers, carers and practitioners who have contributed their stories and wisdom.

1

Introduction to mental health and mental illness: Human connectedness and the collaborative consumer narrative

Nicholas Procter, Amy Baker, Kirsty Grocke and Monika Ferguson

Introduction 2
A narrative approach to mental health 3
Defining mental health
   and mental illness 4
Mental health nursing 13
Mental state assessment 16
Recovery 17

Collaborative practice in mental
   health nursing 18
Chapter summary 21
Critical thinking/learning activities 21
Learning extension 21
Further reading 22
References 22

Learning objectives

At the completion of this chapter, you should be able to:

- Describe the nature and scope of a narrative approach in mental health nursing.
- Identify and discuss the implications of social determinants of mental health such as social, cultural, biological, environmental, employment/work and societal determinants; determinants of inequity; and evidence and population datasets.
- Explain key concepts such as mental health and mental illness; recovery; consumer participation; human rights; vulnerability; promotion, prevention and early intervention in mental health; collaborative practice in mental health; and practical aspects of human connectedness as a means of engaging with people and communities at risk.
- Make real-world links to concepts such as incidence and prevalence; mortality and morbidity; life expectancy; quality adjusted life years; international classification of functioning, disability and health; and potential years of life lost due to mental illness.
- Discuss issues related to the everyday experiences of consumers and carers, including enablers and barriers to meaningful engagement between clinicians and consumers, carers and family members.

Introduction

consumer
a person who uses or has used a mental health service, or who has a lived experience of a mental illness

carer
a person who provides assistance, care and support for someone who has a mental illness

This chapter reflects a coming together of key issues and themes embedded in everyday work with **consumers** and **carers**. Carers include immediate family and friends, and may also include extended family such as grandparents and cousins. In transcultural and other contexts it is important to use humanistic language in line with a recovery approach; for example, the terms 'support person/people' and 'support networks' may be preferable to the term 'carer' in mental health practice and mental health nursing. This approach provides a foundation for human connectedness, and sets the consumer narrative as central to mental health practice and mental health nursing, specifically.

Consumer narrative   Michael's story

My name is Michael. I'm 24 years old and single. I was recently taken to the emergency department of my local hospital, by ambulance. Apparently, my mother was concerned because she could not rouse me. I've been told that on arrival the level of alcohol detected from my breath was pretty high, and I'd also taken some Valium tablets. Once the alcohol level in my system was reduced, I was referred to the hospital's mental health team for assessment. I spoke to a nurse, Melissa, and explained that, although I am aware of the risk of using alcohol with other drugs, I had no intention of trying to hurt myself.

I used to be a sociable, funny guy at school, with loads of friends. When I was 21, I was assaulted during a night out with friends in the city. Since then, everything seems to have been off – completely changed. I've noticed a change in my personality and behaviour. I often feel irritable and tearful, lacking energy and motivation. I feel down most days, and I've given up on finding work after I lost my job last year. I also have nightmares, so I use alcohol to get to sleep. For the past three years, I have been drinking around eight beers a night and up to 16 beers on weekend nights. To help me get to sleep, I take two to three Valium tablets most nights, and I also occasionally smoke cannabis. I know that this isn't helping but I don't know what else to do.

I talked to Melissa about how I often feel isolated from others and hopeless about my situation. At times, I've even thought of ending it all. These kinds of thoughts tend to be worse when I've been drinking and can't sleep. I explained to Melissa that I also have trouble in crowds. I currently live in shared accommodation, and I visit the local supermarket for groceries once per fortnight. My brother visits me weekly; he tries to encourage me to get out of the house, but I find this too stressful. I would really like to get back to being the person I used to be. I'd like to find a job and be able to catch up with my friends again, but I feel so overwhelmed and don't know how to get better.

A narrative approach to mental health

The story of Michael – and many others contained within this book – is central to both the narrative and person-centred approach taken in each chapter. A person-centred approach is concerned with human connectedness: the capacity for feelings to be received and understood, and lives to be revealed. A narrative approach illuminates the needs of the person with a mental health condition, her or his family, carers and clinician through an interactive process of dialogue and information exchange. At a deeper level, narrative is a means of storytelling.

Storytelling is a profoundly human capacity. Meaning is accomplished through an interaction between the teller and the listener. The listener enters into the world of narrator, constructs and helps in the telling of the story; thus, a narrative is jointly accomplished, according to shared knowledge and interaction (Michel & Valach, 2011). Such activity is central to the practice of mental health nursing. This is because the discourse itself involves stories that together become a joint action.

The counterpoint to a narrative approach is application of a structured or mechanistic style of engagement and interaction. Rather than creating a forum for the sharing of various perspectives and possibilities, this approach is largely monologic. In an interview situation (for example) the interviewee is asked a list of questions. Learning is by a predetermined 'case study' that is defined by a distinctive feature, disease or condition. There is a denouement of personhood and, in some instances, it is lost completely. In this situation, a person's life is subjected to being impersonally processed, with little opportunity to contribute a perspective on what actually lies behind his or her situation, life difficulty or aspiration to live a healthy and socially engaged life.

A narrative approach in the context of this book has special meaning. By combining the best evidence in mental health with the opportunity to know and understand the human connections that can and should be made in mental health care, this book adopts an all-encompassing approach to engaging with, responding to and supporting people with mental illness. It signals a change in the nature and context of learning by promoting alternate points of view and lived experience in mental health. Each chapter encompasses relevant information pitched at a level suited to an undergraduate student while simultaneously making sense of the consumer's and/or carer's voice and experience. The consumers, carers and practitioners who have contributed to this book have changed their names to protect their anonymity. Each has had a direct experience in recovering from mental illness, using mental health services or providing mental health support. This form of writing is valuable for both student and academic readers, as it draws from key evidence in the field as well as our relationship to it. The desired outcome of narrative thinking is for the chapters and adjunctive learning materials to reveal a new story through conversational partnership between the student and the text. Dominant themes are examined, discussed and, where necessary, challenged. If the student can empathically put herself or himself in the place of the person with a mental illness, then it will be possible to move beyond current thinking toward new and fresh thinking.

This task can be made more productive through the use of reflective questions and thinking about opportunities for translation to practice.

Defining mental health and mental illness

Mental health

Mental health is the ability to cope with and bounce back from adversity, to solve problems in everyday life, manage when things are difficult and cope with everyday stressors. Good mental health is made possible by a supportive social, friendship and family environment, work–life balance, physical health and, in many instances, reduced stress and trauma.

Mental illness

Mental illness is a clinically diagnosable condition that significantly interferes with an individual's cognitive, emotional or social abilities. The diagnosis of mental illness is generally made according to the classification systems of the Diagnostic and Statistical Manual of Mental Disorders (DSM; American Psychiatric Association, 2012) or the International Classification of Diseases (ICD; World Health Organization (WHO), 2013a). Mental illness affects men, women and children of all ages, nationalities and socio-economic backgrounds, and affects the lives of many people in our community, their families and friends. The experience of mental illness is common, with the most recent national data indicating that 45 per cent of adults (aged 16 years and older) in Australia and 40 per cent in New Zealand have experienced a mental illness at some point in their lives (Australian Bureau of Statistics (ABS), 2007; Oakley Browne, Well & Scott, 2006). Moreover, approximately one in five adults in Australia and New Zealand experience a mental illness each year (ABS, 2007; Oakley Browne et al., 2006). In both Australia and New Zealand, mental illness more commonly influences young people, with prevalence of mental illness typically being highest for those individuals aged between 16 and 24 years. This includes the experience of anxiety and depression, conditions associated with substance misuse and longer-term conditions such as anxiety, chronic and recurrent depression and schizophrenia. Comorbidity (the experience of more than one condition/ disease by an individual) is quite high. For example, of those individuals in New Zealand who experience an illness over 12 months, 37 per cent experience more than one (Oakley Browne et al., 2006). The most likely co-occurrence is of anxiety and mood conditions (Oakley Browne et al., 2006). In both countries, women are more likely to experience mental illness than men, and this is largely accounted for by the higher incidence of anxiety conditions among women (ABS, 2007; Oakley Browne et al., 2006). Despite the relatively high prevalence of mental illness among Australian and New Zealand adults, approximately two-thirds of people with a 12-month or longer mental health condition do not receive treatment for their mental illness (ABS, 2007; Oakley Browne, et al., 2006).

Rates of mental illness among Aboriginal and Torres Strait Islanders are currently undetermined, although recent data from the 2008 Health and Welfare of Australia's Aboriginal and Torres Strait Islander Peoples survey (ABS and Australian Institute of Health and Welfare, 2008) indicate that Indigenous Australians are twice as likely as non-Indigenous Australians to report either high or very high levels of psychological distress, which indicates a higher probability of mental illness. Similarly, the 12-month prevalence of mental illness of Māori and Pacific peoples is 29.5 per cent and 24.4 per cent respectively (compared to 21 per cent for the New Zealand population; Oakley Browne et al., 2006), also indicating a higher incidence of mental illness among these individuals.

Anxiety conditions

Anxiety conditions generally involve feelings of tension, distress or worry. This can include diagnoses of panic, agoraphobia, social phobia, specific phobia, generalised anxiety, obsessive-compulsive conditions and post-traumatic stress. Anxiety is the most common type of mental health condition in Australia and New Zealand, affecting 14 per cent and 15 per cent of people aged 16–85 years, respectively (ABS, 2007; Oakley Browne et al., 2006). In both countries, women are more likely to have experienced anxiety than men (18 per cent compared to 11 per cent in Australia, and 19 per cent compared to 11 per cent in New Zealand; ABS, 2007; Oakley Browne et al., 2006). These conditions are most commonly experienced by women aged 16–54 years in Australia (21 per cent; ABS, 2007) and women aged 16–24 years and 25–44 years in New Zealand (18 per cent each; Oakley Browne et al., 2006).

Affective conditions

Affective or mood conditions involve a disturbance in mood or a change in affect, and diagnoses include major depressive condition, dysthymia and bipolar affective illness. Depression involves signs such as a depressed mood, low self-esteem and reduced energy or activity over a period of at least two weeks. Bipolar illness involves episodes of mania, either alone or with depressive episodes. Manic episodes may be characterised by reduced need for sleep, increased activity or restlessness and disinhibited behaviour. Affective illnesses are experienced by 6.2 per cent of Australians aged 16–85 years, with a slightly higher prevalence in women (7.1 per cent) than men (5.3 per cent; ABS, 2007). Similarly, these conditions are more common among females (9.5 per cent) than males (6.3 per cent) in New Zealand, and are most prevalent in the 16–24-year age bracket (12.7 per cent; Oakley Browne et al., 2006).

Substance misuse

Substance misuse conditions may be defined as dependency or harmful use of alcohol or other drugs. These conditions are slightly less prevalent than other types of mental illnesses, affecting 5.1 per cent of the adult population in Australia and 3.5 per cent in New Zealand (ABS, 2007; Oakley Browne, et al., 2006). In Australia, substance misuse conditions are more common in men aged 16–24 years (13 per cent; ABS, 2007).

Similarly, in New Zealand, these conditions account for 2 per cent of the female and 5 per cent of the male population, and are most common in the 16–24-year age bracket (9.6 per cent; Oakley Browne et al., 2006).

Contemporary approaches

As is sometimes seen in the popular media and cinema, people with a mental illness are portrayed as having an illness only; one that is best managed away from the community, subject to closed institutional care and, in some instances, inhumane treatment. While it is important to communicate factors associated with diagnostic categories, nowadays the practice of mental health care in Australia and New Zealand has a strong emphasis on human rights, personhood, advocacy, care in the least restrictive environment, early intervention and safety for people with a mental mental illness.

Let's take the story of Michael and relate it to recent events in South Australia as an example of a contemporary approach. On 1 July 2010, a new Mental Health Act took effect in South Australia, the *Mental Health Act 2009* (SA), with the broad purposes of: protecting the rights and liberty of people with mental illness; ensuring that their dignity and liberty is retained as far as is consistent with their protection; protecting the public; and the proper delivery of services. The Act also aims to ensure the accessibility and delivery of specialist treatment, care, rehabilitation and support services for people with mental illness, and the creation of more appropriate and effective processes for engagement between consumers and service providers, including transportation and orders for community treatment, detention and treatment. For a person like Michael, the Act means that staff must engage him in a meaningful and collaborative way in the design of a current care plan to enable full recovery with dignity (Mendoza et al., 2013). Michael must also be supported through provision of appropriate transportation should it be required under the Act for him to receive compulsory in-patient treatment.

Mental illness and social determinants

The social determinants of health are the circumstances in which people are born, grow up, live and work, and the systems that are in place to deal with illness (Commission on Social Determinants of Health, 2008). These circumstances are all shaped by wider societal factors, and by the social and economic conditions in which people live. Mental health promotion is therefore not only the responsibility of the health care sector, but also of many other sectors such as housing, education and employment (Keleher & Armstrong, 2005).

The social determinants of mental health can be categorised into four areas:

Individual: These include an ability to manage feelings, thoughts and life in general, emotional resilience and an ability to deal with stress.

Community: These include social supports, and having a good sense of belonging and an opportunity to actively participate in your community. For some people with strong cultural affiliations, understanding and responding to a mental health condition are largely guided and derived from self-identity through community affiliation and cultural belonging.

Organisations: These include factors such as safe housing, employment options and educational opportunities, access to good transport and a political system that enhances mental health.

Whole societies: These include social structures in education, employment and justice to address inequities and promote access and support to those who are vulnerable (Keleher & Armstrong, 2005).

Keleher and Armstrong (2005) suggested that mental health promotion is able to enhance supportive social conditions and create positive environments for the health and well-being of populations, communities and individuals. Mental health promotion can influence determinants of mental health and address inequities through the implementation of multi-level interventions across a wide number of sectors, policies, programs, settings and environments (Keleher & Armstrong, 2005).

The mental health clinician acts as an advocate for people with mental illness accessing services in housing, education and employment, the aim of which is to develop beneficial outcomes in a way that enables the consumer to retain as much control as possible over how it is carried out. The expectation of consumer advocacy is individual empowerment. The mental health clinician stands alongside the consumer, to strengthen her or his voice and to enhance resilience (Department of Health and Ageing, 1998).

Mental illness and life expectancy

Life expectancy from birth of people with serious mental illnesses is between eight and 14.7 years less in men and between 9.8 and 17.5 years less among women than in the general population. In both groups, schizophrenia has been associated with the greatest reduction in life expectancy (Parish, 2011). A recent Australian survey of people living with psychotic illness (n = 1825) (of whom just under 50 per cent had a diagnosis of schizophrenia) found that in the previous month 33 per cent did not have breakfast on any day of the week (Morgan et al., 2011). In the same survey, 41.5 per cent ate only one serving or less of vegetables a day, and 7.1 per cent did not eat any vegetables at all (Morgan et al., 2011).

Since nutrition is inextricably linked to physical health, it is not surprising that the major cause of death for people with a diagnosed serious mental illness is not suicide, as many believe, but cardiovascular diseases. While mental health clinicians are well practised at assessing the risk of self-harm, they are less familiar with assessing the risk of cardiovascular disease. Given that people with a serious mental illness are more likely to be inactive, obese and smoke, compared to the general population, it can be seen that incidents of metabolic syndrome are more common in this population group (Parish, 2011). It must be noted that, collectively, the effects of second-generation anti-psychotic medications, inactivity, overweight and obesity are also the results of psychotropic medication. In this circumstance, poor physical health is associated with the combined elements of the mental health condition as well treatment by psychotropic medication (Saha, Chant & McGrath, 2007).

The largest proportion of non-communicable disease deaths for people diagnosed with a mental illness is caused by cardiovascular diseases (48 per cent), followed by cancers, chronic respiratory diseases and diabetes, which alone are directly responsible for 3.5 per cent of deaths. Behavioural risk factors, including tobacco use, harmful use of alcohol, physical inactivity and an unhealthy diet, are estimated to be responsible for about 80 per cent of coronary heart disease and cerebrovascular disease. Behavioural risk factors are associated with four key metabolic changes: hypertension, obesity, hyperglycaemia and hyperlipidaemia (WHO, 2012). The prevalence of metabolic syndrome in people with a diagnosis of schizophrenia is approximately three times higher than in the general population (De Hert et al., 2009).

The combined and cumulative nature of diet, lifestyle and treatment factors have substantial effects on both quality of life and life expectancy. A recent systematic review covering studies from 25 countries concluded that people with schizophrenia have a standardised mortality ratio for all-cause mortality of 2.58 (Saha et al., 2007). Also important is the knowledge that the physical health care needs of people with a mental illness are often neglected by health care workers, due to stigma. Often, physical complaints are disregarded by clinicians who label the consumer as anxious or somatically focused. Given the vast amount of evidence that people with a mental illness are more likely to suffer poor cardio-metabolic health, clinicians need to listen carefully to the needs of consumers and act to reduce the incidence of cardiovascular disease.

Mental health clinicians work at the intersection of mental and physical health, and have a vital role to play in lifting standards of physical care. Mental health clinicians have an important role in monitoring how medications affect consumers, and their physical health needs. Psychotropic and other forms of medication can cause or at least contribute towards – adverse physical health effects, including premature disability and death. There is tremendous scope to improve the quality of physical care for people with a severe mental illness by having a more direct role, such as assessing physical symptoms, liaising with medical practitioners and specialists, and providing physical health advice on important issues such as diet, exercise and sleep.

At the same time, many people with mental health conditions are not formally engaged with mainstream mental health services in an integrated and sustainable way (Mendoza et al., 2013). Collaborative practice in mental health must be inclusive of this group, and may occur through other health contacts such as primary care and community health services. Health promotion activities, illness prevention and early intervention are all ways in which the mental health clinician, together with the multidisciplinary team, can provide the best care to people with a mental illness who are at risk of developing life-threatening conditions (Happell et al., 2011).

Mental illness and substance misuse

In situations in which mental illness is a factor, there is an emerging picture worldwide suggesting that illicit substance involvement is on the rise (WHO, 2013b). The breakdown of traditional, community based structures such as clubs and societies – which promote a sense of belonging, peer support and valued community involvement – is thought to be linked to boredom among young people and increased exposure to substances such as cannabis, amphetamines and methamphetamine. The co-occurrence of a mental health condition and a substance misuse condition, commonly referred to as 'comorbidity' or 'dual diagnosis', is widespread and complex. It is well established that drug and alcohol misuse is commonly experienced by people with a mental health condition. According to the Australian National Mental Health and Wellbeing Survey (ABS, 2007) 63 per cent of Australians who reported that they misused drugs nearly every day within the previous 12 months had also experienced a mental health condition in the previous 12 months.

Comorbid mental health and alcohol and other drug conditions are more likely to be experienced by young people of refugee background when compared to their Australian-born peers. While it has been established that significant barriers to service engagement and service provision exist for young people of refugee background with one condition, the risk may be higher for those experiencing comorbidity, as they not only face cultural and linguistic barriers, disrupted or fragmented cultural affiliations, but are also often required to navigate two different service sectors (Posselt et al., 2013).

Mental illness and homelessness

Also significant is the prevalence of mental illness among homeless people – thought to be four to five times higher than within the Australian general population. These background factors are often closely associated with a lack of supportive accommodation options available for people with mental health conditions, the transfer of people with unstable mental health conditions to community settings, the episodic nature of mental illness and uncontrolled use of, and access to, illicit stimulants (Schizophrenia Fellowship of NSW Inc., 2008).

Mental illness and violence/aggression

A recent review of the literature examining crime and violence in people with schizophrenia, with and without comorbid substance-use conditions, concluded that increased risk of violent offending in schizophrenia cannot be solely attributed to the effects of comorbid substance misuse, although comorbidity certainly heightens the likelihood of criminality (Short et al., 2013). In addition to offending, people with schizophrenia are more likely than community controls to come to the attention of police through their involvement in family violence incidents. Having a diagnosis of schizophrenia is claimed to be a particularly strong risk factor for violence in females, yet this finding is not conclusive. This situation is made more difficult when we take into account two intersecting and interrelated issues. First, the notion that people with severe mental illness experience significantly more problems in interpersonal relationships, and that family members may often be the targets of violent behaviour (Short et al., 2013). Second, the considerable and continuing stigma and prejudice associated with mental illness in the wider community (Pescosolido, 2013).

Mental illness and risk

Some people are more vulnerable and at higher risk of developing a mental illness than others. The factors that may contribute to a person's risk include trauma and abuse, social isolation, homelessness, socio-economic disadvantage, physical or intellectual disability and genetic predisposition. Harmful use of alcohol and other drugs can significantly increase the occurrence of mental illness. We also know that Aboriginal, Torres Strait Islander and Māori people are more vulnerable to developing a mental illness secondary to intergenerational trauma suffered during European settlement and colonisation (Council of Australian Governments (COAG), 2012; Stewart-Harawira, 2005). Some people with mental illness experience disadvantage such as lowered educational achievement, lack of social connectedness, poverty, poor physical health and reduced life expectancy. These disadvantages may influence whether someone with a mental health condition is able to access the help needed. It is up to clinicians to be aware of these risk factors and how they affect the lives of people with mental illness.

The first signs of mental illness may emerge in childhood, adolescence or early adulthood. Young people at risk of developing a mental illness may be those who have been bullied at school, children of parents with a mental illness, children linked with the criminal justice system, refugees and children brought up in a traumatic environment. These children or young people at risk may already be linked to services offering counselling, or may be part of a youth group. It is therefore important for the wider community, across cultures and across the lifespan, to be able to identify and respond to people in mental distress in order to offer support early and reduce the risk of the person's situation becoming worse and more distressing (COAG, 2012).

Reflective questions

Imagine you are working with a woman who is concerned about her 15-year-old son who is experiencing sadness, irritability, loneliness and withdrawal from others around him. She is seeking information and guidance. Consider the following questions:

- What issues related to this young man's situation would you want to learn more about, and how would you approach this scenario with the young person?
- Why might it be important to focus on his distress and his experience of feeling the way he does?

Mental illness and stigma

Stigma and discrimination are factors that can affect a person's ability to seek help for mental illness. In general, the public – including some health professionals – perceives people who experience mental illness as difficult, dangerous and unpredictable, and those with chronic mental health conditions such as schizophrenia are the most feared (Mental Health Council of Australia, 2011). This perception can result in perpetual discrimination and stigma (Reavley & Jorm, 2011). Stigma can be defined as a spoiled identity that discredits a person in society who possesses an attribute that makes him or her different from others and less desirable; a person who is considered bad, dangerous or weak (Goffman, 1963). These negative attributes are devalued in a particular social context, and are endorsed by a set of prejudicial attitudes and discriminatory behaviours (Corrigan, 2000). According to Australian and New Zealand legislation, discrimination occurs when someone is treated less favourably than another person due to racial, national or ethnic origin; sex, pregnancy or marital status; age; disability; religion; sexual preference; or some other characteristic specified under anti-discrimination or human rights legislation (Australian Human Rights Commission, 2007; *Human Rights Act 1993* (New Zealand)).

Mental health clinicians need to address the issue of stigma, which is so often attached to mental illness. They need to support efforts to prevent mental ill health and promote health, wellness and resilience. Clinicians need to support the rights of people with mental illness, and enable them to participate meaningfully in society. Community awareness from mental health promotion efforts can reduce discrimination and increase opportunities for prevention and early intervention (Commonwealth of Australia, 2009).

Mental health promotion focuses on increasing a person's emotional resilience and reducing vulnerability to mental illness through the development of personal skills and self-esteem, which lead to an increased capacity to cope with life transitions and stresses (Commonwealth of Australia, 2009). Mental illness may cause high levels of stress and a reduced quality of life. Promoting hope and therapeutic optimism in people with a mental illness is an essential skill all clinicians need to practise. The aim is to develop the person's self-confidence, promote belief in her or his own capacity to recover, reach goals and transcend boundaries (Edward et al., 2011).

Reflective question

Imagine you are working with someone who has experienced depression and feelings of hopelessness for many years. This person tells you that his or her life is never going to improve and there is no point talking about the situation.

- What skills or interventions would you use to promote hope and resilience in this person?

Beliefs about mental illness

Another important part of the understanding and experience of working with people who have a mental illness is consideration of the beliefs about what causes or contributes to the onset of mental illness. This has been studied from a diverse range of perspectives, including that of: mental health professionals (Ahn, Proctor & Flanagan, 2009; Marshall et al., 2003); the general public (Adewuya & Makanjuola, 2008; Rüsch et al., 2010; Schnittker, 2008); and others who may have contact with consumers, such as religious leaders (Nguyen, Yamada & Dinh, 2011); family or carers of those affected by mental illness (Marshall et al., 2003; Yang & Wonpat-Borja, 2011); and consumers themselves (Elliott, Maitoza & Schwinger, 2011; Maher & Kroska, 2002; Rüsch et al., 2010).

Different potential reasons or causes for mental illness that have been proposed range from life events such as the loss of significant relationships (Brown & Harris, 1978; Davies, 2001) to genetic factors (Baum et al., 2008), substance misuse (Adewuya & Makanjuola, 2008) and factors such as witchcraft (Adewuya & Makanjuola, 2008) or spiritual possession (Nguyen et al., 2011). Explanations for what origins of mental illness are often clustered into broader categories, such as biological/psychological/social factors (for example, Ahn et al., 2009; Williams & Healy, 2001). Other classifications for causal factors include factors that are considered internal/external (Elliott et al., 2011; Williams & Healy, 2001), or controllable/uncontrollable (Elliott et al., 2011; Maher & Kroska, 2002) to the person. Beliefs about the origins of mental illness are thought to be influenced by various factors, including a person's gender (Maher & Kroska, 2002), cultural background (Schnittker, 2008; Yang & Wonpat-Borja, 2011) or religious views (Nguyen et al., 2011).

Within the biomedical model of psychiatry, mental illness is largely attributed to malfunctioning in the brain. Yet, people who have lived with mental illness propose a much wider range of possible reasons (Elliott et al., 2011). Sandy Jeffs is an Australian writer who has been diagnosed with schizophrenia; in her writing she has pondered the possibilities for what may have been the basis for or contributed to the onset of mental illness in her situation:

> How does one explain the experience of falling into madness, one's mind fracturing? Somewhere in there festers my fraught relationships with my parents, the early experience of sexual assault, a confused attraction to Catholicism, and contradictory feelings of self-loathing and self-aggrandisement … My childhood was awful. I have wondered many times whether its crushing weight was what tipped my fragile mind over the edge. Or was my madness simply a biochemical imbalance that would have developed anyway?
>
> Jeffs, 2009, p. 18

The process of considering these possibilities was an important one for Jeffs, who noted that 'through the process of uncovering and reconstructing my life in sequence and through reflection, I can make sense of it' (2009, p. 18). Making sense of mental illness is a process that often involves moving between – or abandoning – various beliefs, and thus may be marked by movement and uncertainty (Kinderman et al., 2006; Williams & Healy, 2001). The explanations people attribute to mental illnesses are important for a range of reasons. Beliefs about the causes of mental illness may influence preferences and expectations for treatment and engagement (Khalsa et al, 2011). Therefore, beliefs and the understandings people have about the causes of mental illness also carry important consequences for recovery.

Mental health care focuses on consumer recovery as a principle for care delivery that embodies the concepts of consumer self-determination, resilience and self-management in determining nursing interventions. The concept of recovery will be explored in more detail shortly.

Reflective questions

Imagine that you or someone close to you is diagnosed with a mental illness.

- What kind of experiences do you think you/your friend would be having at this point?
- How might these affect your everyday life?
- How might the experience of having a mental illness differ from the experience of a physical illness?

Mental health nursing

Mental health nursing is primarily concerned with responding to people with mental illness. Mental health nursing practice is grounded in the needs of consumers and deployed in support of the person's support and carer network, where this exists. This book seeks to demonstrate this using a range of techniques. In developing each chapter, the authors drew input from people with lived experience of mental illnesses, their families, carers and clinicians at various levels to help illuminate key issues.

The approach taken in this book is consistent with what many believe to be fundamental to mental health nursing. The Australian College of Mental Health Nurses (see www.acmhn.org) believes that mental health nursing is a unique interpersonal process, which promotes and maintains behaviours that contribute to human flourishing for individuals and communities.

Mental health nursing is therapeutic in itself in the caring, honest and trusting relationship it conveys. Mental health nursing embodies the concepts of caring and compassion, by supporting consumers who are unable to maintain mental, social or physical health functioning for themselves, and empowers the consumer to take an active role in self-advocacy and self-care. Caring extends to self and peers, as an active factor in promoting mental health.

The clinician is a non-judgemental, ethically aware person who responds to the needs of the consumer in a flexible and open manner. The clinician works alongside people with a mental illness, empowering, advocating and supporting individuals and their families to find ways of coping with the difficulties they currently face. The clinician helps the person to discover and ascribe individual meaning to her or his experiences and to explore opportunities for recovery and personal growth.

Consumer narrative   Alex: Michael's nurse

Working as a clinical mental health nurse in the city's major emergency department, I received a referral from an emergency department's medical officer for a young man named Michael. Michael had been brought in by ambulance after his mother found him at home, unable to be roused. Michael had consumed alcohol and taken an overdose of

continued ›

40 mg diazepam. On arrival, his breath alcohol provided an estimated 0.32 blood alcohol content (BAC). Michael was referred to me once his BAC had reduced to 0.05.

After approaching Michael in a relatively low-key manner and explaining who I was, he agreed to talk to me about how he had been feeling and why he took an overdose of medication last night.

Michael stated that he has been feeling down 'for ages' and has been using more and more alcohol and marijuana to help him cope. Using his description of the situation, I considered Michael's experiences to be symptoms of trauma and distress, which have developed over the past three years.

I also needed to explore Michael's mental state before this time, so I asked him about his childhood and his experience of school. Michael said that he was a sociable, popular guy at school who enjoyed spending time with friends. Michael said that this all changed after he was assaulted in the city when he was 21 years old.

At this point it was important to assess Michael's risk, so I asked him why he took 40 mg of diazepam last night. He stated that he was intoxicated and wanted to get some uninterrupted sleep, and so took more than the prescribed dose of diazepam. I asked Michael whether he believed this would end his life, which he denied. He appeared to be shocked by the question. He said that he had not thought it would harm him and, although he sometimes has fleeting thoughts of ending his life, he would never intentionally try to hurt himself. He felt upset that his mother had found him in this state. He explained that he wanted help to improve his situation, as he has not spoken to anyone about this before. I reflected back to Michael all that he had told me and asked whether I had missed anything. I thanked Michael for opening up to me and telling me his story. I reassured Michael that his situation could be helped and that his symptoms were treatable with the right support.

I discussed my assessment with the consultant psychiatrist, who agreed to refer Michael to the community mental health team and link him with a cognitive behavioural therapy specialist and psychiatrist who might consider commencement of an anti-depressant. I would also provide Michael with information for community drug and alcohol services to support him in psychosocial activities and other supports to help reduce his alcohol, marijuana and benzodiazepine use. A letter would be sent to Michael's GP with the mental health assessment and a suggested plan for follow-up.

Reflective questions

- How might you engage someone like Michael in conversation so that he feels valued and respected?
- What sorts of behaviours would show Michael that you are engaged in his story and would help him to feel respected and valued?
- What qualities or characteristics, such as compassion, do you think are important to engage effectively with someone like Michael?

Mental health nursing as a specialist field

Mental health nursing is a specialist field of nursing that focuses on meeting the mental health needs of the consumer, in partnership with family, significant others and the community, in any setting. It is a specialised, interpersonal process embodying the concept of caring, which is designed to be therapeutic by:

1 supporting and advocating for consumers to optimise their health status in a manner that is congruent with their explanatory model and life situation;
2 encouraging consumers to take an active role in decisions about their health care;
3 genuinely involving family, significant others and communities in the care and support of consumers;
4 being proactive in the care and support of consumers, in support of citizenship and human rights.

Some of the predominant clinical roles of the mental health clinician are to work collaboratively to assess consumers' mental health needs and provide therapeutic support where possible. The mental health clinician works from a body of knowledge as well as from an experimental basis for which feelings can be received and lives revealed. These combined elements of the consumer narrative and evidence-based care help to ensure that the consumer is provided with the highest possible standard of care, based upon present and future needs.

The importance of trust in mental health nursing

As in most relationships, it is widely acknowledged that trust is a core component of clinical engagement between mental health consumers and clinicians (Gardner, McCutcheon & Fedoruk, 2011; Hellwig, 1993; Junghan et al., 2007; Killaspy et al., 2009; Kirsh & Tate, 2006; Vecchi, Van Hasselt & Romano, 2005). It is also recognised that trust is something that takes time to establish (Addis & Gamble, 2004). There is increasing literature highlighting that mistrust is often a key reason people disengage from mental health services (Priebe et al., 2005; Watts & Priebe, 2002). Trust is a fundamental requirement for effective and contemporary mental health service delivery. Thus, in the mental health context – one that may be characterised with significant human interaction to establish therapeutic relationships – it is important to understand the nature, scope and consequences surrounding how trust is facilitated. From this perspective, we can begin to understand how this contributes to consumer engagement, both in the immediate instance and in the future.

Mental health nurses working with people who are experiencing mental distress may encounter difficult and sometimes complex negotiations and decisions. Such decisions may have to be made at a time when the person is distressed, angry or confused, and when the causes of his or her behaviour are unclear. Being empathetic to consumers' experiences is considered an important means by which to demonstrate 'genuine care'. Without genuine care to facilitate and communicate empathy, the ability to engage in the future may be hindered.

Reflective question

Think of situations when you have felt distressed and/or anxious. Aside from the details of the situation you were in, write down three things that helped you to reduce the feelings you had at that time.

Mental state assessment

The mental state assessment is an important skill for mental health clinicians to have and use in a range of practice settings. Assessment of mental health and mental illness is discussed in extensive detail in Chapter 5. The mental state examination is designed to assess the mental state of a person objectively, and to collect valid data related to the person's current situation and background. It allows the opportunity to develop a therapeutic relationship through building a deeper understanding of the person's experience, and then working to formulate a treatment plan in collaboration with the person and his or her family or carer. During the mental state assessment, the mental health clinician develops a therapeutic connection or alliance with the consumer. The mental health clinician should work in partnership with the person and carer to offer support, treatment and care in an atmosphere of hope and optimism.

Engaging in a therapeutic alliance during the mental state assessment

The idea being advanced here is to consider the assessment interview as an interactive and collaborative process, with opportunities to:

• Develop a relationship with the person.
• Establish trust.
• Promote professional closeness and collaboration.
• Identify and explore issues and concerns relevant to the consumer experience.
• Identify how the person's resources might help him or her to overcome distress.

In deepening our engagement with Michael (see Consumer narrative page 2), the first interview is an opportunity for both parties to experience it as a human-to-human activity. For the nurse, this might mean accepting the need to set aside your professional status, choosing instead to give something of yourself and placing emphasis on attempting to understand 'human crisis' in a 'human way'.

In applying this level of analysis to Michael's situation, the nurse explores:

• Michael's perception of the circumstances that have resulted in him being brought to hospital;
• how Michael sees himself and others within the crisis;
• how it feels to be Michael experiencing his situation;
• how things have changed for Michael and how he feels about this;
• Michael's immediate needs and perceived supports.

This form of relationship engagement will help to build consumers' resilience and aid in their recovery.

Recovery

Recovery is the active process of people with mental illness moving toward achieving well-being and a satisfying life, despite the presence of mental illness. The meaning of this term is in contrast to other understandings of the term 'recovery', such as a return to a previous level of functioning. Recovery is not generally viewed by people with a mental illness as a return to a previous state, since their experiences of living with mental illness, including factors such as treatment, hospitalisation and stigma, have likely changed their lives irrevocably (Davidson, 2003). Thus, recovery has been characterised as a journey that is 'deeply personal' (Anthony, 1993), individual (Jeffs, 2009) or unique (Deegan, 1996). Recovery is often a transformative process (Jeffs, 2009) of accepting the presence of mental illness and in redefining the self as more than a mental illness (Deegan, 1996).

A person seeking to be in recovery assumes responsibility for his or her own mental health, in partnership with family, carers and mental health clinicians. As such, recovery from mental illness does not occur in isolation, but with assistance from key others. Recovery is facilitated by the deeply human responses of others (Anthony, 1993). This means valuing and respecting the lived experience of people with mental illness, their family members and carers.

The importance of hope, resilience and reconnection is paramount. Therapeutic optimism on the part of the clinician is an important factor in this regard, and is defined as a 'clinician's self-reported, specific expectancies regarding client outcomes in a clinical setting' (Byrne & Sullivan, 2006, p. 11). Optimism is made therapeutic as it facilitates the processing of negative information, gives rise to thorough and flexible ways to be supportive and promotes the development of coping and problem-solving skills.

Working collaboratively with consumers, helping and supporting their reconnection with a social life and meaningful activities, in particular social activities outside of the mental health environment, such as gaining employment or volunteering in the wider community, are important to being in recovery. Having roles and routines provide a sense of purpose and goals around which everyday life can be structured. Recovery is not a linear process and continues to occur even when symptoms recur. Therapeutic optimism will help to facilitate resilience and enhance coping skills to manage life's challenges.

Reflective questions

- What do you consider to be the key enablers of helping people achieve optimal recovery?
- What factors or conditions do you think would create challenges to being in recovery?
- How might the idea of therapeutic optimism be developed and deployed in Michael's situation?

Collaborative practice in mental health nursing

Collaborative practice involves taking time and setting the context for a personable relationship with a consumer and her or his family. The approach taken is marked by genuine empathy for the person and belief in the benefits of meaningful engagement. Spending time with Michael requires much more than taking a predefined nursing or medical history. In taking the opportunity to meet with Michael, there is also an opportunity to talk about ways to help him feel connected and safe in his new environment. In preparing to discuss his admission, the nurse enquires about Michael's understanding of his current situation. This means exploring any concerns he may have and the practical steps that can be taken to work together, with dignity and respect, and in partnership with others, to help address these concerns.

Collaborative practice with carers and family members

Collaborative practice also involves working with family members and carers. Mental health carers provide unpaid care and support to family members or friends who have a mental illness. Carers may range from children through to older adults, and may be of any cultural background. Carers are central to the care and support of people with a mental illness, and are the major providers of care in the community (Carers Australia, 2012). The role of caring for someone with a mental illness is not always understood by others, as the tasks undertaken may be quite different to what is generally understood as a 'caring' role (Carers Australia, 2012). For example, tasks associated with caring for someone with a physical disability, such as assistance with bathing or cooking, may not be undertaken to support a person with a mental illness. Instead, the role of caring in this context may include tasks such as providing emotional or social support, helping the person to organise his or her daily schedule or dealing with emergencies.

It is not uncommon that people do not identify themselves as carers, as it is often assumed that carers receive payment for care. Stigma may be another reason for not identifying as a carer of a person with a mental illness. This may be especially pronounced in cultures that view mental illness as having serious, widespread effects on the family of people who have a mental illness; for example, if mental illness is viewed as something that will bring a curse upon family or community members. Therefore, the estimated number of carers for people with mental illness is likely to be largely underestimated. Furthermore, some consumers may not view a family member or friend who provides them with care and support as carers. These issues outline some of the challenges in being a carer for someone with a mental illness.

Carers are a valuable, yet under-utilised source of information about the well-being of a person with mental illness. Carers quite often know the person with a mental illness very well and for a long time. As such, carers may have information that can be useful in supporting the person in his or her recovery. However, due to the many challenges related to being a carer of a person with a mental illness, carers may not seek or receive sufficient support. It is important to ask carers about their own existing support systems, such as family or friends, and whether they require additional help or support, such as counselling or being connected with carer support groups.

Consumer narrative   Zoe's story

My name is Zoe. I'm a 32-year-old engineer, and I'm married with two young children. I am also the carer of David, my older brother. David is 36 years old and has lived with a bipolar condition for the past 15 years. When David was 21 years old, our father died following a gun accident. David was particularly close to our father, often describing him as his best friend. Our parents had divorced prior to our father's passing, and David has had little contact with our mother since they separated.

At the time of our father's death, David was in his final year of study to become a lawyer. David became deeply depressed, refusing to eat or talk. He was hospitalised for three months, where he was given electroconvulsive treatment (ECT). Upon returning home, David found it difficult to continue his studies or socialise. He would spend most of his time watching TV and sleeping, a situation that continued for some years. I would usually visit David every second day, and I would try to encourage him to go for a walk, help me with the shopping, or join in social activities. David's old friends would also ask to visit but he declined. To try and maintain some of his friendships, I helped David to set up a Facebook account, but unfortunately he rarely accessed it.

One day, I noticed David behaving differently – he was very chatty and upbeat, talking about going to a party he had been invited to through Facebook. I thought this behaviour was odd and out of character, but I was relieved that he no longer seemed so down. The next time I visited, David seemed to be a completely different person. He had invited all of the neighbours over and was hosting a martini evening. When he ushered me into the house, I was made to feel like royalty. David was speaking at such a rate that I could barely make sense of what he was saying. He was certainly the 'life of the party', but I couldn't help feeling that I and the other guests were a captive audience. I was concerned about David's behaviour, so I decided to stay until the party finished. The last guests left at 4.00 a.m. At 7.00 a.m., David was still wide awake, singing, cleaning and wearing strange clothes. By midnight the following day, David had still not slept and had become agitated with me and his neighbours, who had asked him to turn the music down. I began to feel increasingly threatened, so I called the police. David repeated that 'the devil would be here to intervene soon'. Instead, the police visited and, shortly afterwards David was taken to the psychiatric hospital.

Reflective questions

- What do you think Zoe might have been feeling or experiencing before and after David was taken to hospital?
- Once David becomes well again, how might he feel about the situation, including Zoe's involvement that led to him being taken to hospital?
- In the long term, what kinds of supports or resources might Zoe need to be able to provide good care and support to David?

Interprofessional connections in mental health nursing

The importance of making meaningful connections with consumers and carers in mental health cannot be overstated. The same can also be said with regard to interprofessional connections. One of the outcomes of mainstreaming mental health services into the community is that nurses working in general health and hospital settings have increased contact with people experiencing mental health issues and mental illness. For this reason, interprofessional care is an increasingly important aspect of clinical practice.

As nurses, we are not expected to take sole clinical or administrative responsibility when responding to a person with mental illness. At the very least we should have fundamental skills to be able to engage therapeutically and to undertake a screening mental state assessment, carefully documenting our findings and talking with colleagues about appropriate support, referral pathways, immediate care and treatment.

It is at this point that we should be aware of our clinical networks, professional strengths and limitations – of what catches our eye, our ear (our senses, really) – and be willing to seek the assistance and support of colleagues for appropriate advice and specialist referral.

The initial contact with a person with mental illness is particularly important, but often it occurs in less-than-ideal circumstances, such as in a busy and noisy emergency room, the unfamiliar surroundings of a person's home, or on the telephone. In some instances, particularly when working with people from diverse cultural and linguistic backgrounds, it may be difficult to speak with the person in private, and confidentiality can be a concern.

It is important to remember that even when people are distressed and facing extreme life circumstances, they may have recently perceived rejection or other negative situations. As such, a considerable degree of expertise and patience may be required in order to establish therapeutic rapport. This can be an effective pathway to establishing safety and dignity for all concerned, and can be achieved by indicating that one wishes to try and understand what is happening to that person and that a certain amount of time has been set aside in order to do so. This approach can help to create a context for human connectedness so that feelings are able to be explored and lives revealed. Such actions are important in their own right, and also are known to favourably shift risk and reduce the likelihood of additional distress and suffering.

Chapter summary

This chapter has presented stories and information, supplemented by activities designed to deepen understanding of:

- The nature, scope and consequences of mental health and mental illness, including social determinants
- The various meanings and understandings of key concepts in mental health; mental illness has been explained through an interaction between the published literature and consumer and carer experiences
- The narrative approach, by making 'real-world links' as we enter into the world of the consumer and carer
- Joint narratives, accomplished through sharing of everyday experiences, knowledge and interaction
- The practice of mental health nursing expressed as a joint activity involving stories through which the consumer, carer and nurse learn together.

Critical thinking/learning activities

1   Consider Michael's story and his experiences. What interventions or services might he need to help him build resilience, to enable recovery with dignity?
2   What does the term 'recovery' mean in the field of mental health? How does this differ from its meaning in other areas of health?
3   What are some of the key roles undertaken by a carer of a person with a mental illness?
4   What are the four key metabolic changes people with mental illness are at risk of developing? How can the risk of these changes be minimised?
5   How does stigma affect the lived experience of a person with a mental illness and his or her family or carers?

Learning extension

The following is a list of terms used to refer to people with a mental illness:

Consumer	Service user	Mentally retarded
Lunatic	Mentally ill	Crazy
Survivor	Client	Mad
Mental health problem	Eccentric	Patient

Write a paragraph answering the following questions:
- How would you feel if these terms were applied to you and/or your family?
- Would any be more or less acceptable to you? Explain your answer.

Further reading

De Leo, **D.** (2011). *Turning Points. An extraordinary journey into the suicidal mind.* Bowen Hills: Australian Academic Press.

Deegan, **P.** (1996). Recovery as a journey of the heart. *Psychiatric Rehabilitation Journal. 19*(3): 91–7.

Mendoza, **J.**, **Bresnan**, **A.**, **Rosenberg**, **S.**, **Elson**, **A.**, **Gilbert**, **Y.**, **Long**, **P.**, **Wilson**, **K.** & **Hopkins**, **J.** (2013). *Obsessive Hope Disorder: Reflections on 30 years of mental health reform in Australia and visions for the future. Summary report.* Caloundra, Qld: CoNetica.

Mental Health Council of Australia (MHCA) (2011). *Consumer and Carer Experiences of Stigma from Mental Health and Other Health Professionals.* Canberra: Author.

O'Hagan, **M.** (2013). *Straight Answers to the Curley Questions in Mental Health.* Retrieved from www.maryohagan.com/publications.php.

References

Addis, **J.** & **Gamble**, **C.** (2004). Assertive outreach nurses' experience of engagement. *Journal of Psychiatric and Mental Health Nursing, 11*: 452–60.

Adewuya, **A.O.** & **Makanjuola**, **R.O.A.** (2008). Lay beliefs regarding causes of mental illness in Nigeria: Pattern and correlates. *Social Psychiatry and Psychiatric Epidemiology, 43*: 336–41.

Ahn, **W.**, **Proctor**, **C.C.** & **Flanagan**, **E.H.** (2009). Mental health clinicians' beliefs about the biological, psychological, and environmental bases of mental disorders. *Cognitive Science 33*: 147–82.

American Psychiatric Association (2012). *Diagnostic and Statistical Manual of Mental Disorders (DSM)* Retrieved from www.psychiatry.org/practice/dsm.

Anthony, **W.A.** (1993). Recovery from mental illness: The guiding vision of the mental health service system in the 1990s. *Psychosocial Rehabilitation Journal, 16*: 11–24.

Australian Bureau of Statistics (ABS) (2007). *National Survey of Mental Health and Wellbeing: Summary of results* (No. 4326.0). Canberra: Author.

ABS & **Australian Institute of Health and Welfare (AIHW)** (2008). *The Health and Welfare of Australia's Aboriginal and Torres Strait Islander Peoples* (No. 4704.0). Canberra: Authors.

Australian Human Rights Commission (2007). *A Guide to Australia's Anti-discrimination Laws.* Retrieved from www.humanrights.gov.au/guide-australias-anti-discrimination-laws.

Baum, **A.E.**, **Akula**, **N.**, **Cabanero**, **M.**, **Cardona**, **I.**, **Corona**, **W**, **Klemens**, **B.** & **McMahon**, **F.J.** (2008). A genome-wide association study implicates diacylglycerol kinase eta (DGKH) and several other genes in the etiology of bipolar disorder. *Molecular Psychiatry, 13*: 197–207.

Brown, **G.W.** & **Harris**, **T.** (1978). *Social Origins of Depression: A study of psychiatric disorder in women.* London: Tavistock Publications.

Byrne, **M.K**, & **Sullivan**, **N.L.** (2006). Clinical optimism: Development and psychometric analysis of a scale for mental health clinicians. *Australian Journal of Rehabilitation Counselling, 12*: 11–20.

Carers Australia (2012). *Carers Australia and Network of Carers Associations National Policy Position Statement: Mental health reform.* Retrieved from www.carersaustralia.com.au/publications/position-statements.

Commission on Social Determinants of Health (2008). *Closing the Gap in a Generation: Health equity through action on the social determinants of health.* Geneva: World Health Organization.

Commonwealth of Australia (2009). *National Mental Health Policy 2008.* Canberra: Author.

Corrigan, **P.W.** (2000). *Mental Health Stigma As Social Attribution: Implications for research methods and attitude change.* United States: American Psychological Association.

Council of Australian Governments (COAG) (2012). *The Roadmap for National Mental Health Reform 2012–2022.* Canberra: Author.

Davidson, **L.** (2003). *Living Outside Mental Illness: Qualitative studies of recovery in schizophrenia.* New York: New York University Press.

Davies, **K.** (2001). 'Silent and censured travellers?' Patients' narratives and patients' voices: Perspectives on the history of mental illness since 1948. *Social History of Medicine, 14*: 267–92.

De Hert, M., Schreurs, V., Vancampfort, D. & Van Winkle, R. (2009). Metabolic syndrome in people with schizophrenia: A review. *World Psychiatry, 8*: 15–22.

Deegan, P. (1996). Recovery as a journey of the heart. *Psychiatric Rehabilitation Journal, 19*: 91–8.

Department of Health and Ageing (1998). *The Kit: A guide to the advocacy we choose to do.* Retrieved from www.health.gov.au/internet/publications/publishing.nsf/Content/mental-pubs-k-kit-toc~mental-pubs-k-kit-kno~mental-pubs-k-kit-kno-und~mental-pubs-k-kit-kno-und-wha.

Edward, K., Munro, I., Robins, A. & Welch, A. (2011). *Mental Health Nursing: Dimensions of praxis.* South Melbourne: Oxford University Press.

Elliott, M., Maitoza, R. & Schwinger, E. (2011). Subjective accounts of the causes of mental illness in the USA. *International Journal of Social Psychiatry, 58*: 562–7.

Gardner, A. McCutcheon, H. & Fedoruk, M. (2010). Therapeutic friendliness and the development of therapeutic leverage by mental health nurses in community rehabilitation settings. *Contemporary Nurse, 34*(2): 140–8.

Goffman, E. (1963). *Stigma: Notes on the management of spoiled identity.* New York: Simon Schuster.

Happell, B., Platania-Phung, C., Gray, R., Hardy, S., Lambert, T., McAllister, M. & Davies, C. (2011). A role for mental health nursing in the physical health care of consumers with severe mental illness. *Journal of Psychiatric and Mental Health Nursing, 18*: 706–11.

Hellwig, K. (1993). Psychiatric home care nursing: Managing patients in the community setting. *Journal of Psychosocial Nursing and Mental Health Services, 31*: 21–4.

Jeffs, S. (2009). *Flying With Paper Wings: Reflections on living with madness.* Carlton North, Vic.: The Vulgar Press.

Junghan, U. M., Leese, M., Priebe, S. & Slade, M. (2007). Staff and patient perspectives on unmet need and therapeutic alliance in community mental health services. *British Journal of Psychiatry, 191*: 543–7.

Keleher, H. & Armstrong, R. (2005). *Evidence-based Mental Health Promotion Resource.* Melbourne: Public Health Group, Victorian Government Department of Human Services.

Khalsa, S., McCarthy, K. S., Sharpless, B. A., Barrett, M. S. & Barber, J. P. (2011). Beliefs about the causes of depression and treatment preferences. *Journal of Clinical Psychology, 67*: 539–49.

Killaspy, H., Johnson, S., Pierce, B., Bebbington, P., Pilling, S., Nolan, F. & King, M. (2009). Successful engagement: A mixed methods study of the approaches of assertive community treatment and community mental health teams in the REACT trial. *Social Psychiatry and Psychiatric Epidemiology, 44*: 532–40.

Kinderman, P., Setzu, E., Lobban, F. & Salmon, P. (2006). Illness beliefs in schizophrenia. *Social Science & Medicine, 63*: 1900–11.

Kirsh, B. & Tate, E. (2006). Developing a comprehensive understanding of the working alliance in community mental health. *Qualitative Health Research, 16*: 1054–74.

Maher, E. J. & Kroska, A. (2002). Social status determinants of control in individuals' accounts of their mental illness. *Social Science & Medicine, 55*: 949–61.

Marshall, T., Solomon, P., Steber, S. & Mannion, E. (2003). Provider and family beliefs regarding the causes of severe mental illness. *Psychiatric Quarterly, 74*: 223–36.

Mendoza, J., Bresnan, A., Rosenberg, S., Elson, A., Gilbert, Y., Long, P., Wilson, K. & Hopkins, J. (2013). *Obsessive Hope Disorder: Reflections on 30 years of mental health reform in Australia and visions for the future. Summary report.* Caloundra, Qld: CoNetica.

Mental Health Council of Australia. (2011). *Consumer and Carer Experiences of Stigma From Mental Health and Other Health Professionals.* Canberra: Author.

Michel, K. & Valach, L. (2011). The narrative interview with suicidal patient. In K. Michel & D. Jobes (eds), *Building a Therapeutic Alliance with the Suicidal Patient* (pp. 63–80). Washington: American Psychological Association.

Morgan, V. A., Waterreus, A., Jablensky, A., Mackinnon, A., McGrath, J. J., Carr, V. & Saw, S. (2011). *People Living With Psychotic Illness 2010: Report on the second Australian national survey.* Canberra: Commonwealth of Australia.

Nguyen, H. T., Yamada, A. M. & Dinh, T. Q. (2011). Religious leaders' assessment and attribution of the causes of mental illness: An in-depth exploration of Vietnamese American Buddhist leaders. *Mental Health, Religion & Culture, 15*: 511–27.

Oakley Browne, M. A., Well, J. E. & Scott, K. M. (2006). *Te Rau Hinengaro: The New Zealand Mental Health Survey.* Wellington: Ministry of Health.

Parish, C. (2011). Mental illness reduces life expectancy: Research finds. *Mental Health Practice, 14*: 5.

Pescosolido, B. (2013). The public stigma of mental illness: What do we think; what do we know; what can we prove? *Journal of Health and Social Behavior, 54*: 1–21.

Posselt, M., Galletly, C., de Crespigny, C. & Procter, N. G. (2013). Mental health and drug and alcohol comorbidity in young people of refugee background: A review of literature. *Mental Health and Substance Use*. Retrieved from www.tandfonline.com/doi/pdf/10.1080/17523281.2013.772914.

Priebe, S., Watts, J., Chase, M. & Matanov, A. (2005). Processes of disengagement and engagement in assertive outreach patients: Qualitative study. *British Journal of Psychiatry, 187*: 438–43.

Reavley, N.J. & Jorm, A.F. (2011). *National Survey of Mental Health Literacy and Stigma*. Canberra: Department of Health and Ageing.

Rüsch, N., Todd, A.R., Bodenhausen, G.V. & Corrigan, P.W. (2010). Biogenetic models of psychopathology, implicit guilt, and mental illness stigma. *Psychiatry Research, 179*: 328–32.

Saha, S., Chant, D. & McGrath, J. (2007). A systematic review of mortality in schizophrenia: Is the differential mortality gap worsening over time? *Archives of General Psychiatry, 64*: 1123–31.

Schizophrenia Fellowship of NSW Inc. (2008). *Accommodation*. Retrieved from www.sfnsw.org.au/Mental-Illness/Quality-of-Life/Quality-of-Life-Accommodation#.Uh7KObxvSQk.

Schnittker, J. (2008). An uncertain revolution: Why the rise of a genetic model of mental illness has not increased tolerance. *Social Science & Medicine, 67*: 1370–81.

Short, T., Thomas, S., Mullen, P. & Ogloff, J.R.P. (2013). Comparing violence in schizophrenia patients with and without comorbid substance-use disorders to community controls. *Acta Psychiatrica Scandinavia*. Retrieved from http://onlinelibrary.wiley.com/doi/10.1111/acps.12066/pdf.

Stewart-Harawira, M. (2005). *The New Imperial Order: Indigenous response to colonisation*. Wellington: Huia Publishers.

Vecchi, G.M., Van Hasselt, V.B. & Romano, S.J. (2005). Crisis (hostage) negotiation: Current strategies and issues in high-risk conflict resolution. *Aggression and Violent Behavior, 10*: 533–551.

Watts, J. & Priebe, S. (2002). A phenomenological account of users' experiences of assertive community treatment. *Bioethics, 16*: 439–454.

Williams, B. & Healy, D. (2001). Perceptions of illness causation among new referrals to a community mental health team: 'Explanatory model' or 'exploratory map'? *Social Science and Medicine, 53*: 456–76.

World Health Organization (WHO) (2012). *World Health Statistics. Part II: Highlighted topics*. Retrieved from www.who.int/gho/publications/world_health_statistics/EN_WHS2012_Part2.pdf.

WHO 2013a. *International Classification of Diseases (ICD)*. Retrieved from www.who.int/classifications/icd/en.

WHO 2013b. *Substance Abuse*. Retrieved from www.who.int/topics/substance_abuse/en.

Yang, L.H. & Wonpat-Borja, A.J. (2011). Causal beliefs and effects upon mental illness identification among Chinese immigrant relatives of individuals with psychosis. *Community Mental Health Journal, 48*: 471–6.

2

Learning through human connectedness on clinical placement: Translation to practice

Denise McGarry

Introduction 26
Mental health (nursing) education:
  An overview 26
Attitudes, expectations and positive
  engagement within practice 28
Application of interpersonal skills within
  the mental health practicum placement
  and other, non-mental health settings 31
Power relations involved in the therapeutic
  relationship 31
Development of emotional competence 34
Reflective practice as a critical thinking
  process 34
Clinical supervision for the beginning/novice
  nursing student within mental health
  nursing 35

Developing objectives for clinical
  placements 38
The process of self-assessment and personal
  problem solving 40
Reflection, self, in-action and
  post-placement 40
Ethical and political influences on care 41
And off to clinical placement: Pragmatic
  strategies for learning 42
Chapter summary 47
Critical thinking/learning activities 47
Learning extension 47
Further reading 48
References 48

Learning objectives

At the completion of this chapter, you should be able to:

- Develop strategies to prioritise and personalise learning objectives when undertaking mental health study as an undergraduate student.
- Recognise opportunities and responsibilities to develop your existing learning to meet the needs of the clinical practice environment.
- Describe ways to support the recovery model through alliance with those experiencing mental illness and their carers, to achieve goals developed collaboratively.
- Develop self-reflective emotional competence to support therapeutic interactions skills applicable across a range of mental health and non-mental health practice settings.
- Practise with skill in the environment of health services, utilising evidence-based approaches.

Introduction

This chapter explores a range of challenges for students as they learn to apply interpersonal skills within the mental health practicum placement and other non-mental health settings. Exploration of the student's own attitudes, expectations and positive engagement within practice begins the chapter. This is followed by discussion of power relations characterising the therapeutic relationship, including the development of emotional competence. The chapter outlines reflective practice as a critical thinking process and clinical supervision for the beginning/novice nursing student within mental health nursing. How to go about developing objectives for practice, and the process of self-assessment and personal problem solving are discussed in the context of various clinical settings. Reflection, self in-action and post-placement will also be explored as they relate to learning in mental health. Throughout this chapter, critical examination of the ethical and political influences on care that extend beyond individual engagement with the person experiencing mental illness will be highlighted.

Mental health (nursing) education: An overview

It is probably fair to suggest that not everyone who undertakes studies in mental health has planned to do so or to work in this field. However, a large number of people experience a mental health condition during their lifetime, and it is likely that you will encounter such people in your personal life, or experience mental health challenges yourself. In preparing for a career in the health professions, adequate education to be able to help with mental health conditions is vital.

Studies have shown that there are more people experiencing mental illness in the population of general health services than in the general population (Happell & Platania-Phung, 2005). This challenges all health practitioners, and especially nurses, who represent the largest sector of the health workforce, to be capable of responding to this need. The World Health Organization (WHO) studied the health care needs of people accessing 14 different types of primary health services, in a range of countries and cultures. They found that almost a quarter (24 per cent) of participants had a mental illness (WHO, 2001). Clearly, the need for mental health services is highly prevalent and encountered in a range of settings, including some in which the mental illness may not be the problem that precipitated the initial encounter with the health service. This recognition has influenced the formats of current health education, especially that of nurses, in order to ensure their capacity and skills to recognise the need for mental health services and to be able to respond appropriately. Consider that in Australia, it has been suggested that perhaps as many as 66 per cent of adults and 75 per cent of children and young people with a mental illness do not receive treatment of any form (Department of Health and Ageing, 2005). Discussion elsewhere in this text explores the consequences of this.

Education curricula in mental health education conform broadly with those taught elsewhere in health: theoretical instruction and clinical application. The actual implementation of the curricula varies across different education programs, but increasingly the preparation of undergraduate nurses shares fundamental minimum characteristics. This is partially because national regulatory authorities require every beginning practitioner in nursing to have undertaken a set number of hours of theoretical study in mental health and clinical placement in mental health.

There are increasing pressures being experienced in Australia in the provision of the clinical placement component. Competition between different health disciplines for placement and a reduction in suitable placements have both intensified. This has resulted in clinical placements being made across a broad range of services that are now involved in the provision of care for those experiencing mental illness. Thus, the public in-patient mental health service is no longer the dominant setting for clinical placement by nurses in their preregistration education. Forensic, community, non-government and general health services are increasingly being utilised as clinical placement settings for mental health nursing.

The theoretical component of nursing education also varies according to the different university providers. This variation goes to the extent of mental health in the curriculum, its placement in the program and the background of those teaching the curriculum (Mental Health Workforce Advisory Committee, 2010).

Not all theoretical curricula for mental health nursing are designed exclusively to prepare nurses to work in this field. Nursing shares many skills and understandings across the specialist fields of health, especially at the beginning health practitioner level. Communication skills are a good case in point, as are infection control principles. Therefore, not all theoretical preparation for mental health nursing will be labelled as such. At times, the relevance and contribution of these fields of study to your beginning practice in mental health nursing can be challenging to recall and recognise.

This may contribute to an often-reported phenomenon: the self-perceived lack of preparation for clinical placement in mental health reported by nursing students. In turn, this may contribute to the fear reported by many nurses prior to their first placement in a mental health service. This fear is often described as arising from three major concerns:

1 the assumed unpredictable nature of behaviour associated with mental illness;

2 expectations of high levels of violence associated with mental illness; and

3 concern that failure to speak or respond in a 'correct' manner may cause harm to a consumer (Hayman-White & Happell, 2005).

It is important, first, to acknowledge that some of these ideas and beliefs are remnants of unexamined **stigma** and **stereotyping**. Health practitioners, including nurses, ordinarily

stigma
a form of prejudice against people with a mental illness that involves inaccurate and hurtful representations of them; in some instances those representations might be as violent, comical or incompetent. This form of stigma is dehumanising and makes people with a mental illness the object of fear or ridicule

stereotype
a taken-for-granted assumption about a person, based on the presumed qualities of the group to which she or he belongs; stereotypes can lead to inaccurate assessments of people's personal qualities and characteristics

have a range of socially determined beliefs about the nature of mental health problems (Mental Health Council of Australia, 2011). Even direct instruction or education may not alter these, as this teaching is filtered through the lens of prior beliefs and constantly reinforced by many prominent social institutions, such as the media.

Also, the nature of therapeutic interventions in mental health nursing can be in stark contrast to the procedural delivery model applicable elsewhere in health care. Therapeutic use of self has prominence that can be unsettling (Edwards & Burnard, 2003). It is, however, what those experiencing mental illness most value, but are not always accorded by mental health nurses (Rydon, 2005; Shattell, Starr & Thomas, 2007).

Attitudes, expectations and positive engagement within practice

The ability to engage in a positive manner within mental health nursing draws on the therapeutic use of 'self'. The aim of this type of practice is to establish a therapeutic alliance with the person experiencing mental ill health, to help in achieving her or his desired recovery goals. It is part of the central tradition of caring in nursing, but has some different features and emphases in the domain of mental health nursing.

The therapeutic relationship is the foundational component of mental health nursing care, which facilitates any other interventions or therapies. Its ascendancy in mental health nursing is often attributed to the work of Peplau (1952, 1997), especially in the United States. However, the details of how to use the therapeutic relationship in mental health nursing are complex and are sometimes contested (Hurley & Rankin, 2008).

Empathy, collaboration and alliance have been suggested as critical elements of the therapeutic relationship (Norcross, Beutler & Levant, 2006), and these are explored more closely in this chapter. However, the claims for the importance of the therapeutic relationship must be judged by the effect it has on recovery for people experiencing mental health problems. Norcross and colleagues have suggested that although much of the variation in therapeutic outcomes is related to the severity of mental illness and characteristics of those experiencing them, the remaining unexplained variance is understood to be attributable not to a particular intervention, but to the therapeutic relationship itself (Norcross & Lambert, 2006, pp. 208–18).

Empathy

This construct is central to all the helping professions, including mental health nursing, and comprises two aspects: a cognitive and an affective component. It is sometimes characterised as feeling 'with' rather than 'for' the person experiencing mental illness. This rough characterisation attempts to emphasise the importance of understanding the other person's situation and his or her feelings about the situation. This is often contrasted with the emotion of sympathy, which is concerned with how the nurse responds personally to the consumer's situation. Although empathy is considered a central component in facilitating positive outcomes for consumers, it has not been frequently and rigorously studied or demonstrated to be responsible for such results (Kunyk & Olson, 2001).

Collaboration

Collaboration refers to a mutual endeavour by the nurse and consumer. This endeavour is the engagement of both in the (therapeutic) relationship. Mutual goals are able to be established for the relationship when agreement is reached about the problems of the person experiencing mental illness.

Therapeutic alliance

The nursing literature exploring this element of the therapeutic relationship is not extensive, particularly when compared with other disciplines (Perraud et al., 2006). Much of the understanding in mental health nursing has been drawn from studies in psychology of psychotherapy (Norcross et al., 2006). Essentially, the therapeutic alliance refers to the strength of goal-directed activity between nurse (or other health care practitioners) and consumer. If a person-centred negotiation of goals is undertaken, the therapeutic alliance is reinforced (Horvath & Bedi, 2002).

Table 2.1 Therapist contributions to the therapeutic alliance

Therapist contributions	References
Make the development of the alliance the highest priority early in therapy.	Horvath & Bedi, 2002, pp. 60–1
Foster a collaborative partnership.	Hubble, Duncan & Miller, 1999, pp. 430–1
Listen to the consumer's theory of illness and avoid reinterpreting it to match your own theory.	Hubble et al., 1999
Allow the consumer to direct therapeutic choices.	Hubble et al., 1999
Attend to and address what the consumer considers is important and relevant.	Hubble et al., 1999
Agree on interventions – only use those that you feel confident will work.	Hubble et al., 1999, p. 417
Find out what the consumer thinks would represent improvement.	Hubble et al., 1999, p. 419
Ask consumers to notice and record improvements between sessions.This conveys an expectation that the therapy will work.	Hubble et al., 1999, p. 431
Tailor interventions and homework to accomplish goals set by the consumer.	Bachelor & Horvath, 1999, p. 152
Recognise attitudes and behaviours that cause consumers to react negatively. Avoid them.	Bachelor & Horvath, 1999, p. 152
Explore consumer hostility when it is directed towards you.	Friedlander, 1993

continued >

Table 2.1 (continued ›)

Therapist contributions	References
Engage in (clinical) supervision to explore relational difficulties	Horvath & Bedi, 2002, p. 61
Be in touch with your own experience of the consumer. Consider it relevant to use in therapy.	Klein et al., 2001
Respond honestly and sincerely	

Source: Perraud et al., 2006, p. 221.

Professional boundaries

Counter-transference is a phenomenon that may occur in any field of health care, and is also evident in mental health nursing. Defined as an unconscious response to a consumer's **transference**, it may be a significant factor requiring explicit monitoring. It may be a support to the therapeutic relationship or it may affect it detrimentally, but it risks being a factor in transgression of **professional boundaries**.

The key to maintaining professional boundaries and avoiding the potential for harm to consumers and oneself is the development of self-awareness by mental health nurses. This helps to highlight counter-transference and other factors that may affect the maintenance of a therapeutic relationship that incorporates empathy, alliance and collaboration. Developing an understanding of how a consumer's behaviour affects you and why helps to ensure that interactions remain focused on the consumer's needs and goals. This can be achieved by reflective practice, most usefully by clinical supervision or personal therapy. As a student this may be difficult to achieve, yet it is perhaps a time when it can be most critical. The **mentor**, **preceptor** or **clinical facilitator** can be an excellent source for this support.

counter-transference
the response that is elicited in the recipient (therapist) by the other's (client's) unconscious transference communications

transference
the phenomenon whereby we unconsciously transfer feelings and attitudes from a person or situation in the past onto a person or situation in the present; the process is at least partly inappropriate to the present

professional boundaries
limits that protect the space between the professional's power and the consumer's vulnerability; the borders that mark the edges between a professional, therapeutic relationship and a non-professional or personal relationship between a nurse and a person in her or his care

mentor
a teaching–learning process acquired through personal experience within a one-to-one, reciprocal, career-development relationship between two individuals diverse in age, personality, life cycle, professional status and/or credentials

preceptor
a clinical staff member – as opposed to a faculty member – who provides supervision and clinical instruction to new practitioners, undergraduate or newly registered, or new to a specific clinical environment

clinical facilitator
a registered nurse employed on a sessional basis by a school of nursing to work with a group of students allocated to a designated health facility while on their clinical placement; the clinical facilitator, who performs many linking roles between the school of nursing and the clinical facility, works with the facility's staff to ensure clinical learning opportunities for students and to assess their attainment of learning objectives for the placement

Debriefing discussion, either alone with the facilitator or with a group of fellow students, can serve as a proxy.

Application of interpersonal skills within the mental health practicum placement and other, non-mental health settings

Learning to use interpersonal skills is a daunting challenge for all health practitioners. What do I do differently to practise these skills? Often, students feel confounded by how to achieve an opportunity to rehearse and master these elusive skills, which take on a mysterious and reified nature that contributes to these difficulties.

Primarily, courteous curiosity may be a sound manner to start exploring how to use interpersonal skills in your mental health nursing practice. Observe the manner and methods of your colleagues. What do you admire about they ways in which they communicate? What do you feel falls short of skilful interpersonal communication? Take note of these observations – how can you ensure that you do not replicate the communication and interpersonal skills that you find wanting? If you are able to analyse those aspects of interpersonal communication that are less helpful, can you understand why they are sometimes used? If you gain this insight, perhaps you may be able to devise alternate strategies to replace the less-helpful interpersonal skills that you have observed.

Encountering a nurse with admirable interpersonal skills offers a great opportunity for learning. Approach this individual and request a chance to discuss your observations. She or he may be able to give you an in-depth understanding of how to develop skilful interpersonal abilities. Discuss these observations with your peers and clinical facilitator, mentor or preceptor. Additional strategies are discussed in Chapter 15.

Finally, request feedback from your peers, clinical facilitator, mentor or preceptor about your interpersonal skills. This may be difficult and confronting, but these observations may highlight your strengths and weaknesses in ways that are difficult to discern on your own. Remember that you are a student: this is an acceptable time to make mistakes and try different approaches. Take advantage of this.

Power relations involved in the therapeutic relationship

Power is a pervasive and multifaceted aspect of mental health nursing that affects the therapeutic relationship. It has origins in many of the contextual elements of the delivery of nursing practice, including the physical environment, knowledge, interprofessional teams, the law and models of holistic nursing care.

debriefing
a process frequently employed in nursing as a means by which to provide support and ensure learning possibilities are realised from clinical (real or simulated) experiences; it is often facilitated by teaching staff and encourages critical reflection and contribution from nursing students in a shared space removed but adjacent in time and place to the clinical experience

power
a complex and multifaceted construct that in health care and other social environments centres on the ability to influence people's behaviour; closely associated with constructs such as coercion, authority and influence

Its effects may be both limiting and empowering within the therapeutic relationship, where judicious use by the nurse may support a consumer to regaining his or her resilience in recovery (Pieranunzi, 1997).

Knowledge – both having and lacking knowledge – contributes to the power differential in the therapeutic relationship. A nurse has knowledge of all manner of things that may be mysterious, confusing and not self-evident to consumers. What is wrong with me? What will happen to me? Who are the people in the treatment team and of what significance are they? Nurses may have knowledge of such matters, whereas consumers may not. The knowledge in question may be quite prosaic – what is the layout of the venue, what is the timetable of events (meals, visits, appointments)? However, the imbalance undercuts an otherwise equal relationship, as the consumer is dependent upon the nurse to provide information about such matters.

The therapeutic relationship between a person with mental health problems and the nurse occurs in limited contexts. These contexts are frequently those characterised by greatest need or distress and, in certain organisational arrangements, such as assessment interviews. A nurse rarely knows a person with a mental illness beyond the role of recipient of care; for example, as a sibling, co-worker, fellow student or friend. The nurse constructs the therapeutic relationship within the limits of the 'nurse–consumer' relationship that denies the person's history, future and achievements, and this is limited to the period when mental health need is highest (May, 1992).

pathologising
the interpretation of beliefs and behaviours as evidence of an underlying disease condition, regardless of whether these constitute agreed evidence; in the field of mental health services, unusual beliefs for example, may be more likely to be seen as evidence for the illness than accepted as legitimate (although perhaps mistaken) variation in worldview, and often this is be applied to normal behaviours and is suspected in the understanding of some grief experiences

It may be argued that this is less the case in mental health practice than in other areas of nursing endeavour because of the wide range of environments in which mental health nursing occurs and its engagement in both primary and secondary preventative activities. This could be so, but mental health nursing – even within community and non-government organisational settings – defines the therapeutic relationship in terms of the mental health problems being experienced. Development of strengths-based models of nursing care, with their emphasis on resilience, continue to regard these facets of the consumer in a traditional, objectifying manner, through the lens of mental illness.

Maintaining professional boundaries also serves to establish power differentials between the nurse and consumer. Mutual sharing of confidences, personal thoughts and information are not regarded as being therapeutic and potentially are detrimental, by removing the focus of the relationship from the needs of the consumer. This also helps avoid any potential for the misuse of person power such that there is a power differential between the nurse and the person with mental illness and her or his family.

Consumers cannot be seen to have a legitimate right to insist on the disclosure of the nurse's personal world in the same manner that a nurse may ask of the consumer. Indeed, failure to 'play the patient game' and comply with a nurse's expectation of self-disclosure may have the undesired consequence of the **pathologising** of the behaviour (Foucault, 1986). What is accepted in ordinary social discourse may be regarded as evidence of problems in the context of a mental health service. A person who refuses to divulge intimate information or who demands that the nurse reveals personal information is poorly regarded. Yet, these behaviours may be defining characteristics of egalitarian relationships. The nurse, further, is involved in reinterpreting the consumer's experience, an exercise of power that effectively invalidates the consumer's personal experience.

Legal framework of practice

Establishing a therapeutic relationship in a context in which treatment is legally determined, whether as an involuntary in-patient or under involuntary provisions in a community setting, clearly skews power relationships from the initial encounter. The existence of a legal framework of compulsion for treatment within which the therapeutic relationship is engaged is problematic. A subtext, frequently unacknowledged, is that the failure to comply with the nurse's construction of the relationship may incur a legal consequence. The consumer who has engaged voluntarily in treatment may lose his or her voluntary status, or someone being treated in a community setting may have this freedom curtailed. Clearly, the law vests significant power in nurses in this regard, either formally, for example, as accredited persons under a Mental Health Act, or informally, as a discipline whose professional assessment will have weight in determining a consumer's treatment.

Cleary (2003), in a study of the changes brought to in-patient mental health nursing by the *Mental Health Act 1990* (NSW) and other changes in service provision emerging from this philosophical change, quoted a nurse's reflection on the nature of the power allocated by the legislative framework:

> It basically gives us the power to take control over [some]one's (a consumer's) life and that's very scary in a way because for us to want to do that, we really must believe that a client's lost control of their life and they need it.
>
> Cleary, 2003, p. 141

This is a very clear acknowledgement of the legislative origin of some of the differences in power that influence the therapeutic relationship. As further noted, '… nurses enforce aspects of the Mental Health Act, thus influencing patients' perceptions in relation to what they assume to be the nurses' power' (Cleary, 2003, p. 141).

As Anthony and Crawford (2000, p. 432) have stated:

> If a nurse is at one moment facilitating client choices and involvement in care and in the next required to enforce compulsory Mental Health Act sections, this is likely to confuse and discourage both parties from engagement in active working alliances.

Reflective question

Consider the dual roles for mental health nurses of care and control. Aggressive behaviour and administration of medication are two areas in which conflict may evolve. Discuss the characteristics of the conflict of these role components as manifested by aggressive behaviour management and administration of medication.
- How might the nurse maintain a therapeutic alliance in these circumstances?

Development of emotional competence

The notion of emotional intelligence (EI) is an idea with special resonance in working within mental health services. It is important for both the effectiveness of the care offered and the interprofessional nature of this work, and also for the self-care that is important in mental health nursing and health care more generally (Freshwater & Stickley, 2004; Montes-Berges & Augusto, 2007).

Some of the seminal work in this field is associated with Peter Salovey and John Mayer (1989–90) and Daniel Goleman (1996). These authors challenged traditional views that emotions were a countervailing force to intelligence that required firm control to ensure rational behaviour. An alternate early view did credit emotion as a motivating force that serves to galvanise and focus subsequent action.

Salovey and Mayer (1989–90, p. 189) defined emotional intelligence as:

> … the ability to monitor one's own and others' feelings and emotions, to discriminate amongst them and to use this information to guide one's thinking and actions.

Emotional competence therefore refers to the ability to recognise, interpret and respond constructively to emotions in oneself and in others (Beaumont, 2005). This can be recognised in empathetic responses to other's emotional reactions in health care, which is dependent upon an ability to recognise feelings and appreciate their nature.

How to achieve this ability is challenging, but it is proposed that it is a skill that can be developed with practise (Hurley & Rankin, 2008). It has been suggested that EI might affect the quality of student learning, ethical decision-making, critical thinking, evidence and knowledge use in practice (Bulmer Smith, Profetto-McGrath & Cummings, 2009). However, Bulmer Smith and colleagues (2009, p. 1626) in their review of EI literature in nursing noted that:

> The following three key criticisms limits scientific knowledge development related to emotional intelligence: emotional intelligence is poorly defined and measured, emotional intelligence is an old idea for constructs previously identified and measured, and the importance of emotional intelligence is exaggerated and not supported by research.

So, essentially evidence supporting the value and utility of EI is the subject of contention and debate.

Reflective practice as a critical thinking process

The way in which one might approach the work of mental health nursing can be unclear. What is it that mental health nurses 'do'? How do they set priorities?

Mental health nursing shares with all fields of nursing certain habits of mind and ways of thinking, albeit with some aspects at different levels of importance. The familiar cycle of clinical reasoning in nursing (also known as the nursing process) is applicable to mental health nursing (Levett-Jones et al., 2009). This six-step process developed from the work of Ida Jean Orlando, and progresses through the following predictable phases: assessment, problem identification, outcome of problem identification, planning, implementing and assessment (Funnell, Koutoukidis & Lawrence, 2009). In this context, a nurse undertakes a predictable series of activities when determining a course of action in clinical practice. Ordinarily, this starts with consideration of the consumer's mental health condition and experiences, in collaboration with the consumer and the collection of cues and information relevant to the consumer. This information requires processing to understand the relevant factors for the consumer and through the synthesis of these to establish the definitive problem for support or resolution. The outcome or goal of resolving the problem requires clarification prior to taking action, by selecting between alternatives. Following this action – perhaps an intervention – an evaluation is made of the outcomes achieved. The final component of the nursing process is reflection directed at the process undertaken and discerning the possible learning achieved.

A component of this clinical reasoning cycle of the nursing process is the utilisation and development of a habit of critical thinking. Heaslip (2008) has suggested that nursing requires a questioning disposition and a reflective capacity, to ensure that safety and high standards are achieved. Critical thinking contributes to this by supporting an ability to think in a systematic and logical manner that is non-judgemental. It acts as the guide to establishing beliefs and courses of skilful action.

Critical thinking can be understood to be part of a reflective process, in which both actions and emotions are considered. Reflection examines assumptions, particularly those underlying opinion, actions and beliefs. Its aim is to deepen the understanding of the clinical situation and of the self (Scheffer & Rubenfeld, 2000; Rubenfeld & Scheffer, 2006).

Clinical supervision for the beginning/novice nursing student within mental health nursing

Clinical supervision is an important component of professional practice in mental health. It is a concept that can be confusing and is at times spoken of interchangeably with the practices of mentorship and preceptorship. It is does differ from those practices, and it is helpful to understand the distinction between these three supportive practices (Mills, Francis & Bonner, 2005).

Mentorship

This is a broad-based relationship that is entered into by a less experienced nurse with a more expert nurse. It is usually a relationship selected by the novice, with a view to supporting personal and career development through qualities in the expert nurse's practice that the novice may seek to emulate. The relationship is negotiated between the two parties and will ordinarily occur outside of working hours. It may be a long-term relationship in which the novice seeks advice from the mentor on a range of practice matters over periods of time. The frequency of these consultations may reflect the needs of the novice or may be more formally convened at regular intervals. Sometimes these mentor relationships may last a career lifetime!

The mentoring relationship differs from the admiration one may hold for an esteemed expert nurse and her or his practice. It is an exclusive relationship that acknowledges the role of the expert nurse in the provision of advice to the novice. Although the management of the relationship may in many ways be the responsibility of the novice, there is mutuality in the concern and commitment to the development of the novice nurse.

Preceptorship

A preceptorship may be distinguished as a relationship that occurs within the bounds of the work environment. Ordinarily, a particular skill or set of skills forms the focus of the relationship. The preceptor is appointed to support the novice in attaining mastery of these skills or procedures. The duration of the relationship is usually limited to the period that it takes to achieve this mastery.

While on clinical placement, the term preceptorship is commonly used to describe the particular staff member assigned to support the student's learning while on placement. At times this will take the form of 'buddying' or working entirely with this staff member. At other times, working arrangements cannot support such a consistent and exclusive relationship over the period of clinical placement. In such instances, the preceptor may have responsibility to negotiate the learning opportunities for the student in her or his absence. It is common for a preceptor also to have a role in the assessment of skills.

Clinical supervision

The term clinical supervision has often been criticised as being prone to misunderstanding. Supervision has a managerial connotation that is the antithesis of the relationship of clinical supervision. In fact, the frank and confidential nature of the clinical supervision role precludes the conflict of interest inherent in any attempt to develop such a relationship with one's manager.

Clinical supervision is a supportive relationship that is focused on the development of improved clinical practice. It may occur under the guidance of a specifically educated supervisor (who also engages in her or his own clinical supervision to maintain a good standard in the supervisory role) or between peers. It may occur on an individual basis between a single supervisee and clinical supervisor, or as part of a group.

The frequency of meetings varies, but research has established that in order to be most effective, it should occur at no less than monthly intervals (White & Winstanley, 2011a). It is usually acknowledged that the duration of the meetings should be 60 minutes. There is increasing use of innovative means to access clinical supervision, especially by nurses who practice in rural, isolated or remote environments. Video conferencing and other media and information technologies are used to facilitate participation.

Participation in clinical supervision is supported by health authorities such as the state or territorial Ministry of Health (NSW Health, 2007; Queensland Health, 2009) and professional associations (Australian College of Mental Health Nurses Inc, 2010). The Australian College of Mental Health Nurses and the New Zealand College of Mental Health Nurses are active advocates for clinical (or professional) supervision. The standards of practice for mental health nurses explicitly nominate clinical supervision as a core component of professional mental health nursing, irrespective of the role performed or amount of time a nurse has practised in mental health (Australian College of Mental Health Nurses Inc, 2010). The Australian Health Minister's Advisory Council recommended access to clinical supervision be made available for mental health nurses (Whitstanley & White, 2003).

In the United Kingdom, clinical supervision was introduced in the 1980s and has become an established part of public health systems, with the intention of improving clinical governance and quality improvement. Uptake of clinical supervision in Australia has been traditionally greater in mental health nursing (Mills et al., 2005). However, in the past 10 years there has been renewed interest in other areas of nursing and in midwifery.

The form of clinical supervision that has been most frequently adopted in nursing contexts for the past 25 years has been that developed by Bridget Proctor (Proctor, 1986; White & Winstanley, 2011a). This model conceptualises clinical supervision as having three functions: the so-called Normative, Formative and Restorative domains. Normative functions are those that aid in developing and maintaining standards for clinical practice and clinical review. Developing knowledge and skills are those represented by the Formative domain. Personal well-being of participants is the Restorative function. There is some evidence that these domains become effective at differing rates (White & Winstanley, 2010). Changes are first seen in Normative and Restorative domains. It is later that the Formative domain shows change, suggesting that improvements for consumers may become possible when organisational culture responds to the benefits of the Normative and Restorative domains (White & Winstanley, 2010).

Evidence for the effectiveness of clinical supervision has been difficult to establish. Design of robust tools to measure relevant and agreed outcomes is challenging. But there is emerging evidence that clinical supervision contributes to both improved consumer outcomes by improvements in clinical skills as well as improved wellness and therapeutic orientation of nurses involved with clinical supervision (White & Winstanley, 2011b).

Overall rates of clinical supervision in mental health nursing have been low in Australia, despite support from health authorities and professional associations (White & Roche, 2006). This presents a challenge for novice nurses who wish to access this form of structured professional support and development. As a newcomer to the workforce, the novice nurse may find it difficult to persevere to secure access to clinical supervision in the absence of overt and explicit managerial support.

Reflective questions

- By what means could clinical supervision be secured by a novice mental health nurse?
- How might student nurses utilise clinical supervision?
- What reasons would you suggest to explain the low clinical supervision participation rates in mental health nursing in Australia and New Zealand?

Developing objectives for clinical placements

Setting learning objectives for clinical placement is dependent upon three factors:

1 Knowledge of the learning objectives of the unit of study associated with the placement
2 Knowledge of the opportunities available within the clinical placement setting at that point in time
3 Knowledge of one's own learning needs based on the objectives to be accomplished in the formal unit of study and personal objectives arising from reflection on one's areas of weakness or challenge in this area of nursing practice.

Achieving alignment of these three factors may be difficult. However, it offers an opportunity to rehearse negotiating skills as you attempt to achieve these objectives. Negotiation with clinical staff of the placement setting may help to determine the objectives that may be supported during the placement, and negotiation with the university's clinical facilitator is required to achieve this. Additionally, the self-scrutiny of what you do well, what you might improve upon and what you may not as yet be able to perform can help you to develop the habit of critical questioning and prioritising of your own learning objectives.

Sometimes, clinical placements may appear to be restricted in what they offer for learning. This may be a first impression and based on a misunderstanding of the nature of and experience of people with mental illness, mental health nursing or mental health services associated with the placement. Learning may need to be considered in a different manner than in other domains of nursing. If you have concentrated on achieving skills in clinical procedures, the relatively low profile of these skills in mental health nursing may be unsettling. Although such aspects of nursing practice form part of mental health nursing, pursuit of these learning opportunities may be misplaced. Utilisation of such clinical skills may, however, prove a valuable way to engage in the more central activities of mental health nursing.

Another aspect of mental health nursing that is arguably in contrast with other fields of nursing is a further feature of the relationship between mental health nurse and consumer. Nurses work 'with' consumers to achieve the recovery goals established by the consumer. This may be contrasted with other fields of nursing, where the work is about doing 'for' or 'to' the recipients of nursing care. Procedures are a clear example of this contrast. In medical and surgical fields of nursing, these have a high profile in mediating the relationship between the nurse and the consumer of her services.

It is probably fair to characterise most, if not all, mental health placements as offering opportunities to spend time with those experiencing mental illness and perhaps their carers as well. This feature, and the associated documentation opportunity, gives an excellent chance to develop a deeper appreciation of the lived experience of mental illness. This is something that can only be approximated in other learning opportunities or settings. Books, films, documentaries and simulation are a pale attempt to replicate the authentic experience.

The time in clinical placement serves to help rehearse and deepen communication skills. These skills will be valuable across the entire range of nursing practice, and are also helpful in one's personal life. These communication skills may include developing an ability to tolerate uncertainty and ambiguity in communication, and improving the ability to recall the content and features of communication for documentation at a later time. Rehearsing communication skills that enhance the ability to respond in a therapeutic manner and tolerating silence is an important learning opportunity. Clinical placement will also help to develop an ability to recognise alterations in speech form and the relevant descriptive terms for these. All these communication skills are useful learning to accomplish during early placements.

It is sometimes tempting to listen to accounts from peers and assume that their placements offer superior learning opportunities. While there are certainly occasions when this might be an accurate assessment, changing placement location frequently in pursuit of a 'better' learning opportunity can be counter-productive. The experiences may be elusive and may only offer themselves by dint of your own effort and growing familiarity with the environment in which you are placed.

The therapeutic relationship is central to work in mental health nursing. Time can be a very helpful factor in establishing such a relationship. Clinical placement that allows for your presence on a continuing basis and an opportunity to persevere in this regard is valuable. Take it!

Students frequently identify boredom as a feature of clinical placement, especially at in-patient services. This can present a particular difficulty, but may be a time to reflect deeply on what contributes to the boredom experienced by students. It is possible that explanations are multifactorial and may include factors such as that:

1 The nature of mental illness presenting in the placement context may have features that reduce people's motivation and enjoyment of everyday social interaction, and increase preoccupation with the experiences of the condition.
2 The medications frequently have sedative side-effects that reduce people's interest and capacity to interact.
3 The environment may have features of bureaucracy that render mental health consumers disempowered and unable or unwilling to be active agents in their own recovery.
4 The student's desire to 'keep busy' may be acting as a way to manage anxiety associated with a mental health placement.

Reflective questions

- List the features of a bureaucracy in health care. Link these features with the disempowering experiences of a consumer. This may not be limited to the mental health environment, so consider the situation of consumers of health services across a broad range, and then think about what features may be common to mental health services as well.
- Examine commonly prescribed mental health medications for their sedative side-effects. How can these effects be used to enhance recovery, or minimised to avoid over-sedation?
- Consider the term 'negative symptoms'. What are these? How can they influence a mental health consumer's recovery? What strategies may be developed to ameliorate them?

The process of self-assessment and personal problem solving

Understanding one's learning needs and devising ways to address these can be a challenging task. What do I know? How do I ensure my understanding is accurate and comprehensive? How do I respond to gaps I am aware of?

Utilising a personal learning plan is a useful device. This log of learning objectives and possible courses of action may take a variety of forms that is best suited to your own style. A plethora of online tools are available, many of which will be available through your university. Professional nursing groups often have these available, too, as all nurses are now required to keep an ongoing log of their professional development. Commencing this process by utilising a learning plan on clinical placement will start habits that will be valuable in your later career.

One approach to determining your learning objectives is by keeping a diary during your placement and then reviewing it for evidence of aspects of the placement that are challenging. Learning objectives are useful if they are constructed to address this identified weakness.

Reflection, self, in-action and post-placement

Your conceptualisation of the experience and your learning from mental health clinical placement will develop over time. As you consider your experiences, both within the clinical placement and through theoretical preparation, fresh understandings will develop. Reflection about your prior attitudes and understanding of mental health and how these may have changed as a result of these experiences will deepen and expand your potential capacity to provide therapeutic care.

Many students report greater appreciation of the prevalence of mental illness among people throughout health care services following their education in mental health nursing.

As you also consider consumers from other areas in which you have practised, perhaps the full implications of consumer-centred and holistic care will take on deeper meaning.

Reflective questions

- How might you incorporate mental health care in nursing practice in other clinical domains?
- What ethical considerations are relevant?
- What implications might there be for the characteristics of practice that are required to change?

Ethical and political influences on care

Mental health services have been the focus of a reform agenda since the early 1990s in Australia. The manner in which mental health services have changed, moving from predominantly separate in-hospital services to services delivered primarily in community settings and 'mainstream' health settings. These services now employ a broader range of providers, including non-government organisations.

In addition, different types of workers have joined the mental health workforce, contributing a variety of skill sets. Some groups of workers now joining the mental health workforce have less formal education than has been usual in the past, leading some to question of the adequacy of their preparation.

Some political factors have had some unforeseen and unfortunate consequences for consumers. It has been common for people with mental illness to find it difficult to get adequate living arrangements. Homelessness and involvement in criminal and justice systems have seen significant rises following these political decisions about health care. These changed circumstances represent challenges to mental health nursing, not only in the provision of services but in ethical dimensions as well. Mental health nurses may feel that their professional practice is compromised by some of the circumstances of care delivery. Their delivery of care may be constrained by limitations in resources, especially when working with some of the most vulnerable groups, such as homeless people and asylum seekers.

Some may argue that these types of circumstances call for a fresh range of skills for mental health nurses – those of political action to achieve advocacy. Many may find this confronting. It might not sit easily with prior or traditional understandings of the nurse's role.

Reflective questions

- How can the role of advocacy be undertaken in an ethical manner?
- What consent should be obtained? Where might mental health nurses undertake advocacy?
- What conflicts might arise in adopting this role?

And off to clinical placement: Pragmatic strategies for learning

A number of approaches are available to help you make the best of your clinical placements in mental health services. These can be summarised as preparation, communication and self-care. The following sections give some direction and suggestions.

Preparation

- Find out about the service prior to the commencement of your placement. To whom does it offer help? Who runs the service? How big is the service – does it offer a range of services? A website may available that will provide this type of overview, or your university may supply some information. It is probably not advisable to ring the service as it may provide a great deal of clinical placements that makes repeated provision of this type of information a burden. However, it is often true that a show of interest and initiative on the part of students is very well regarded.
- Be clear about meeting venues and times for your first day. It may be advisable to visit the service prior to your placement, to ensure you are clear as to the location of the mental health service and the meeting venue.
- Clarify dress codes. Some mental health services discourage the wearing of uniforms because of their potential to stigmatise people with mental illness, especially in rehabilitation and community services. In other services, uniforms are seen as helpful to identify your role to staff and consumers.
- Make sure that your requisite vaccinations, police checks and student identification documentation are in order prior to commencing your placement.
- Wear comfortable and safe footwear.
- Review the theory subject that has prepared you for this placement. Clarify the learning objectives expected from the placement and your university's specific requirements. Consider what you have researched about the placement and develop personal learning objectives for the placement.

Communication

- Identify your facilitator/preceptor/mentor and her or his contact details. Ensure you keep the relevant staff of the health facility and university apprised of any variation in your attendance.
- Introduce yourself to staff and consumers in a friendly and courteous manner.
- Make an effort to get to know the members of the team and the consumers of the service.
- Request feedback on your performance. This is a valuable learning opportunity, and as a student you are allowed to make mistakes.
- Avoid gossip.
- Spend your time engaged with the consumers of the service as much as you can. The service exists to help these people, and you are there to learn how to make

your contribution. Meetings, case notes and university assignments can be completed in many other venues – time spent with people who are experiencing mental illness will be invaluable to your learning.

- Anticipate that some services may not be structured for your needs as a student, but rather to meet the needs of consumers as a priority. Additionally, consumers may not wish to interact with you because of their experiences of mental health disorders. Be patient, be present. Do not seek to 'sight-see' by requesting to visit other services as a panacea for 'feeling bored', as this approach is both superficial and disrespectful. Perseverance can bring unexpected insight and opportunities.
- Maintain professional boundaries. Do not keep confidences for consumers and do not divulge personal details such as your phone number or address. Do not arrange to meet socially with consumers you meet on your clinical placement.

Looking after yourself

- Ask questions, seek clarification about the things you observe on clinical placement.
- Actively engage in tutorials or meetings arranged by your clinical facilitator, preceptor or mentor. It can be helpful to make a note of the topics you wish to talk about.
- If you experience difficulties or feel emotionally affected by your experiences, make sure that you report this to your clinical facilitator and ward staff. Actively prepare a plan of action to re-establish your equilibrium.
- Exercise, eat and sleep well. This advice may seem clichéd but it does help.
- Avoid excessive consumption of caffeine or alcohol (see above).
- Have fun, get involved, enjoy your experience – this is your education.

Consumer narrative   Angie: A paramedic's story

I am an undergraduate paramedic student who recently attended my first clinical placement. After reading for two years, I could barely contain my excitement to start applying my knowledge in a rush of lights and sirens. I had come prepared with an arsenal of objective protocols – mental recipes – designed to help me save lives and make a difference.

Prior to my time on the road, I had thought that my understanding of how the body works and what to do when it goes wrong was the most critical element of being a good paramedic. However, when I found I was spending most of my time talking to people, I realised the relief of suffering is not always straightforward.

I recall a particular incident on a busy night in the emergency department (ED) when we brought in 19-year-old Dolores (not her real name) after she had threatened suicide. The triage nurse rolled her eyes in exhaustion: F****** mental health [patients] … I wish we could just put them all in a room and end them …' After seeing the shocked expression on my face, she looked down at my student ID before continuing 'Ahh, no wonder you don't understand. They come in every f****** day with the same f****** problem …'

continued ›

Dolores had an extensive history of schizophrenia, depression and suicidal ideation, and was known to police and paramedics for being hostile and aggressive. It was almost amusing to think that this slight and softly spoken girl was brought here involuntarily in handcuffs. We were in bed block and she hadn't spoken a word for over an hour.

Having a sister her age, I felt a surge of compassion that drove me to find out Dolores's story. I started by gently cleaning the blood off her hands, commenting how her finger nails were just like my sister's, short and down to the quick: 'Haha, are you a biter, too?!' This broke the silence and, after some small talk, Dolores began to open up about her life and the tragic circumstances that had led her here.

Some time passed and Dolores asked to go to the toilet. When she came back, it became clear that she was getting restless. I actually felt sorry that I couldn't let her wander around or go outside for a smoke. When she asked to go to the toilet again 10 minutes later, Dolores tried to abscond, punching another patient in her path towards the door.

In seconds, there were three of us pinning her face down on the ground. Dolores was angry, swearing at us to let her go. When I explained the situation to her again, she started to bang her head on the floor. I instinctively put my hand between her forehead and the hard surface, as I recalled the number of times I've done that to protect my autistic sister. My heart sank; I knew what was going to happen next. Two burly security guards took over, tying her to a bed as the doctor prepared a sedative. As I watched on, Dolores was thrashing at her restraints, glaring at me.

I didn't cry but I could have, as I suddenly realised the difficulty of building genuine rapport without taking a betrayal of your trust personally. I had been quick to judge the apparent callousness of the professionals around me, yet in light of my own emotional exhaustion, I started to see it as a form of self-protection. While we're taught to fix things with drugs and interventions, I've learned that there are times when 'making a difference' requires something of yourself. Beyond the clinical element of being a paramedic, it has dawned on me that the experience of suffering and our response to it are inherently human.

Reflective questions

Angie is studying to be a paramedic.
- How is her experience relevant to learning to be a nurse working in mental health services?
- What implications does it have for other professions?
- How might Angie respond to the derogatory comments of the nursing staff?
- How might Angie ensure she maintains her own well-being?
- What role did transference and counter-transference play in Angie's experience with Dolores?

Consumer narrative

James's thoughts: The value of education

I was asked to write a piece on why education is so important to me. This is a difficult question, but my overall response is that I enjoy it. While I thought about this I remembered all the times education had been valuable to me. The first of which and the most obvious are my position and my opportunities in life, but this is not interesting. With deeper thought the most rewarding thing about my current profession is solving the problems that wouldn't have been solved without additional education.

In my current role my primary objective is to assess clients and identify the management needed. While there have been many cases in the past, this one is memorable as it was the first instance when I knew that my additional education had made the difference and that without it I would have made a very different choice.

The story is of a woman in her mid-20s. Her initial presentation included symptoms of nausea, with a suspicion of organic origins. The client came to our attention when treatments seemed not to be benefiting her, and a psychosomatic component to the presentation was suspected. The client was assessed with a primary consideration that her experience of nausea may have been caused by anxiety. She had some neuro-vegetative features of depression but did not meet the full diagnostic criteria. She was questioned about possible mood changes, but denied any irregularity. Her family history of depression was also queried but there was not any evidence of its existence.

After this further assessment it became clear that the client was unusually concerned about appearing competent. This was explored and it appeared the client felt a need to be the strong leader in her family. She stated this was due to financial concerns about the family farm, concerns that are not uncommon in rural areas. After some discussion, an approach was taken that allowed the client to admit to diurnal mood variation, and her concern with appearing competent was explored for a psychotic nature.

There were several very subtle indicators that would have been otherwise easily missed in the presentation and that ultimately led to the conclusion that the client was actually very unwell. It was identified that she had a psychotic depression, with an atypical presentation which, combined with the need to appear competent, increased the difficulty for her to accept help. During my education regarding psychotic depression I had learned that the rate of successful suicides, regardless of treatment, could be as high as one in four. I undertook extensive questioning of the client regarding suicide. She admitted to having suicidal ideation, and was later hospitalised voluntarily. During her hospitalisation the client did not respond to the initial antidepressant administered, and required a course of electroconvulsive treatment (ECT). In this situation, identifying the high suicide risk could easily have been overlooked, potentially with fatal consequences. This was a case where I felt that without the further education I had undertaken, I would not have pursued this direct line of questioning. Thus a potentially tragic outcome was averted.

Reflective questions

James's thoughts about the value of education are framed as an experienced clinician who has undertaken continuing education.

- What benefit does he recognise from continuing education?
- How might one practise safely as a novice mental health nurse?

Interprofessional connections   Denise's experience

As a nurse manager for education in mental health services for many years, a major part of my responsibilities was to ensure student health professionals were facilitated in their clinical placements. This experience was a constantly evolving role that encompassed changing formalities and requirements by the many groups involved. Nursing placements were largely routine, and the clinical placements of other traditional mental health professions had long-established patterns. However, the desire to include a broader range of students from professions making increasing contributions to mental health services prompted a revision of the usual clinical placement patterns within one mental health service (a 200-bed, long-term residential facility).

Establishing these extended student clinical placement arrangements required an extensive range of collaborative work with the consumers of the services, the staff of the service, the regulating authorities, the management of the service and broader health services authorities, the course coordinators for the exercise physiology and speech pathology courses, and with the students of these courses. It was necessary to make sure that the students had appropriate learning opportunities, and that the service consumers were not over-burdened by the presence of yet more students. Regulating authorities and the health services undertook vaccination and criminal check requirements for students. The staff of the services needed to understand the learning required for students during their placements. Both groups had successful pilot placements, with consumers benefiting from an increased range of personalised services, and existing staff from a deepening of interprofessional understanding.

Chapter summary

This chapter has presented stories and information, supplemented by activities designed to deepen understanding of:

- The role of the nurse from other areas of health care in mental health nursing and the skills required;
- The opportunities available for students on mental health clinical placements, requirements of their program of study and their own personal learning objectives, and the potential to reconcile and meet these;
- The opportunities available for students to spend time with consumers of mental health services during clinical placements;
- Strategies to support student well-being, which include a range of different activities that should be self-initiated at all times; and
- The fact that mental illness may be experienced by students themselves or their friends, or in a variety of health environments, and therefore the skills developed in mental health nursing will have wide-ranging applicability.

Critical thinking/learning activities

1 How do the standards for mental health nursing attempt to reconcile the inherent conflict between mental health nursing's dual roles of control and care?
2 What constraints affect learning on clinical placement in mental health nursing?
3 Many factors interfere with self-care. List factors in your daily life that stop you meeting ideal standards of self-care. What other issues might arise when you begin your nursing career? What methods can be used to ensure that you employ self-care strategies throughout your nursing career?

Learning extension

When you complete your nursing education you will be required to undertake continuing professional development to maintain your registration as a health practitioner. Research what these requirements are. What happens if you do not practice for an extended period?

Prepare a learning portfolio that can set your learning objectives for your mental health nursing placement, record evidence of meeting these objectives and provide a record that will meet the requirements of registration.

Utilising the framework outlined in Heron's (1989) therapeutic interaction model, undertake a series of process recordings. During your clinical placement, record interactions with people experiencing mental illness following these conversations. This exercise supports the development of improved recall abilities. Explore the interaction using the framework suggested by Heron, which will help you reflect on the therapeutic intention of your communication and the alternative responses that might have been used.

Further reading

Heron, J. (2001). *Helping The Client: A Creative practical guide*. London: Sage.
This book outlines a method that is easy to apply to one's practice and helpful in analysing its characteristics. The guide focuses on alternative ways of responding to consumer conversations that can be helpful in achieving and maintaining the therapeutic alliance.

Mental Health Workforce Advisory Committee (2010). *Mental Health in Pre-registration Nursing: Progress report and full survey results*. Melbourne: Author.
This report itemises features of mental health nursing preparation in Australia and sets an agenda for the future characteristics of preparation.

References

Anthony, P. & Crawford, P. (2000). Service user involvement in care planning: The mental health nurse's perspective. *Journal of Psychiatric and Mental Health Nursing*, 7: 425–34.

Australian College of Mental Health Nurses Inc. (2010). *Standards of Practice for Australian Mental Health Nurses 2010*. Canberra: Author.

Bachelor, A. & Horvath, A. (1999). The therapeutic relationship. In M. A. Hubble, B. L. Duncan & S. D. Miller (eds), *The Heart and Soul of Change: What works in therapy* (pp. 133–78). Washington, DC: American Psychological Association.

Beaumont, L. R. (2005). Emotional Competency website, www.emotionalcompetency.com.

Bulmer Smith, K., Profetto-McGrath, J. & Cummings, G. G. (2009). Emotional intelligence and nursing: An integrative literature review. *International Journal of Nursing Studies*, 46(12): 1624–36.

Cleary, M. (2003). The challenges of mental health care reform for contemporary mental health nursing practice: Relationships, power and control. *International Journal of Mental Health Nursing*, 12(2): 139–47.

Department of Health and Ageing (2005). *National Mental Health Report 2005: Summary of Ten Years of Reform in Australia's Mental Health Services under the National Mental Health Strategy 1993–2003*. Canberra: Commonwealth of Australia.

Dickson, C., Walker, J. & Bourgeois, S. (2006). Facilitating undergraduate nurses clinical practicum: The lived experiences of clinical facilitators. *Nurse Education Today*, 26(5): 416–22.

Edwards, D. & Burnard, P. (2003). A systematic review of stress and stress management interventions for mental health nurses. *Journal of Advanced Nursing*, 42(2): 169–200.

Foucault, M. (1986). Afterword: The subject and power. In H. L. Dreyfus & P. Rabinow (eds), *Beyond Structuralism and Hermeneutics* (pp. 208–27). Brighton: Harvester.

Freshwater, D. & Stickley, T. (2004). The heart of the art: Emotional intelligence in nurse education. *Nursing Inquiry*, 11(2): 91–98.

Friedlander, M. L. (1993). Does complementarity promote or hinder client change in brief therapy: A review of the evidence from two theoretical perspectives. *The Counseling Psychologist*, 21(3): 457–86.

Funnell, R., Koutoukidis, G. & Lawrence, K. (2009). *Tabbner's Nursing Care*, 5th edn. Port Melbourne: Elsevier.

Goleman, D. (1996). *Emotional Intelligence: Why it can matter more than IQ*. New York: Bantam Books.

Happell, B. & Platania-Phung, C. (2005). Mental health issues within the general health care system: The challenge for nursing education in Australia. *Nurse Education Today*, 25(6): 465–71.

Hayman-White, K. & Happell, B. (2005). Nursing students' attitudes toward mental health nursing and consumers: Psychometric properties of a self-report scale. *Archives of Psychiatric Nursing*, 19(4): 184–93.

Heaslip, P. (2008). *Critical Thinking: To think like a nurse*. Kamloops, BC: Thompson Rivers University.

Heron, J. (1989). *Six Category Intervention Analysis* (3rd edn). Surrey, UK: Human Potential Resource Group, University of Surrey.

Horvath, A. O. & Bedi, R. P. (2002). The alliance. In J. C. Norcross (ed.), *Psychotherapy Relationships That Work: Therapist contributions and responsiveness to patients* (pp. 37–70). New York: Oxford University Press.

Hubble, M. A., Duncan, B. L. & Miller, S. D. (1999). Directing attention to what works. In M. A. Hubble, B. L Duncan & S. D. Miller (eds), *The Heart and Soul of Change: What works in therapy* (pp. 407–47). Washington, DC: American Psychological Association.

Hughes, P. & Kerr, I. (2000). Transference and countertransference in communication between doctor and patient. *Advances in Psychiatric Treatment, 6*: 57–64.

Hurley, J. & Rankin, R. (2008). As mental health nursing roles expand, is education expanding mental health nurses? An emotionally intelligent view towards preparation for psychological therapies and relatedness. *Nursing Inquiry, 15*(3): 199–205.

Klein, M., Kolden, G. & Michels, J. & Chisholm-Stockard, S. (2001). Congruence or genuineness? *Psychotherapy: Theory, Research, Practice, Training, 38*(4): 396–400.

Kunyk, D. & Olson, J. K. (2001). Clarification of conceptualizations of empathy. *Journal of Advanced Nursing, 35*(3): 317–25.

Levett-Jones, T., Hoffman, K., Dempsey, Y. Jeong, S. Y-S., Noble, D., Norton, C. A., Roche, J. & Hickey, N. (2009). The 'five rights' of clinical reasoning: An educational model to enhance nursing students' ability to identify and manage clinically 'at risk' patients. *Nurse Education Today, 30*(6): 515–20.

May, C. (1992). Individual care? Power and subjectivity in therapeutic relationships. *Sociology, 26*(4): 589–602.

Mental Health Council of Australia (2011). *Consumer and Carer Experiences of Stigma From Mental Health and Other Health Professionals.* Canberra: Author.

Mental Health Workforce Advisory Committee (2010). *Mental Health in Pre-registration Nursing: Progress report and full survey results.* Melbourne: Author.

Mills, J., Francis, K. & Bonner, A. (2005). Mentoring, clinical supervision and preceptoring: clarifying the conceptual definitions for Australian rural nurses. A review of the literature. *Rural and Remote Health, 5*(410) (online).

Montes-Berges, B. & Augusto, J. M. (2007). Exploring the relationship between perceived emotional intelligence, coping, social support and mental health in nursing students. *Journal of Psychiatric and Mental Health Nursing, 14*(2): 163–171.

Neill, M. A. & Wotton, K. (2011). High-fidelity simulation debriefing in nursing education: A literature review. *Clinical Simulation in Nursing, 7*(5): e161–8.

Norcross, J. C., Beutler, L. E. & Levant, R. F. (2006). *Evidence-based Practices in Mental Health: Debate and dialogue on the fundamental questions.* Washington, DC: American Psychological Association.

Norcross, J. C. & Lambert, W. G. (eds) (2006). *The Therapy Relationship.* Washington, DC: American Psychological Association.

NSW Health (2007). *NSW Drug and Alcohol Clinical Supervision Guidelines.* Sydney: Author.

Nursing and Midwifery Board of Australia (2013). *A Nurse's Guide to Professional Boundaries.* Retrieved from www.nursingmidwiferyboard.gov.au/Codes-Guidelines-Statements/Codes-Guidelines. aspx#professionalboundaries.

Peplau, H. E. (1952). Interpersonal relations in nursing. *American Journal of Nursing, 52*(6): 765.

Peplau, H. E. (1997). Peplau's theory of interpersonal relations. *Nursing Science Quarterly, 14*(2): 162–7.

Perraud, S., Delaney, K. R., Carlson-Sabelli, L., Johnson, M. E., Shephard, R. & Paun, O. (2006). Advanced practice psychiatric mental health nursing, finding our core: The therapeutic relationship in 21st century. *Perspectives in Psychiatric Care, 42*(4): 215–26.

Pieranunzi, V. R. (1997). The lived experience of power and powerlessness in psychiatric nursing: A Heideggerian hermeneutical analysis. *Archives of Psychiatric Nursing, 11*(3): 155–62.

Proctor, B. (1986). Supervision: A cooperative exercise in accountability. In M. Marken & M. Payne (eds), *Enabling and Ensuring: Supervision in Practice* (pp. 21–34). Leicester: National Youth Bureau and Council for Education and Training in Youth and Community Work.

Queensland Health (2009). *Clinical Supervision Guidelines for Mental Health Services.* Brisbane: Author.

Rubenfeld, M. & Scheffer, B. (2006). *Critical Thinking Tactics For Nurses.* Boston: Jones and Bartlett.

Rydon, S. E. (2005). The attitudes, knowledge and skills needed in mental health nurses: The perspective of users of mental health services. *International Journal of Mental Health Nursing, 14*(2): 78–87.

Salovey, P. & Mayer, J. D. (1989–90). Emotional intelligence. *Imagination, Cognition and Personality, 9*(3): 185–211.

Scheffer, B. & Rubenfeld, M. (2000). A consensus statement on critical thinking in nursing. *Journal of Nursing Education, 39*: 352–9.

Shattell, M. M., Starr, S. S. & Thomas, S. P. (2007). 'Take my hand, help me out': Mental health service recipients' experience of the therapeutic relationship. *International Journal of Mental Health Nursing*, *16*(4): 274–84.

White, E. & Roche, M. (2006). A selective review of mental health nursing in New South Wales, Australia, in relation to clinical supervision. *International Journal of Mental Health Nursing*, *15*(3): 209–19.

White, E. & Winstanley, J. (2010). A randomised controlled trial of clinical supervision: Selected findings from a novel Australian attempt to establish the evidence base for causal relationships with quality of care and patient outcomes, as an informed contribution to mental health nursing practice development. *Journal of Research in Nursing*, *15*(2): 151–67.

White, E. & Winstanley, J. (2011a). Clinical supervision for mental health professionals: The evidence base. *Social Work and Social Sciences Review*, *14*(3): 77–94.

White, E. & Winstanley, J. (2011b). Clinical supervision for mental health professionals: The evidence base. Commissioned for Special Edition 'Current Trends in Mental Health Services'. *Social Work and Social Sciences Review*, *14*(3): 73–90.

Whitstanley, J. & White, E. (2003). Clinical supervision: Models, measures and best practice. *Nurse Researcher*, *10*: 7–38.

World Health Organization (WHO) (2001). *The World Health Report 2001: Mental health–new understanding, new hope*. Geneva: Author.

3

The social and emotional well-being of Aboriginal Australians and the collaborative consumer narrative

Debra Hocking
Consumer narratives by Barbara O'Neill and Sandra Murphy

Introduction 52
Social and emotional well-being versus
    mental health 52
Culture 53
Colonisation 54
Aboriginal worldviews 55
Government policies 56
The incidence of trauma 62

The concept of healing 65
Chapter summary 68
Critical thinking/learning activities 68
Learning activity 68
Acknowledgement 69
Further reading 69
References 70

The glossary definitions provided in this chapter have been developed with the idea that readers should be open to further exploring terms with people in the Aboriginal context, taking into account consumer narrative and history. Also important is taking into account that some of the terms are interpreted based on the lived experience of the person and family concerned.

Learning outcomes

At the completion of this chapter you should be able to:

1 Describe the context of social and emotional well-being.
2 Analyse the historical, sociological and political forces that are important in mental health care provision.
3 Analyse the degree of trauma experienced by Aboriginal Australians.
4 Discuss the concept of trauma-informed practice.
5 Describe the concept of healing.

Introduction

This chapter is not designed to invoke guilt but to tell a story based on fact and lived experiences. Readers may find it challenging and may even feel a sense of responsibility, but responsibility in contemporary terms is to provoke empathy and understanding from an historical misguidance of people who were ignorant of the actions governments and individuals had taken that would have such a negative effect on Aboriginal people, and with devastating effects. Two examples of government policy directed at Aboriginal people that may be seen to have the greatest effects on mental and physical health were the **Assimilation** policy and the Child Removal Policy.

> **assimilation**
> to attain the same manner of living as other Australians
>
> **colonisation**
> the forced act of establishing a colony or colonies, taking full political, social and economic control, with complete disregard for existing peoples and cultures
>
> **resilience**
> strength of spirit

The contributors to this chapter are Aboriginal women who, while they have led diverse lives, have in common certain similarities that can be drawn from the effects of **colonisation** and the challenges that have shaped many lives. Many Aboriginal Australians live with the challenges that stem from the colonisation process (that is, past government policies) on a day-to-day basis, and it is not us who live in the past, but rather the past that lives in us.

'Aboriginal' is a term used to refer to individuals of Aboriginal descent and who are recognised by the community in which they live, or who identify as Aboriginal. While there is a scarcity of national data that specifically measure the social and emotional well-being of Indigenous Australians, data that are available paint a consistent picture: one of much higher rates of use of mental health services by Indigenous Australians, compared to other Australians (Australian Institute of Health and Welfare, 2009). To gain an understanding as to why Aboriginal people have higher incidence of mental distress we must examine the historical and cultural factors that have and continue to affect the lives of Aboriginal Australians.

This chapter sets the context for further discussion regarding Aboriginal people and explores issues relating to social and emotional well-being and mental health. Colonisation and its history are discussed, as well as the subsequent decimation/ devastation that followed and continues today. Government policies that were specifically designed to control the lives of Aboriginal people are discussed and the effects revealed. The **resilience** and struggle that has taken place, along with cultural recognition and renewal, ultimately shapes the present. While the present is explored in this chapter, the complexity and effects of colonisation on Aboriginal people are so monumental that not all aspects are able to be covered within this chapter. For this reason, additional online resources are provided for further reading.

Social and emotional well-being versus mental health

In 2004, the Social Health Reference Group (SHRG) for the National Aboriginal and Torres Strait Islander Health Council and the National Mental Health Working Group – responsible for developing the National Strategic Framework for Aboriginal and Torres Strait Islander Peoples' Mental Health and Social and Emotional Well Being 2004–2009 – articulated a distinction between the concepts of 'social and emotional well-being' used in Aboriginal settings and the term 'mental health' used in non-Aboriginal settings:

> The concept of mental health comes more from an illness or clinical perspective and its focus is more on the individual and their level of functioning in their environment. The social and emotional wellbeing concept is broader than this and recognises the importance of connection to land, culture, spirituality, ancestry, family and community, and how these affect the individual.
>
> SHRG, 2004, p. 9

Health is a multifaceted concept that has been defined and shaped most strongly by a non-Indigenous, biomedical discourse on health. It is a model of health framed with reference to disease or how a person presents according to her or his symptomatology. The focus is also on a curative framework rather than on attending to the whole person (Van Loon, 2001). For Aboriginal people, the biomedical model of health continues to be informed by the legacy of colonisation. This means that the lived experience of health and well-being within colonist traditions and the paradigm of understanding of Aboriginal people are culturally reframed. Non-Indigenous understandings of health hold 'knowledge about'... are spoken about – rather than being actively engaged with Aboriginal people (Anderson, 2004). The net result is that, despite best intentions, social and emotional well-being programs treat *clients* as though they are *sick* and need *experts* to help them with their *illnesses* (Aboriginal and Torres Strait Islander Healing Foundation Development Team, 2009).

While it is difficult to elaborate on the specific effects of historical and contemporary circumstances on the social and emotional well-being of all Indigenous people, this informs our discussion of Indigenous mental health. That such a synopsis could be made belies both the historical and contemporary diversity of Indigenous people. That it is requested is perhaps indicative of perceptions to the contrary that are remnant of relationships between Indigenous and non-Indigenous people since colonisation (Zubrick et al., 2005).

Culture

When I ask my nursing students how they would define **culture**, they usually answer 'religion', 'cuisine', 'dance', 'art' and 'dress code'. Even more interesting is the definition of Australian culture, suggested as barbeques, thongs, beer, sport and music. These are lifestyle choices rather than expressions of culture.

> **culture**
> a way of understanding and interpreting tradition, belief, custom, worldview and values

In thinking more deeply about culture and how it is viewed differently for Aboriginal Australians, Rose (2000) reminded us to conceptualise or perceive culture as meaning different things for each group and section of our society. This takes into account the collective thoughts, experiences and actions of a group in society. Rose's definition is important as it opens up the meaning of culture within groups and that there may be cultures within cultures – some with common understandings or beliefs.

Aboriginal cultures are among the oldest surviving cultures in the world. Aboriginal cultures are numerous and diverse, made up of hundreds of different kinship and language groups that have adapted to diverse living conditions throughout Australia over many thousands of years. Aboriginal cultures remain dynamic and are evolving and, for Aboriginal individuals and communities, form the context for the development of health policy (NATSIHC, 2003).

Reflective questions

In small groups, discuss your own culture.
- What aspects/influences of it determine the way you live?
- Have you ever felt confronted by aspects of other cultures and, if so, what were they and why did you feel confronted?

Colonisation

The likely Aboriginal population in 1788 was around 750 000, or even more than a million (Thompson, 2001). Henry Reynolds has stated that:

> … Australians are so familiar with the events of January and February 1788 that they have lost sight of the ability to see how extraordinary the claim was … As many as half a million people, living in several hundred tribal groupings, in occupation of even the most inhospitable corners of the continent, had, in a single instant, been dispossessed. From that apocalyptic moment forward they were technically trespassers on Crown land even though many of them would not see a white man for another thirty, another fifty years … It was a stunning takeover. It would have dazzled even the lions of the business world.
>
> Reynolds, 1992, p. 8

The basis in (European) international law for the progressive take-over of the Australian continent was the doctrine of *terra nullius* – land belonging to no one (Hollinsworth, 2006). This meant that Aboriginal lands were considered to be Crown lands according to British law. This idea that Australia belonged to no one was not because the British did not see the Aboriginal people who were living here, but because Aboriginal people did not cultivate land or build permanent dwellings as Europeans did. *Terra nullius* meant that the land was considered not to have a sovereign owner, and it was on this basis that Britain took possession of Australia without a treaty. It is also the basis for the prevailing belief that colonisation was peaceful 'settlement'.

In fact, Australia was inhabited by sovereign peoples for whom the land had great cultural, spiritual and economic significance. The settlement of the continent by the British was not peaceful, and is increasingly accepted as having been a countrywide invasion. As the British colonies spread across the continent, traditional lands were taken over and Aboriginal peoples became viewed as trespassers on their own lands. Across Australia there was Aboriginal resistance, but this was written out of history (Hollinsworth, 2006).

Colonisation and the appropriation of Aboriginal land ensured that little value was placed on Aboriginal culture. It began a history of indifference towards Aboriginal people, and attempts were made to eradicate Aboriginal people by military force and by poisoning them (Macdonald, 2010).

The effects of colonisation and the imposed changes that came with it had a dramatic effect on the worldviews of Aboriginal Australians. The loss of access to land resulted in an inability to continue normal economic activity and the loss of access to traditional sacred sites, ceremonial sites and to the relationship between land and **identity**. As the Aboriginal population declined, totemic structures and marriage patterns also came under stress. Small residential groups were forced to live in large communities on government settlements or missions, which dramatically restructured traditional social relationships (Hollinsworth, 2006).

> **identity**
> a distinctive characteristic belonging to any given individual or shared by all members of a particular social category or group

Aboriginal Australians now had to deal with elements of life that were not a part of their original worldviews. The challenge was to adjust (quickly) to new people who looked different, had no connection to the land and could not be fitted into existing structures of kinship. There were now new commodities, such as flour, sugar, tea, metal, blankets, cotton and alcohol. There was also the arrival of animals such as sheep, cattle, rabbits, horses and foxes. Guns were introduced. The foundations of Aboriginal spirituality were shaken, in much the same way that Christianity was shaken by scientific discoveries about how the world was created.

The removal of people from their land to reserves or missions, high death rates due to violence and disease, and lack of access to ceremonial sites precipitated a process of cultural breakdown, and the massive changes that directly affected individual worldviews and their place in it.

Reflective question

- Why is it important for mental health professions to 'know the past'?

Aboriginal worldviews

> In losing our land, we also lost our health.
>
> Flick, 1995, p. 5

The above quotation is a concise view of how Aboriginal people perceive the relationship between health and country.

There are some pertinent differences between Aboriginal and non-Aboriginal worldviews, and how these are contexualised in relation to health and land. There is also a fundamental understanding and belief about well-being that is maintained by being linked body to country, and by virtue of maintaining a continuous connection with the land in performing songs and ceremony (Taylor & Guerin, 2010). Broadly speaking, an Indigenous Australian worldview on health is likely to be framed within a well-being perspective to include concepts such as being 'strong, healthy, happy, knowledgeable ('smart'), socially responsible ... beautiful, clean and safe, both in the sense of being within the Law ... of being cared for' (Anderson, 2004, p. 85).

Reflective question

- How would you describe your worldview, and what/who do you think has influenced it?

Government policies

Assimilation

In 1937, the Australian government convened a conference with the states, where it was agreed that the aim for those Indigenous people not of 'full blood' should be their ultimate absorption in the general population, with some form of protection for the 'semi-civilised' people of the north and centre of Australia. Two recommendations were tabled at the conference:

1 The destiny of the native of Aboriginal origin but not the full-blood lies in their ultimate absorption by the people of the Commonwealth, and ... all efforts should be directed to that end.

2 Efforts by all state authorities should be directed towards the education of children of mixed blood at white standards, and their subsequent employment under the same conditions as whites with a view to taking their place in the white community on an equal footing with whites. (Bell, 1959)

In 1951 this policy was extended to all Aboriginal people. The aim of assimilation policies for the 'Aboriginal problem' ultimately to disappear – Aboriginal people would lose their identity within the wider community. The introduction of the Assimilation policy did not mean that Aboriginal people had equal citizenship rights. The policy was promoted through a continuation of restrictive laws and paternalistic administration.

The Assimilation policy was clearly defined. It stated that all Aboriginal people should attain the same manner of living as other Australians, enjoying the same rights and privileges, accepting the same responsibilities, observing the same customs and being influenced by the same beliefs, hopes and loyalties (Lippman, 1981).

Over time, this policy also led to a further policy to remove Aboriginal children from their families. In 1997, *Bringing Them Home* (BTH), the Report of the National Inquiry into the Separation of Aboriginal and Torres Strait Islander Children from Their Families, was released. This report told the tragic story of how Aboriginal children were forcibly removed – 'stolen' – from their parents and placed in public institutions or private homes. The hidden stories were exposed as these 'stolen children' told the Inquiry about the painful experiences of Aboriginal parents and children subjected to the misguided government policy of racial assimilation. The children who were specifically targeted by this policy were the so-called 'half-castes', of mixed heritage. The government's aim was to 'make' them white by assimilating the children into white society. It is important to note that some people who saw the policy as evil opposed it or found a way to negate it.

Fifty-four recommendations were included in the BTH report and, to date, only a few have been implemented. One recommendation relevant to this chapter was:

> **Mental health worker training**
> Recommendation 35 – *That all State and Territory Governments institute Indigenous mental health worker training through Indigenous-run programs to ensure cultural and social appropriateness.*
>
> Human Rights and Equal Opportunity Commission, 1997, p. 43

Reflective question

- If you were forced to assimilate into a new culture, language and governance that would have negative consequences, how would you react?

The effects of child removals

It is difficult to over-estimate the traumatic and harmful effects of the child removal policies of Australia between 1910 and the 1970s. Haebich (2000) described this era as perhaps the most brutal of government policies bestowed upon Indigenous Australians. The term 'Stolen Generations' was coined in the BTH report. The fact that 'generations' is in the plural implicates that this misguided government policy was not just relative to a particular period of Australia's history, but has had a continuing effect on the lives of undoubtedly most, if not all, Aboriginal people of Australia. The overwhelming evidence is that the effects do not stop with the children removed; their children and families inherit them. The effects on family and structure have been documented in the context of war-related trauma, or even family terrorism. The effects of trauma on Aboriginal Australians have therefore been widespread and enduring, recurring across generations (Bessarab and Crawford, 2013).

As a survivor of the Stolen Generations, there were many layers of **trauma** that affected my own social and emotional well-being for many years. Attempting to seek assistance with this from health professionals was extremely difficult. I was passed on from one professional to another. Thankfully, things have changed in the sense that now there is a lot more known regarding the traumatic events Aboriginal Australians have endured, and this is improving all the time. I use the term 'survivor' because for many years I remained in a 'victim' state until I began my journey of **healing**, which incorporated the capacity to forgive. It was not an easy process but I could no longer carry the burdens of others, and forgiveness brought release and a sense of empowerment; it freed me from hatred and bitterness.

> **trauma**
> an emotional shock following a single or recurring stressful event; for Aboriginal people, trauma must be understood in the context of land, connection with country, identity, family and community
>
> **healing**
> a uniquely personal experience comprising forgiveness, self-acceptance and, as far as possible, an absence of mental distress

There are many Aboriginal people who have not yet begun this journey and simply do not know where to start. Being able to disclose your feelings of pain, helplessness and grief is a great place to begin.

Formal apology to Indigenous people

On 13 February 2008 Prime Minister Kevin Rudd delivered a speech to the nation with a formal apology to the Stolen Generations of Australia. The word 'sorry' was uttered many times, and responsibility was finally taken and accountability was evident. The fact that it was not Mr Rudd's government that was responsible for the Child Removal Policy and the actions that followed showed true leadership and sincerity on his part. The previous government, led by John Howard, had refused to apologise to Aboriginal people on the grounds that these events had not happened in his generation and therefore the government of that day was not responsible.

The speech delivered by Mr Rudd is reproduced here:

> I move:
>
> That today we honour the Indigenous peoples of this land, the oldest continuing cultures in human history.
>
> We reflect on their past mistreatment.
>
> We reflect in particular on the mistreatment of those who were Stolen Generations – this blemished chapter in our nation's history.
>
> The time has now come for the nation to turn a new page in Australia's history by righting the wrongs of the past and so moving forward with confidence to the future.
>
> We apologise for the laws and policies of successive Parliaments and governments that have inflicted profound grief, suffering and loss on these our fellow Australians.
>
> We apologise especially for the removal of Aboriginal and Torres Strait Islander children from their families, their communities and their country.

For the pain, suffering and hurt of these Stolen Generations, their descendants and for their families left behind, we say sorry.

To the mothers and the fathers, the brothers and the sisters, for the breaking up of families and communities, we say sorry.

And for the indignity and degradation thus inflicted on a proud people and a proud culture, we say sorry.

We, the Parliament of Australia, respectfully request that this apology be received in the spirit in which it is offered as part of the healing of the nation.

For the future we take heart; resolving that this new page in the history of our great continent can now be written.

We today take this first step by acknowledging the past and laying claim to a future that embraces all Australians.

A future where this Parliament resolves that the injustices of the past must never, never happen again.

A future where we harness the determination of all Australians, Indigenous and non-Indigenous, to close the gap that lies between us in life expectancy, educational achievement and economic opportunity.

A future where we embrace the possibility of new solutions to enduring problems where old approaches have failed.

A future based on mutual respect, mutual resolve and mutual responsibility.

A future where all Australians, whatever their origins, are truly equal partners, with equal opportunities and with an equal stake in shaping the next chapter in the history of this great country, Australia.

(Rudd, 2008)

I was in Sydney's Martin Place that day. Huge screens had been erected for everyone to crowd around, separate, alone. They were symbolic of the fair-skinned babies and children who were the Stolen Generations. The dark-skinned Aboriginal people stood together in strong groups. They were symbolic of the families from whom these children had been taken. There were many non-Aboriginal Australians who were obviously distressed and who also needed to hear the Apology for their own healing.

by Barbara

Reflective question

The concept of Stolen Generations has become a topical issue now in Australia.

- What has prompted this and why did it not receive consideration before now?

Aboriginal identity

The issue of identity has been one of the most problematic issues confronting members of the 'Stolen Generations'. When the debilitating government policy of assimilation was announced in 1937, the principle of identity became extremely significant. The expected outcome from implementing this policy was that Aboriginal people would lose their identity within the wider community; hence the 'Aboriginal' problem would disappear. The Child Removal Policy was a huge part of this process, and the children who were victims of this process were referred to as 'half-castes', presumably because of their British heritage. This was a reflection of emerging theories of the mixing of races.

The BTH report stated that:

> By the late nineteenth century it had become apparent that although the full descent Indigenous population was declining, the mixed decent population was increasing. In social Darwinist terms they were not regarded as near extinction. The fact they had some European 'blood' meant that there was a place for them in non-Indigenous society, albeit a very lowly one.
>
> Human Rights and Equal Opportunity Commission, 1997, chapter 2

Although assimilation policies had been used in earlier colonial practices shaped around nation-building projects intended to develop a 'uniform' Australia, in the issue of assimilation of Aboriginal people there was a serious intention to abandon race-based politics and practices and therefore to create a place for Aboriginal people within mainstream Australia. These assimilation projects were directed at families, not just children.

It was believed that by placing Aboriginal children in non-Aboriginal homes, and preventing contact with their families their Aboriginality (Aboriginal identity) would cease to exist. It was thought that this process would eventually 'breed out' the cultural inheritance and identity of the children. In many cases this worked, but there were also a good percentage that resisted this process, and retained their heritage under the most extreme attempts to remove it. This was indeed true resilience.

> Due to a European approach to religion, family, inheritance and breeding, the policy in the long term failed due to the unique, non-deity spirituality of Aboriginal people; our ancestors are still singing us home.
>
> by Barbara

What was not taken into account was the inherent cultural knowledge and understanding that could not be visualised by the white authoritarians and so were not considered to be relevant. To understand Aboriginality, one must understand the significance of cultural identity, what it is made up of and what it stems from.

To restore personal and cultural identity can be one of the most hurtful and painful parts of healing. The question many Stolen Generations ask is 'Where do I fit in?' After perhaps being raised by a non-Aboriginal family and your life having been shaped by the values, understandings and knowledge within that family, sometimes the individual strength and spirituality of Aboriginal identity is suppressed for a long time.

It is not only the fact of accepting your own inherent identity, but that people sometimes look to others for approval. I have seen it in my community – some individuals who have had their Aboriginality challenged are so intent on 'proving' their Aboriginality. There are some who have taken their case to the High Court for such proof. What is it that creates this urge to prove one's identity? Some people believe they can take remove a person's identity simply with a few words. Intracultural rejection plays a role in many Aboriginal people's lives in Australia. It is one thing to suffer rejection of your identity by the wider community, but to experience it from within the Aboriginal community can be devastating. However, it is a very personal decision as to whether you restore your identity as an Aboriginal person. Some people chose not to do so, as they may be quite happy living with the identity that they already have.

The issue of being 'fair-skinned' at times poses a problem, not necessarily for Aboriginal people but for non-Aboriginal people. It may be that fair-skinned Aboriginal people are a stark reminder of the colonisation process and the fact that they have not assimilated.

> That day of the Apology in Martin Place, I saw some dark-skinned Aboriginal women I worked with in an Aboriginal organisation. I stood in a group photo with them; a week later at work the photo was put up on screen and I had been photo shopped out of the group. I must have been too fair-skinned for acceptance.
>
> by Barbara

> You spend your whole life wondering where you fit. You're not white enough to be white and your skin isn't black enough to be black either and it really does come down to that.
>
> Human Rights and Equal Opportunity Commission, 1997, p. 21

The above quotation sums up in a few lines what many of us experience in our everyday lives, simply trying to fit in somewhere and calling a place home.

In this huge human experiment I have no doubt that identity was the last thing on the minds of governments when removing the children from their families and communities. The practice of Britain sending its convicts to Australia in the hope that they would be rid of the 'criminal class' – and if possible to forget about them, too – was similar to the situation in Australia and the Stolen Generations. The difference was that most of the children removed could not be sent to another country, but had to be displaced within their own country.

It may be difficult for the Australian public at large, who live in what some consider 'the lucky country', to understand the trauma and suffering of Aboriginal people. This may have been caused by the denial or omission of Aboriginal Australians when exploring issues such as colonisation, assimilation and child removal policies. The exclusion of Aboriginal Australians from Australian history was dubbed 'the great Australian silence' by the anthropologist W.E.H. Stanner. The notion he was conveying was of the incompleteness of Australia's history.

With this in mind, it is important to note that with this silence, Aboriginal Australians to a certain degree may have no understanding of their own history, which could contribute to the loss of identity of many Aboriginal people. To plan for the future, we need to understand our past, and if there are many missing links, sometimes we are starting anew.

The incidence of trauma

The traumatic experiences of introduced infections and diseases, physical violence, rape, starvation, torture and death are not those of the individuals alone. Rather, these traumas are at once individual and collective. Furthermore, any one of these disasters as a traumatic event could be passed from the adult and child survivors to their children and grandchildren. Today, the trauma remains in the hearts, minds and souls of Aboriginal families whose ancestors survived these times (Atkinson, 2002).

> The psychological impact of the experiences of dispossession, denigration and degradation are beyond description. They strike at the very core of our sense of being and identity ... Throughout Aboriginal society in this country are seen what can only be described by anyone's measure as dysfunctional families and communities, whose relationships with each other are very marked by anger, depression and despair, dissention and divisiveness. The effects are generational ... I recognised all the things that had happened to me through my grandparents, and their parents; their brothers and sisters whom I had known as a child; through my mother and her siblings; through my cousins and my siblings. I recognised the things that happened to the thousands of other Aboriginal families like our family, and I marveled that we weren't all stark raving mad.
>
> O'Shane, 1995, 151–3

> We are still hurting; colonisation commenced 200 plus years ago after 40 000–150 000 years of uninterrupted existence; within context, the indigenous Irish people are still recovering from their British colonisation experience 800 years later. We are still grieving our losses, it is still relatively early; we are still unwell.
>
> by Barbara

According to the Healing Forum Working Group (2009), there are four types of unresolved trauma affecting the lives of Aboriginal and Torres Strait Islander people, which stem from the process of colonisation and the repercussions of government policy. These are:

1 *Situational* trauma – specific situations such as death or forcible removal produce traumatic responses;
2 *Ecological* trauma – chaotic environments contribute to trauma;

3 *Cumulative* trauma – traumas such as daily experiences of racism, abuse or violence or poverty are repeated; and

4 *Intergenerational* trauma – trauma left unresolved in one generation is often unwittingly handed down to the next generation through, for example, fear, shame, violence or abusive behaviour.

While there have been many attempts to address social and emotional well-being over the years through policy interventions, the lack of success has been due to taking a symptomalogical approach rather than addressing causative factors. Many disciplines in the health sector tend to 'band-aid' mental health distress, which allows for these issues to continue.

Consumer narrative   Sandra

One of the major effects on Aboriginal people due to the dispossession of our land was the introduction of alcohol. The real problems began with the white invasion, which contributed to, and still contributes to, the breakdown of Aboriginal society. Alcohol has and still does contribute to major issues facing Aboriginal people today, such as, health, relationships and parenting practices, to name a few. I have been a victim of the white man's introduction of alcohol into Aboriginal society.

I was raised by both my parents until the age of nine, when I was removed from their care and went to live with my grandmother, because the presence of alcohol and violence was a major part of my upbringing. I then watched my mother fall victim to the disease of alcoholism. Unfortunately for me, no matter what I tried to do to get her help, the damage had been done and I lost my mother early last year. Since then I have continued to lose more people in my community because of the poisonous effects of alcohol.

Unfortunately, the story recounted by Sandra is common among Aboriginal families across Australia. Through this writing comes a sense of hopelessness and trauma. Sandra's frustration at not being able to assist her mother must have affected her greatly. The devastation alcohol causes in some Aboriginal families is well documented, albeit from a biomedical perspective. Simply dealing with the symptoms is not enough, and investigating causative factors is imperative. Alcohol may be used as self-medication to attempt to 'block' trauma and the associated thoughts. It may also be used as a slow method of suicide. To assess someone with such an alcohol-related condition, it is important to encourage the person to disclose traumas she or he has experienced in a safe, non-judgemental environment, without fear of prejudice. Understanding trauma experienced by Aboriginal Australians due to colonisation is imperative for any health care worker. There may be multiple traumas present, caused through loss of connection to land, family or community. This is not an easy process as some traumas are deeply entrenched, but dealing with them one at a time is suggested. This, of course, will take time but it will provide meaningful care with hopefully positive outcomes.

Trauma-informed practice – what does this mean?

According to the Aboriginal and Torres Strait Islander Healing Foundation Development Team (2009, p. 4):

> … many of the problems prevalent in Aboriginal and Torres Strait Islander communities today – alcohol abuse, mental illness and family violence … have their roots in failure of Australian governments and society to acknowledge and address the legacy of unresolved trauma still inherent in Aboriginal and Torres Strait Islander communities.

> It is as though the non-Aboriginal health practitioner has sole access and knowledge to the illness because of his or her academic knowledge, whereas with Aboriginal people, the ill person is the healer with support from a knowledgeable other person.
>
> by Barbara

Trauma-specific care consists of the specific actions taken to address the consequences of trauma on individuals, and to facilitate their healing. These actions need to focus more on developing understandings of and appropriate responses to the complex psychobiological and social reactions to trauma, and less on recounting and categorising the traumatic events (Brier & Scott, 2006; Scaer, 2001).

> The white man seems to always ask the questions of: how do I connect with Aboriginal people, how do I engage with them? What I say to the white man is: you can't, you never will be able to, and for an Aboriginal person the effects of our past will always be in our present. Part of Aboriginal tradition is storytelling. Our stories have been told for generations, knowledge passed by our ancestors, stories of our history, culture and land, and so multiple generations later we will never forget or forgive the suffering our people have and continue to endure in this land that belongs to the Indigenous peoples of Australia.
>
> by Sandra

> Aboriginal people don't necessarily accept non-Aboriginal processes and worldviews, but on the surface, it is cultural to do so. This does not mean they are accepting or they are in rapport with them. Sometimes there is complacency regarding this from the non-Aboriginal health worker.
>
> As long as Aboriginal sovereignty (the land Australia belongs to Aboriginal people) is not recognised, this problem will remain.
>
> by Barbara

The concept of healing

Healing means encouraging different thought processes in different people, which may depend on historical factors, spiritual/religious and cultural beliefs.

According to Atkinson (2012):

> Aboriginal peoples, as individuals and within their families and communities, have been profoundly hurt across generations by layered historic, social and cultural (complex) trauma. 'Closing the Gap' on Aboriginal 'disadvantage', must acknowledge that where there is hurting, there has to be a healing. In healing, people's Trauma Stories become the centrepiece for social healing action, where the storyteller is the teacher and the listener is the student or learner.

> I created Biz Sisters, a start-up business development program that mentors economically disadvantaged Aboriginal women into social and private entrepreneurship, focusing on the psychological and practical aspects of business. I also facilitate the Learning Circles program for severely disengaged women. The aim and expected outcomes of both programs is to empower Aboriginal women towards economic independence.
>
> by Barbara

As stated by the Aboriginal and Torres Strait Islander Healing Foundation Development Team (2009, p. 11):

> Healing is about bringing feelings of despair out into the open, having your pain recognized and, in turn, recognizing the pain of others. It is a therapeutic dialogue with people who are listening. It is about following your own personal journey but also seeing how it fits into the collective story of Aboriginal and Torres Strait Islander trauma.

BORROWED LAND

We are living on borrowed land

The land we once called home

The white man repossessed it

And reclaimed it for their own

We no longer hold the power

Or the rights to this great land

We come underneath their headings

Of the socially disadvantaged

We must not give up fighting though

Because if we do they win

It's time to stand together

And let the unity begin

Give our people back power

Let their voices be heard

Get the message out there

Let the truth be spoken

Through our words

by Sandra Murphy

Interprofessional connections

My name is Fay, and I am a social and emotional well-being worker and have just accepted a position to work at a remote clinic east of Darwin. One of my clients is Anna, who is an Aboriginal Elder of the community.

One day the nurse on duty (Dianne) approached me and informed me that Anna wanted to talk to the social and emotional well-being worker, adding that she did not think that Anna had a 'mental problem'. She said that Anna was a frequent attendee at the clinic, a 'big worrier' and that the biggest worry was her adult children.

Anna looked about 60 years of age, but was, in fact, a decade younger.

'Fay, it's my daughter Melissa and her man, Edward," she explained, adding, 'I want someone to tell them they got to stop this fighting and drinking.'

After talking with Anna, I discovered that her real concerns were for her granddaughter, Milly, whom she has raised for the most part and has recently started to hang out with a group of young males and females who use marijuana heavily. Several have already been evacuated to the regional hospital with acute psychotic episodes. Last year, Milly had been seen at the clinic on one occasion after an episode of petrol sniffing.

As the interview continued I asked, 'Why did you stop drinking, Anna?'

'I was sick, Fay, with high blood pressure and diabetes and all sorts of things. Dr Lavery, he was a very good doctor, he cared about people and spent time with them, like you – he told me straight. He talked to me hard, but I knew it was because he was worried. He showed me all those tests and things. Showed me how grog was causing me to be sick, just like my husband, who died from stroke. I listened to that doctor; he changed my life.'

Indeed, Anna seemed to have settled and appreciated my willingness to listen and to allow silence rather than pushing with questions or rushing to recommendations.

I organised for a local medical officer to undertake a full physical examination of Melissa and Edward, including a psychological assessment. I also contacted the alcohol, tobacco other drug services worker to also provide an assessment and suggest appropriate information for all the family involved.

continued ›

Interprofessional connections continued ›

At the next staff meeting at the clinic I reported on this case and informed my colleagues of the initial assessment and how this approach is needed for Aboriginal people. I advised the clinical staff that while it may take longer to allow people to tell their story and what is happening, it is worthwhile because emotional well-being is equally, if not more important than physical health.

Chapter summary

This chapter has presented the lived experiences of Aboriginal people and information and activities designed to deepen the understanding of:

- Social and emotional well-being in an Aboriginal context;
- Worldviews: understanding your own and how the worldviews of Aboriginal Australians have had to accept the non-Aboriginal domain and adjust under forced circumstances;
- The effects colonisation continues to have in the form of loss of land, culture, language and identity;
- The concept of Aboriginal identity, and how the blending of cultures has affected Aboriginal Australians;
- The importance of understanding the mental distress experienced by Aboriginal Australians, by appreciating the trauma they have experienced due to the losses incurred by colonisation;
- How this will affect assessment of Aboriginal Australians in a mental health context, using trauma-informed practice;
- The healing process for Aboriginal Australians at different stages, and that it is an individual process; and
- Consumer narratives: the importance of listening to the stories.

Critical thinking/learning activities

1   Aboriginal communities in Australia are diverse by history, culture and worldviews. Although this is the case, the effects of colonisation bring similar themes affecting the social and emotional well-being of Aboriginal people, regardless of geographical location. The much larger incidence of mental distress for Aboriginal Australians currently may be seen as a reflection of the significant disruption and decimation to Aboriginal society and has a strong perspective of social and emotional deprivation. How would the significant changes to Aboriginal Australians' cultures and worldviews since European occupation have led to changes in patterns of mental illness?

2   There are increasing concerns that the assessment tools used to evaluate mental distress in Aboriginal Australians do not provide a true diagnosis of the extent of trauma that individuals, families and communities experience. The lack of understanding of Australian Aboriginal culture and worldview, the potential cultural bias and monoculturalism, the transgenerational effects of government policy and the differing contexts of mental health make it difficult to find easy solutions. Reflect on past and present mental health assessment and think about how this process could be improved for the mental distress assessment for Aboriginal Australians.

Learning extension

Imagine losing your right hand, or your dominant hand by some tragic accident. This hand has followed your neural responses, been in some ways the most important part of your body for survival. Then, one day it is gone. What happens now? Your hand is not retrievable so a transplant is an option.

However, we do not know how easy it will be to find tissue donors for this purpose. There are so many different colours and textures of skin, so it might be hard to find a perfect match.

Normally, the body's immune (protective) system treats any new organ or tissue as an invader, like a germ, and tries to destroy it. Transplant drugs, however, partially shut down the immune system so that the body can accept the new organ or tissue. Transplant patients have to take strong drugs for the rest of their lives to prevent rejection of the transplant.

What problems, both clinical and psychological, do you see as potential barriers to successful recover following transplant?

In small groups discuss the following considerations.

Key words for discussion: Rejection, infection, trauma, loss, adaptation, acceptance.

- What happens to the thinking and feeling processes after the loss of a limb?
- Even after a successful transplant, there is a realisation that life will never be the same again. What do you think life will be like after transplant for a person in this situation? Would there be an expectation of things in the person's life being either the same or different?
- What if you simply couldn't get a match and had to have a hand that doesn't look or feel the same? How would you adjust?

This analogy is used to explain the feelings of loss and confusion that Aboriginal people faced with the onset of colonisation, and the traumas to follow.

Acknowledgement

I would like to sincerely thank Barbara and Sandra for their generosity in sharing their experiences and insight in contributing to this chapter. Debra Hocking.

Further reading

Online

Aboriginal and Torres Strait Islander Healing Foundation: http://healingfoundation.org.au/.

Aborigines Protection Act 1909 **(Cth)**: www.austlii.edu.au/au/legis/nsw/num_act/apa1909n25262.pdf

Animated Dreaming Stories: www.abc.net.au/dustechoes/

Australian Indigenous Psychologists Association:www.indigenouspsychology.com.au/Assets/Files/Defining%20 Indigenous%20Social%20and%20Emotional%20Wellbeing%20and%20Mental%20Health.pdf

Australian Institute of Family Studies: www.aifs.gov.au/institute/pubs/fm1/fm35yw.html

Close the Gap Clearinghouse: www.aihw.gov.au/uploadedFiles/ClosingTheGap/Content/Publications/2013/ ctgc-rs19.pdf

Deaths in Custody: www.abc.net.au/news/2013-05-24/death-in-custody-report-alarms-indigenous- leaders/4712056

Mental Health Coordinating Council: www.mhcc.org.au/learning-and-training/trauma-informed-aboriginal- healing.aspx

Native title: www.nntt.gov.au/Information-about-native-title/Pages/default.aspx
Social and emotional wellbeing workers: www.healthinfonet.ecu.edu.au/other-health-conditions/sewbworkers
Stolen Generations' Testimonies: http://stolengenerationstestimonies.com/
Working together – Aboriginal and Torres Strait Islander Mental Health and Wellbeing Principles and Practice: http://aboriginal.childhealthresearch.org.au/media/54847/working_together_full_book.pdf

Film

Bran Nue Dae (2010) – Directed by Rachel Perkins
Jindabyne (2006) – Directed by Ray Lawrence
The Last Wave (1977) – Directed by Peter Weir
Mabo (2012) – Directed by Rachel Perkins
Rabbit Proof Fence (2002) – Directed by Phillip Noyce
Samson and Delilah (2009) – Directed by Warwick Thornton
Ten Canoes – Directed by Rolf de Heer
The Tracker (2002) – Directed by Rolf de Heer

References

Aboriginal and Torres Strait Islander Healing Foundation Development Team (2009). *Voices from the Campfires: Establishing the Aboriginal and Torres Strait Islander Healing Foundation*. Canberra. Commonwealth of Australia.

Anderson, I. (2004). Aboriginal health. In **C. Grbich** (ed.), *Health in Australia: Sociological concepts and issues*, 3rd edn (pp. 75–100). Sydney: Pearson Longman.

Atkinson, J. (2002). *Trauma Trails Recreating Song Lines: The transgenerational effects of trauma in Indigenous Australia*. North Melbourne: Spinifex Press.

Atkinson, J. (2012). *An Educaring Approach to Healing Generational Trauma in Aboriginal Australia*. Retrieved from www.aifs.gov.au/institute/seminars/2012/atkinson/index.php.

Australian Institute of Health and Welfare (2009). *Measuring the Social and Emotional Wellbeing of Aboriginal and Torres Strait Islander Peoples*. Cat.No. IHW24. Canberra. Author.

Bell, J. (1959). Official policies toward the Aborigines of NSW. *Mankind*, 5(8): 345–55.

Bessarab, D. & **Crawford, F.R.** (2013). Trauma, grief and loss: The vulnerability of Aboriginal families in the child protection system. In **B. Bennet, S. Green, S. Glibert** & **D. Bessarab** (eds), *Our Voices: Aboriginal and Torres Strait Islander Social Work*. (pp. 93–113). Melbourne: Palgrave Macmillan.

Brier, J. & **Scott, C.** (2006). *Principles of Trauma Therapy: A guide to symptoms evaluation and treatment*. Thousand Oaks, CA: Sage.

Flick, B. (1995). Spiritual healing, land and health. *Aboriginal and Islander Health Worker Journal*, 19(1): 3–5.

Haebich, A. (2000). *Broken Circles Fragmenting Indigenous Families, 1800–2000*. Fremantle: Fremantle Arts Centre Press.

Healing Forum Working Group (2009). *A Healing Foundation Discussion Paper*. Retrieved from http://aboriginalhealth.flinders.edu.au/Newsletters/2009/Downloads/Development%20Team%20Discussion%20Paper.pdf.

Hollinsworth, D. (2006). *Race and Racism in Australia*. South Melbourne: Thompson Social Science Press.

Human Rights and Equal Opportunity Commission (1997). *Bringing Them Home: A guide to the findings and recommendations of the National Inquiry into the separation of Aboriginal and Torres Strait Islander children from their families*. Canberra: AIATSIS.

Lippmann, L. (1981). *Generations of Resistance: The Aboriginal struggle for justice*. Melbourne: Longman Cheshire.

Macdonald, G. (2010). Colonising processes, the reach of state and ontological violence: Historicising Aboriginal Australian experience, *Anthropologica*, 52(1): 49–66.

NATSIHC (2003). *National Strategic Framework for Aboriginal and Torres Strait Islander Health*. Canberra: NATSIHC.

O'Shane, P. (1995). The psychological impact of white colonialism on Aboriginal people. In J. Atkinson (ed.), *Trauma Trails Recreating Song Lines: The transgenerational effects of trauma in Indigenous Australia.* Melbourne: Spinifex Press.

Reynolds, H. (1992). *The Law of the Land*, 2nd edn. Ringwood, Vic.: Penguin.

Rose, D. B. (2000). *Dingo Makes Us Human: Life and land in an Australian Aboriginal culture.* Oakleigh, Vic.: Cambridge University Press.

Rudd, K. (2008). Apology to Australia's Indigenous Peoples, House of Representatives, Parliament House, Canberra, 13 February. Retrieved from http://australia.gov.au/about-australia/our-country/our-people/apology-to-australias-indigenous-peoples.

Scaer, R. (2001). *The Body Wears the Burden: Trauma, dissociation and disease.* New York: The Howarth Press.

Social Health Reference Group (2004). *National strategic framework for Aboriginal and Torres Strait Islander peoples' mental health and social and emotional well being 2004–2009.* Canberra: National Aboriginal and Torres Strait Islander Health Council and National Mental Health Working Group.

Taylor, K. & Guerin, P. (2010). *Health Care and Indigenous Australians Cultural Safety in Practice.* South Yarra: Palgrave Macmillan.

Thompson, N. (2001). Indigenous Australia: Indigenous health. In J. Jupp (ed.), *The Australian People: An encyclopedia of the nation, its people and their origins.* Port Melbourne: Cambridge University Press.

Van Loon, A. (2011). Contexts of community nursing. In D. Kralik & A. Van Loon (eds), *Community Nursing in Australia*, 2nd edn. (pp. 46–84). Brisbane: John Wiley & Sons Australia.

Zubrick, S. R., Silburn, S. R., Lawrence, D. M., Mitrou, F., Dalby, R., Blair, E., Griffin, J., Milroy, H., De Majo, J. A. & Cox, A. (2005). *The Social and Emotional Wellbeing of Aboriginal Children and Young People: Summary booklet.* Perth: Telethon Institute for Child Health Research.

4

Māori mental health

Jacquie Kidd, Kerri Butler and Reina Harris

Introduction 73

Kawa whakaruruhau (cultural safety) 75

Whānau ora 77

Hauora (health) and oranga (wellness) 78

Engagement with tangata whai i te ora:
The Ten Commitments 80

Chapter summary 86

Critical thinking/learning activities 86

Learning extension 87

Further reading 87

References 87

Learning objectives

At the completion of this chapter, you should be able to:

- Understand the different ways of being Māori, and the importance of accurately identifying Māori mental health and cultural needs.
- Consider how a nurse's own ethnicity might influence her or his care of Māori *tangata whai i te ora*.
- Explore how historical trauma and current health care practices have affected the mental health of Māori, and how health professionals can help to improve Māori health outcomes.
- Develop skills in culturally safe assessment, including *whanaungatanga*.
- Develop skills in facilitating the culturally safe care of *tangata whai i te ora* and *whānau*.

Whakatauki

Mā te rongo, ka mōhio; Mā te mōhio, ka mārama; Mā te mārama, ka mātau; Mā te mātau, ka ora.

Through resonance comes cognisance; through cognisance comes understanding; through understanding comes knowledge; through knowledge comes life and well-being.

Mihi

This chapter has been written by three women, each with different experiences of mental health, mental distress and being Māori.

Ko te mea tuatahi me mihi ki te Atua nana nei nga mea katoa

Tuarua me mihi ki nga mate

Ko Maungataniwha te maunga

Ko Tapapa te awa puta atu ki te wahapū o Hokianga Whakapau Karakia

Ko Ngatokimatawhaorua te waka

Ko Ngapuhi te iwi

Ko Te Uri Mahoe te hapū

Ko Mangamuka te marae

Ko Reina Tuai Harris ahau

No reira, tena koutou tena koutou tena koutou katoa

The first thing is to acknowledge God the creator of all things.

Secondly, I acknowledge those who have passed on.

My mountain is Maungataniwha.

My river is Tapapa, which flows into the many subtribes in Hokianga of the wasted incantations.

My tribe is Ngapuhi.

My subtribe is Te Uri Mahoe.

My name is Reina Tuai Harris.

Formal greetings to you all.

> **mihi** a speech, formally acknowledging, among other things, people you meet, the purpose of the meeting and the place (where the meeting is being held), through protocols set by the **iwi**.

Introduction

There are many ways of being Māori. Ethnicity in New Zealand historically has been based on biology and a caste system, but has now moved to a more contemporary approach that assumes ethnicity is not static and predetermined. Instead, ethnicity and culture are viewed as intertwined aspects of a person's identity that are influenced by our social environment and therefore can change as we mature and our context shifts (Cormack, 2010; Kukutai & Didham, 2009). This means that any combination of physical features and cultural beliefs can be found in people who self-identify

tangata whaii te ora
a person moving
towards well-being;
ora is a part of the
word *oranga*
(to be well)

as Māori. In short, it is not possible to assume that someone is Māori or non-Māori based on her or his appearance or lifestyle. Asking the **tangata whaii te ora** (person on his or her recovery journey) is the only way to be certain about someone's ethnicity, and is a vital part of the first nursing assessment.

For Māori, health and culture are intricately linked, so when a person identifies as Māori there are vital aspects of *te ao Māori* (the Māori worldview) that must be incorporated into her or his mental health experiences in order to provide safe and effective care. In this chapter we discuss how nurses from all cultural backgrounds can develop practices that engage with *tangata whaii te ora* and *whānau* in mental health and addiction settings. The chapter will be helpful for people practising in the New Zealand context, as well as those who encounter people of Māori background and culture in Australia. It will also assist nurses to consider how institutional racism might influence their ability to care for Māori, and will encourage the exploration of personal cultural beliefs to transcend this. The Tidal Model's Ten Commitments (Buchanan-Barker & Barker, 2006) will be presented as a framework for developing culturally safe practice.

> I recall during one of my admissions being told by a Māori nurse that I had no right to talk about culture. She spoke to me in Māori and demanded that I translate it. I turned to her and said 'You know I wasn't bought up in a Māori environment; I don't have to speak *Te Reo* to feel Māori'.
>
> by Kerri

Background

The Māori population in New Zealand comprised more than one in seven people in 2006, with this number projected to increase rapidly during the decade to 2015 (Ministry of Health, 2008). Māori is a young population, with high proportions of young Māori people in every region of New Zealand.

Māori are disproportionately represented among those with the highest socio-economic need, which means that Māori have higher risks associated with poor mental health than non-Māori. Māori are also less likely to receive health care than people from other cultures (Ministry of Health, 2008).

The New Zealand national mental health survey of more than 12 000 households found that more than 50 per cent of Māori people experienced illnesses affecting their mental health at some time during their lives (Oakley Browne, Well & Scott, 2006). The most common disorders were anxiety (31.3 per cent), substance use disorders (26.5 per cent) and mood disorders (24.3 per cent), and many Māori had more than one problem (Baxter et al., 2006). The most common reasons for Māori to be hospitalised are schizophrenia and bipolar disorder. More than half of Māori who have a serious mental illness and about three-quarters who have a moderate illness also had no contact with health care providers for their mental health needs (Oakley Browne et al., 2006). Māori access to mental health care is often through the court and justice systems, with higher rates of overall hospitalisation and a higher likelihood of admission to forensic or secure units than non-Māori (Baxter, 2008). In 2010 the suicide rate for Māori young people (aged 15–24 years) was more than 2.5 times higher than for non-Māori young people. The suicide rate for Māori across all age groups was more than twice that of non-Māori (Ministry of Health, 2012).

An explanation for these health outcomes is that Māori in New Zealand have been subjected to a continuous process of colonisation since 1840, whereby land, language and traditions have been systematically removed and resulting in many Māori being displaced from the economic and social structures that had historically supported them. The consequences of colonisation can be seen in the continuing high levels of socio-economic deprivation and poor health status of many Māori (Stewart-Harawira, 2005).

While these statistics show a disturbing picture of Māori mental health, this is not the whole story. *Te ao Māori* provides an holistic approach to health and well-being that aligns with the philosophy of recovery. Effective mental health nursing requires nurses to move beyond the deficit approach (a perspective that focuses on the negative aspects of health) towards a way of understanding *tangata whai i te ora* and *whānau* as individuals who have unique experiences, needs, strengths and stories of personal success (Barker & Buchanan-Barker, 2004). In the next section we discuss the potential of nursing to respond to Māori needs for health and wellness.

Kawa whakaruruhau (cultural safety)

The Nursing Council of New Zealand sets out competencies that require nurses to practise in a manner that *tangata whai i te ora* and *whānau* determine as being culturally safe, and to demonstrate the ability to apply the principles of the Treaty of Waitangi to nursing practice (Nursing Council of New Zealand, 2007).

The historical component of cultural safety is found in the Treaty of Waitangi (1840), which underpins the government and legislation of New Zealand. It is viewed as the foundational document for mental health service planning and delivery (Mental Health Commission, 2012). In summary:

- Article One requires the Crown to consult and collaborate with iwi (tribes) and hapū (subtribes) regarding the functions and operations of 'good government'. This includes the development and delivery of health services.
- Article Two guarantees Māori rights of ownership, including non-material assets such as *te reo Māori*, **hauora** Māori and

iwi
a tribe with particular geographical boundaries

hapū
a division of a Māori *iwi* (tribe), often translated as 'subtribe'; membership is determined by genealogical descent; a *hapū* is made up of a number of *whānau* (nuclear/extended family) groups

hauora
health, including social, emotional, spiritual and physical health

tikanga Māori (language, health and customs). It establishes the principle of *tino rangatiratanga* (self-determination), ensuring that Māori communities and organisations can manage their own property, assets and resources.

- Article Three guarantees Māori the same rights of citizenship and privileges as British subjects, including the rights of equal access to mental health and addiction services, to equal health and well-being outcomes and to access of mainstream mental health and addiction services that meet the needs of Māori.

Over time, these articles have been simplified into three principles; partnership, participation and protection (Durie, 1994). For mental health nurses, these principles highlight the need to work together with Māori to improve health outcomes, support Māori participation in their own health care, recognise that health is a *taonga* (treasure) that is worthy of protection and facilitate equitable access to health care. The Treaty of Waitangi principles, along with Māori health education, form the basis for *kawa* **whakaruruhau**, or cultural safety within the Māori context (Nursing Council of New Zealand, 2011).

There are two particular challenges that can interfere with the delivery of culturally safe care. One is that, as nurses and people, we are often not good at recognising how our culture influences our everyday attitudes and activities. Increased personal awareness is a way of opening our eyes to the cultural differences *tangata whaii te ora* and *whānau* might experience when they accept mental health care.

The second challenge is known as 'institutional racism', which means that culturally specific attitudes, processes and routines are embedded

within the health system and create barriers that are detrimental to other cultures (Jones, 2000). Examples of institutional racism include policies that stop *whānau* from staying to support *tangata whaii te ora*, buildings that cannot accommodate *powhiri* and **whanaungatanga** processes (greeting and connection processes, both of which are discussed below), professional codes of conduct that forbid the sharing of personal histories and the lack of provision of trained and acceptable translators.

One of the key things that I can say in regards to working with Māori is having an understanding of different worldviews. Essentially, the predominant worldview in the health world is Eurocentric and with this worldview comes the tendency to place lesser emphasis on things that other cultures consider as extremely relevant. For Māori one of the key things that is relevant to well-being is spirituality.

by Reina

Reflective question

- What barriers to cultural safety can you identify in the education and health organisations of which you are a part?

Whānau ora

riki
en

ātua
e elder who is traditionally a
an of genealogy, spirituality
āori knowledge

ale elder who is traditionally a
an of genealogy, spirituality
āori knowledge

Whānau is the central structure for Māori society, so prioritising the health of *whānau* is a way of improving Māori health outcomes. The concept of *whānau ora* has been used widely within the public sector to describe an overarching goal in the development of Māori-specific programs, strategies and policies. *Whānau ora* happens when Māori families are supported to achieve their maximum health and well-being within both Te Ao Māori and New Zealand society, and have control over their own destinies (Ministry of Health, 2002, 2008). The function of *whānau* is to provide strength, security, identity and nurturing.

A *whānau* can have many shapes. A familiar one consists of **tamariki** (children), *rangatahi* (youth), *pakeke* (adults) and **kaumātua/kuia** (grandparents/elders). *Whānau* can also include formal or informal adoptees, or arise from social structures such as school or church groups.

> I remember my overnight stay in Sunnyside hospital after being at a conference. It sticks in my mind how amazing the staff were at involving my brother and sister-in-law. Instead of shunting them off with a 'Thanks, we'll take care of her now', they asked them to stay with me and to help them to encourage me to take the medication. I lay down and went to sleep with them beside me. It was in vast contrast to having my husband removed from the room and four to five staff lined up against a wall ready to restrain and administer medication less than a week later in a different unit.
>
> by Kerri

Reflective questions

- What shape is your *whānau?*
- Do you belong to more than one?

Whānau is the base structure from which *hapū* (wider *whānau* or subtribes) and *iwi* (tribes) are built, with the processes for connecting individual, *whānau*, *hapū* and *iwi* as important as the structures themselves. Focusing on *whānau ora* has the potential to create ripples of health and well-being that improve health outcomes at every level of Māori society (Whānau Ora Taskforce, 2009).

When working with *tangata whaii te ora* and *whānau*, it is also important to recognise that *tangata whai i te ora* have individual voices. Some *tangata whai i te ora* have spoken of the distress they feel when their individual voice becomes 'lost' in the collective voice, especially if the *whānau* adopt a caregiving role that focuses on symptom identification and management, and 'pathologises' normal responses to distress. Just as we identify the key roles a clinician plays in recovery, we need to ensure that *whānau* are clear about the roles they can play in their loved ones life, and that the *tangata whai i te ora* feel empowered to have a say in how that looks. Relationships can be severely damaged when the roles intersect and sometimes collide with one another, and mental distress can become an even lonelier existence when *everyone* seems to be taking care of you.

> I can remember an incident of walking around the open, low-stimulus area asking if someone could please contact my mum. I can recall feeling like my head was fragmenting and the only thing I knew that would ground me was my mum. To be told 'We are not contacting her, she knows you are in here' was really distressing. I spoke to my mum about that and she said 'I never said that, I had no idea'.

> I think about my own children and know that I would want to be there no matter what time of night if they needed me. First and foremost, *whānau* have to take care of themselves, but part of taking care of their own *wairua* is being there for their loved ones. There is a disjointedness that comes from being separated and left helpless when your loved ones are sick. This can damage relationships; whilst one is left dealing with the mental illness, the other is the *whānau*, who are left feeling like they failed and let their loved one down.
>
> by Kerri

wairua
spirit, soul, spirit of a person which exists beyond death

It must also be acknowledged that not all *whānau* are healthy; some contribute to distress for the *tangata whaii te ora*. The principles of trauma-informed care can help to guide nurses when this is identified (see below).

Hauora (health) and *oranga* (wellness)

oranga
well-being, in both material and non-material senses, including food, livelihood, welfare, health and living well; it may also refer to safety

Hauora and *oranga* represent social, emotional, spiritual, and physical health for Māori. With all these in a healthy balance, the *whānau* and individuals are able to participate in and enjoy their language, spirit and land. These are the cornerstones of a flourishing people (Blisset, 2011). These four concepts have been drawn together in a model called *te whare tapa wha* (Durie, 1994), which views each concept as the side of a house. Each side is important to the structure and stability of the house; if one aspect of life is missing or unhealthy, the entire structure is at risk.

> In the Hokiangaarea, Māori cultural values are interlinked with the provision of health services. Why this works for *tangata whai i te ora* is that the service recognises the spiritual dimension of healing. *Mirimiri* is part of the 'package of care' wrapped around *tangata whai i te ora*. *Mirimiri* literally translates as 'massage', but it really means that a connection has to be made between the healer and the *tangata whai i te ora* on a spiritual level for the treatment to have a greater effect … a connection between energies … I was not in a good place when I began *mirimiri*,. I had my first session when my son was four days old, when things began to whirlwind out of control for me … I remember walking blankly into the room and I just sat there with baby in my arms and I just could not stop the tears. The healer just started to *mirimiri* me … when I left I felt lighter and centred.
>
> by Reina

Te Whare Tapa Wha (the four-sided house)

- *Te Taha Wairua* (spiritual) is associated with more than religion. It also encompasses how a person is connected to the environment; land, language, history, mythology and heritage. *Wairua* includes how a person communicates with his or her world, and what she or he has faith in.

> The way that I was taught is that the spirit world is closely connected to the living world. Māori will always acknowledge spirits as the essence of things. This worldview allows for little distinction between the world of the living and the spirit world. The reason I am talking about this is because for me when I am more 'sick' my connection with *te ao wairua* is more pronounced. I see things and hear things and am more aware of things. The irony is that I am less able to participate fully in today's society. The point is that people who are 'mentally ill', although they may not be able to cope well in society, they may not be able to hold down a job, or function according to societal expectations of education, housing, timeframes, relationships and commitments, their link to *te ao wairua* may be stronger, and because of that, from a Māori perspective they are unique and gifted.
>
> by Reina

- *Te Taha Whānau* (family) involves being close to people, sharing experiences, beliefs and decision-making. It also encompasses the wider social context. *Whānau* is the essential structure for belonging through connecting to the past, flourishing in the present and looking to the future.

Within six weeks of the birth of my daughter all of my immediate family decided to go and live in Australia in search of wealth and prosperity. This affected my well-being greatly because I had lost my connections and my support; I had lost my *whānau*. It is important for Māori *whānau* to take note of what we do have, and what we do have is strong families, and retaining and remaining a strong connected *whānau* who see each other and support each other often is important. We don't work well when we are separated. Equally important is that service providers recognise the central nature of *whānau* for Māori to function well. If people have *whānau*, encourage those connections and include them in care. If people are estranged from their *whānau*, understand the effect on the *tangata whai i te ora* and help them recognise and deal with that trauma. If I had been able to access the support that I needed for my postnatal depression. I believe that someone would have been able to help me understand how the loss of my *whānau* contributed to my illness.

by Reina

- *Te Taha Hinengaro* (thoughts and emotions) includes how we see ourselves in the world, how we communicate with others, and how we connect our mind, body and soul.
- *Te Taha Tinana* (physical) encompasses all of our physical experiences, including our future potential.

Te whare tapa wha provides a way of understanding the devastating effects of colonisation on the health of Māori. The loss of land through war, confiscation or subterfuge meant that *whānau*, *hapū* and *iwi* lost the means to support themselves and lost places of great spiritual significance. These losses, in turn, affect the sense of *whānau* identity and the individuals' ability to express themselves as belonging to a secure social structure. The transition from self-determination to powerlessness and poverty, in addition to the introduction of new strains of disease, reduced physical health further and affected the resilience of *whānau* (Jackson, 1992). The interconnectedness of the four sides of health now has a vital role to play in the recovery of *tangata whai i te ora* and *whānau*.

Engagement with *tangata whai i te ora*: The Ten Commitments

The common understanding of an initial nursing assessment includes the nurse having a list of questions that the person in care will answer. The initial assessment of *tangata whai i te ora* and *whānau* requires a different approach, with a focus on achieving engagement and understanding first, before any probing questions are asked. It is important to note here that these processes are also quite likely to benefit *tangata whai i te ora* who do not identify as Māori. Culture is often presented as a boundary that divides people

(Maddalena, 2009), but in fact people across the world have a similar need for connection and security. The processes we are describing here are taking a Māori worldview that is specific to meeting the needs of Māori, but need not be exclusive to Māori.

The Ten Commitments are the essential values embedded in the Tidal Model (Barker, 2001), a person-centred, empowering approach to recovery in mental health settings. They were initially framed as the moral, ethical and philosophical bases for mental health nursing care, but have since also been framed as a way for nurses to work with *tangata whai i te ora* and *whānau* in a way that upholds *kawa whakaruruhau* (Kidd, 2010).

The Ten Commitments have been grouped into three waves or levels of engagement.

The first wave incorporates the Māori process of the *powhiri* (welcome and greeting). This is a formal practice in an environment that is familiar to *tangata whai i te ora* and *whānau*, and involves getting to know each other and bringing our history, social context and professional qualifications to share. Known as **manaakitanga**, this is a caring, nurturing process that opens up a space for respectful communication to occur, and affirms the willingness of the health professionals to work in culturally safe ways. The commitments in this wave are 'valuing the voice', 'respecting the language' and 'developing curiosity'.

> **manaakitanga** involves treating other people in a respectful, hospitable manner, especially when the other people are visitors; it is important that such hospitality is acknowledged and reciprocated

When people are able to articulate their stories in a way that makes sense to them it creates a sense of empowerment. It communicates to them that their story matters, where they have come from matters and their sense of identity and 'self' matters. It is important to remember that we all experience things differently.

Challenges for nurses during this wave of interaction include buildings that have not been designed for large groups of people to meet, the pressures of time for all health professionals and the need to produce large amounts of documentation within a very short period of the initial contact with mental health services.

The second wave begins once people are known to each other. In this wave, the needs of the *tangata whai i te ora* and *whānau* are explored through inviting and respecting their stories. Nurses and other health care professionals have a tendency to search for symptoms in people's stories, disregarding accounts of personal achievements and their explanations about why they are distressed right now.

It is important to remember that for Māori people 'storytelling' is a big part of the process of *whanaungatanga*. Being too quick to explain what is happening and to ask questions can stop the storytelling process, and the opportunity for connection may be lost. In our experience, giving *tangata whai i te ora*, the 'gift of time', usually means that people are more receptive to ongoing contact with nurses.

Working with the commitments to 'become the apprentice', 'use the available toolkit' and 'craft the step beyond' enables us to listen carefully to the whole of the story without needing to reframe or edit it. Becoming the apprentice and using the available toolkit involves putting aside our professional expertise in order to hear about the strengths, solutions and unmet needs of *tangata whai i te ora* and *whānau*. They allow *whānau* to be prioritised rather than marginalised through the expression of the *whānau* story, and give us the tools to provide trauma-informed care.

Trauma-informed care (see Chapter 10) for Māori includes awareness of the dispossession and alienation associated with colonisation, as well as knowledge of the effects of socio-economic deprivation on rates of interpersonal violence, including sexual abuse (Marie & Fergusson, 2008). Re-traumatisation occurs when an already traumatised person and/or *whānau* has her or his pain recreated through experiences in health settings (Herman, 1997). Having a respectful and caring process for listening to stories can help to create the profound human connection that allows the work of recovery from trauma to begin.

Crafting the step beyond encourages nurses, *tangata whai i te ora*, *whānau* and other health professionals to recognise that involvement with mental health and addiction services is not a lifelong sentence. This commitment supports us to understand what needs to be done now to reduce distress, and what recovery looks like for this person and her or his *whānau* (Barker & Buchanan-Barker, 2004). It is the first step in planning for discharge, and it takes place in the very beginning of the relationship.

The third wave of engagement refers to the work of the entire health care team, including *tangata whai i te ora*, *whānau* and health care professionals. The commitments to 'give the gift of time', 'reveal personal wisdom', 'know that change is constant' and 'be transparent' collectively create an environment of support, expertise, shared insights and hope. This is the work of recovery.

The notion that change is 'constant' provides a challenge to nurses to adapt to the adjustments and transformations experienced by *tangata whai i te ora* and *whānau* as distress resolves and new discoveries are made. Change for some people is a rapid process of revelations and new knowledge, while for others it is a slow progression that can span several years. During this time it is easy for nurses to become discouraged and either withdraw from care or become harsh (Caldwell et al., 2006), so being aware of our own mental health and job satisfaction is an important feature of being able to deliver culturally safe care.

A well-known Māori *Tohunga* (expert) wrote about the connected nature of God, Man and Universe and, indeed this is what I have been taught. Everything is connected and it is vital to make connections in regards to identifying yourself, your connections with the environment, mountains, rivers, land and your connections to people, tribes and subtribes. It is these connections that can build or impinge on well-being. When I think back to the time when I became unwell (or depressed, as is the clinical term), I believe it is directly related to my loss of connections. I was brought up close to my tribal land and I became unwell in the city, where I was estranged from my land. I am not saying that you can't move from your tribal area and be well, but I am saying that in my case I feel that being estranged from my tribal area contributed to my unwellness. Conversely, when I have difficulties I have to go home; the water is very important to me so I go to this special place, a river where my ancestor healed his battle wounds.

by Reina

Consumer narrative   Mare's story part one

I was the primary nurse for Mare, a young Māori woman who had developed puerperal psychosis following the birth of her first child, four weeks prior to her admission. Mare had been brought to hospital by the police after a member of the public had noticed the baby lying unattended on the front lawn. Mare believed that her child was sick and that she needed to be surrendered to Papatuanuku (Goddess of the Earth) for healing. From a Māori worldview, Mare's beliefs were consistent with a strongly traditional way of managing illness; however, the baby appeared to be healthy and meeting developmental milestones.

Mare's involvement with police, a mental health in-patient unit and social workers who were concerned with the welfare of the baby had increased her anxiety and separated her from her partner, mother and wider *whānau*. The processes of assessment and admission had removed from her the very people who could have explained her thought processes and relieved her anxiety.

I proposed that a *whānau hui* (meeting) be held and, in consultation with Mare's mother, organised a *hui* for Mare, her female relatives and a female psychiatrist. Mare's male relatives stepped back from this process because issues relating to childbirth are *tapu* (sacred) and are the domain of women. Mare's grandmother, a *kuia* (elder), opened the *hui* with a *karakia*, then provided support and spiritual protection for the *whānau* as they discussed what had happened.

> *karakia*
> a prayer or incantation for a specific purpose, such as spiritual guidance or protection

An important process in this *hui* was for the psychiatrist and I to introduce ourselves with a high level of personal disclosure. I shared my *whakapapa* (genealogy), my nursing background and some information about my childbirth experiences, including that I had experienced severe postnatal depression following all my children's births. From this sharing of stories, the *whānau* came to see that I had a professional and personal history that enabled me to understand what Mare and the *whānau* might be experiencing.

by Jacquie

Reflective questions

- How does it make you feel to think about sharing personal information?
- How much is too much?

Consumer narrative   Mare's story part two

The women of the *whānau* wanted to take responsibility for Mare and the baby, by taking them home and staying with them while Mare's symptoms resolved. The *whānau* revealed that Mare had been trying to get pregnant for almost two years before conceiving, and that even before the birth of her child had been terrified that some harm would befall her baby. They felt that her anxiety had increased after the birth, and had been exacerbated by a long labour and severely interrupted sleep over the previous month. She was getting up many times each night to check that the baby was breathing and warm. Mare's symptoms appeared to the *whānau* as a logical consequence of combining high levels of anxiety and fear with physical trauma from the birth and postpartum period, and a Māori worldview. They understood her desire to put her baby in close connection with the Earth mother to assist with healing, although they were concerned about why and how she chose to do this, and the potential for harm to the baby.

The *whānau* discussed taking turns to stay with Mare and the baby, including Mare's mother taking leave from work to be available. In total, four of the women in the *whānau* committed to a roster, so that someone would be present in the house with Mare to support, monitor and help her with care of the baby.

Daily visits from the Māori mental health service were organised, as well as weekly meetings with the psychiatrist to monitor Mare's progress. Social support services agreed to step back from the *whānau* on the condition that they received regular reports about Mare's care and the baby's progress. Mare's general medical practitioner was brought onto the care team to provide care for the *whānau* and to monitor the baby's health.

Mare and her baby were discharged from the mental health unit that day, and I had no further involvement in their care. Recovering from puerperal psychosis takes time and ongoing treatment; for Mare and her *whānau* it took more than three months of care and support. Mare and her mother came to visit me six months after our meeting, and brought the baby for me to see.

by Jacquie

Consumer narrative   Kerri's story

I never grew up with an attachment to my Māori roots, yet when I become unwell there is a connection there. I seem to sense my grandmother around me.

When I was back in the community after a particularly traumatising seclusion when I was six-and-a-half months pregnant, I knew all I wanted to do was to get back up north to where my grandmother was buried. I felt if I did then everything would

continued ›

come right for me. The ward staff involved the Māori cultural team and I was given the most amazing support. They used to come and get me off the ward whenever I rang and take me to the *whare*, which was a place of healing and sanctuary for me. More importantly, they helped me make connections and links to the people back 'home' in the north, so that when my baby girl was born we were able to take a trip back up north to bury her placenta at my grandmother's feet.

There was a huge sense of belonging. To this day, during times of turbulence and extreme distress I want to link back to my *turangawaewae* (land to which I belong). There's a feeling and sense of safety in 'coming home'.

> **turangawaewae**
> 'a place to stand'; places where we feel especially empowered and connected; our foundation, our place in the world, our home

During my last admission it was really important to me have the seclusion rooms blessed, and to have a *taonga* (treasured object or idea). I was fortunate that the *Kaumātua* said 'Get your partner or *whānau* to bring something in for you'. I chose a football. My football was blessed and affectionately became known as 'Harry Hippo' to both me and fellow patients. I was allowed to dribble it around the unit sometimes, and I even slept with it. I became distressed and difficult to manage at times it was taken from me. It was a way I had of disconnecting from the trauma I was experiencing at being away from my *tamariki* (children) and my *whānau*. That ability to hold myself in the moment and create my own safe world was a powerful source of recovery/grounding for me.

by Kerri

Reflective questions

Kerri has identified some important cultural needs in her story, including feeling her grandmother around her when she's distressed, wanting to have the seclusion room blessed and keeping a *taonga* close to her. Changing the language of a story can completely change its meaning.

- Try rewriting Kerri's story from a medical perspective. How has it changed? What might those changes in language and meaning mean for your practice?
- Advocacy is an important part of our clinical role. Would you be brave enough to advocate for Kerri's football? What strategies could you use to gain acceptance from the rest of the clinical team?

Chapter summary

- *Kawa whakaruruhau* comes from a combination of understanding your own cultural position and how it shapes your thoughts and behaviour, the principles of the Treaty of Waitangi and Māori health needs.
- An important part of the initial nursing assessment is to discover what is important to the *tangata whai i te ora* and her or his *whānau*.
- Colonisation and ongoing socio-economic deprivation have a significant effect on Māori mental health. Contributing to an improvement in Māori health outcomes requires thoughtful and respectful engagement with *tangata whai i te ora* and *whānau*.
- The Ten Commitments that underpin the Tidal Model can contribute to a framework for engagement with *tangata whai i te ora* and *whānau*.
- It takes time and effort to facilitate culturally safe care. Nurses need to take care of their own mental health to do this over the long term.

Critical thinking/learning activities

1 In small groups, discuss the following:
   - When you think of your own ethnicity or culture, what are the most important aspects for you? These could include particular relationships, ceremonial occasions such as birthdays, weddings or Christmas, foods, or special places.
   - How often do these aspects of culture show up in your everyday life? Consider books, music, television, slang, and jokes.
   - Discuss how your own cultural outlook might manifest itself in your nursing practice.
2 In small groups, list the benefits that come from having a regular, long-term source of income and place to live. Once you have completed your list, use *Te Whare Tapa Wha* to discuss the effects of losing these.
3 Role-play possible ways of working with the *whanaungatanga* wave of engagement. Consider how to arrange the environment, who should be present, who should speak and what should be shared.
4 In pairs, take turns to tell a story about a time in your life when you have been distressed or traumatised. For the listener, how does it feel to listen to a story without interrupting, sharing your own story or providing solutions? For the storyteller, did you feel comfortable sharing this story? Why or why not?
5 In small groups, discuss your response to part two of Mare's story. What risk factors can you identify? Were all of these risk factors acknowledged in Mare's plan of care? What could have been done differently?

Learning extension

New Zealand has a diverse cultural population, including people who are indigenous to other lands but who live here by choice or necessity. There are several more Māori health models, some of which appear in the 'further reading' section of this chapter. Choose one more model that describes a Māori worldview and one from each of two other indigenous cultures that are present in the region in which you live. Compare the similarities and differences in the approaches. Consider whether providing care that meets the competencies for *kawa whakaruruhau* might assist you in providing culturally safe care to people from these other cultures.

Further reading

* Te Rau Matatini, to access the latest in Māori mental health research and projects: www.matatini.co.nz
* *The Insatiable Moon* is a book and film. Sometimes magic happens in the most unlikely of places. Arthur claims to be the second son of God. The rest of the world calls him mad. But he knows who he is, and gets on with the work he needs to do. www.theinsatiablemoon.com
* The Tidal Model website is where you will find resources and ideas to challenge your nursing practice and engage with people: www.tidal-model.com
* *Te wheke* is a traditional Māori model of health that acknowledges the link between the mind, the spirit, the human connection with *whānau*, and the physical world in a way that is seamless and uncontrived. www.health.govt.nz/our-work/populations/maori-health/maori-health-models/maori-health-models-te-wheke
* Te PaeMahutonga is a Māori health model that brings together elements of contemporary health promotion. www.health.govt.nz/our-work/populations/maori-health/maori-health-models/maori-health-models-te-pae-mahutonga

aroha
love and empathy; an attitude and an important cultural value

mana
respect and dignity

References

Barker, P. (2001). The Tidal Model: Developing an empowering, person-centred approach to recovery within psychiatric and mental health nursing. *Journal of Psychiatric and Mental Health Nursing*, 8(3): 233–40.

Barker, P. & Buchanan-Barker, P. (2004). Beyond empowerment: Revering the story teller. *Mental Health Practice*, 7(5): 18–20.

Baxter, J. (2008). *Māori Mental Health Needs Profile Summary: A review of the evidence*. Palmerston North, New Zealand: Te Rau Matatini.

Baxter, J., Kokaua, J., Wells, J. E., McGee, M. A. & Oakley Browne, M. A. for the New Zealand Mental Health Survey Research (2006). Ethnic comparisons of the 12 month prevalence of mental disorders and treatment contact in Te Rau Hinengaro: The New Zealand Mental Health Survey. *Australian and New Zealand Journal of Psychiatry*, 40(10): 905–13.

Blisset, W. (2011). *He Puawaitanga Mo Tatou Katoa. Flourishing for All in Aotearoa: A creative conversation to explore a Māori world view of flourishing*. Wellington: Mental Health Foundation.

Buchanan-Barker, P. & Barker, P. (2006). The Ten Commitments: A value base for mental health recovery. *Journal of Psychosocial Nursing and Mental Health Services*, 44(9): 29–33.

Caldwell, B. A., Gill, K. J., Fitzgerald, E., Sclafani, M. & Grandison, P. (2006). The association of ward atmosphere with burnout and attitudes of treatment team members in a state psychiatric hospital. *American Journal of Psychiatric Rehabilitation, 9*: 111–29.

Cormack, D. (2010). *The Politics and Practice of Counting: Ethnicity in official statistics in Aotearoa/New Zealand.* Wellington: Te Rōpū Rangahau Hauora a Eru Pōmare.

Durie, M. H. (1994). *Whaiora: Māori health development.* Auckland: Oxford University Press.

Herman, J. L. (1997). *Trauma and Recovery.* New York: Basic Books.

Jackson, M. (1992). The treaty and the word: The colonisation of Māori philosophy. In G. Oddie & R. Perrett (eds), *Justice, Ethics and New Zealand Society* (pp. 1–10). Auckland: Oxford University Press.

Jones, C. P. (2000). Levels of racism: A theoretic framework and a gardener's tale. *American Journal of Public Health, 90*(8): 1212–15.

Kidd, J. (2010). Cultural boundary surfing in mental health nursing: A creative narration. *Contemporary Nurse, 34*(2): 277.

Kukutai, T. & Didham, R. (2009). In search of ethnic New Zealanders: National naming in the 2006 Census. *Social Policy Journal of New Zealand, (36)*: 46–62.

Maddalena, V. P. (2009). Cultural competence and holistic practice: Implications for nursing education, practice, and research. *Holistic Nursing Practice, 23*(3): 153.

Marie, D. & Fergusson, D. M. (2008). Ethnic identity and intimate partner violence in a New Zealand birth cohort. *Social Policy Journal of New Zealand, 33*(March): 126–45.

Mental Health Commission (2012). *Blueprint Ii: How things need to be.* Wellington: Author.

Ministry of Health (2002). *He Korowai Oranga: Māori health strategy.* Wellington: Author.

Ministry of Health (2008). *Te Puawaiwhero: The second Māori mental health and addiction national strategic framework 2008–2015.* Wellington: Author.

Ministry of Health (2012). *Suicide Facts: Deaths and intentional self harm hospitalisations 2010.* Wellington: Author.

Nursing Council of New Zealand (2007). *Competencies for the Registered Nurse Scope of Practice.* Wellington: Author.

Nursing Council of New Zealand (2011). *Guidelines for Cultural Safety, the Treaty of Waitangi and Māori Health in Nursing Education and Practice.* Wellington: Author.

Oakley Browne, M. A., Well, J. E. & Scott, K. M. (2006). *Te Rau Hinengaro: The New Zealand Mental Health Survey.* Wellington: Ministry of Health.

Stewart-Harawira, M. (2005). *The New Imperial Order: Indigenous response to colonisation.* Wellington: Huia Publishers.

Whānau Ora Taskforce (2009). *Whānau Ora: A whānau-centred approach to Māori wellbeing. A discussion paper.* Retrieved from www.msd.govt.nz/about-msd-and-our-work/publications-resources/planning-strategy/whanau-ora/index.html.

5

Assessment of mental health and mental illness

Terry Froggatt and Susan Liersch-Sumskis

Introduction 90

The meaning of mental health and mental health conditions within assessment 90

Therapeutic communication within the assessment process 92

The assessment process 95

Mental status examination 98

Strengths-based assessment 104

The Tidal Model 106

Aboriginal mental health assessment 107

Assessment in the context of forensic psychiatry 107

Diagnosis of mental illness 110

Chapter summary 113

Critical thinking/learning activities 113

Learning extension 114

Further reading 114

References 114

Learning objectives

At the completion of this chapter, you should be able to:

- Identify and consider common assessment and diagnostic processes in mental health.
- Identify and consider issues that relate to effective professional–consumer interpersonal communication.
- Identify and consider the assessment process in terms of its history and culture, various conceptual models, issues of validity and reliability, and the expertise necessary to conduct an assessment.
- Develop an awareness of and understand the application of four current assessment and diagnostic systems.
- Discuss issues and experiences related to assessment and diagnosis of mental health conditions from the perspectives of the consumer, the carer and the clinician.

Introduction

mental health
a state of well-being in which each individual realises his or her own potential, is able to cope with the normal stresses of life, to work productively and to make a contribution to her or his community

mental illness
a clinically diagnosable condition that significantly interferes with an individual's cognitive, emotional or social abilities

assessment
an holistic assessment of a person to identify areas of unmet need, symptoms of a mental illness and the supports to be utilised in collaborative care and treatment planning

diagnosis
the cause, nature and manifestation of a condition; diagnosis is reached on the basis of signs, symptoms and associated information from the consumer and others, including family members and carers

In this chapter we discuss contemporary, evidenced-based approaches to the assessment of **mental health** and **mental illness** from multiple perspectives, including a section on forensic mental health. We discuss a range of themes, principles and concepts within the **assessment** of mental health, and these are underpinned by personal experiences, contemporary, evidence-based research and a range of other literature. The personal accounts of consumers, their families and carers, and of nurses practising in a mental health context are used to contextualise assessment as it relates to mental health and mental conditions.

Assessment of a person who is experiencing a mental illness is the first step in the nursing process; further steps are **diagnosis**, planning, implementation and evaluation (Barry, 2002). Most health service providers utilise structured documentation to record assessment data; however, nursing assessment is not simply a matter of sitting down with the person and filling out forms in a question-and-answer format. It is a process of genuine therapeutic engagement between the person, as expert in her or his own situation, and the nurse, as a skilled facilitator of health care solutions. Through a process of engagement to hear the person's story, and with the aid of notes jointly created to facilitate shared understanding, the nurse is later able to complete the structured organisational documentation.

The meaning of mental health and mental health conditions within assessment

Within the literature, mental health and mental illness are distinctly different concepts, despite the fact that they are frequently used as de facto descriptors for each other (Keyes, 2005). Mental illness is referred to within this work. However, within diagnostic criteria, the term 'mental disorder' is used, and within the majority of Mental Health Acts within Australia the term 'mental illness' is used.

Mental health and mental illness are not considered to be two ends at polar opposites of the same continuum, but rather as two distinctly different trajectories (Manderscheid et al., 2010; Westerhof & Keyes, 2010; World Health Organization (WHO), 2005). In contrast to the term 'mental illness', the concept of mental health has rarely been researched. Interest in 'mental health' as a distinct concept emerged in the 2000s, with the main aim of improving the mental health of populations (Westerhof & Keyes, 2010). A state of mental health has been defined by the WHO (2005, p. 100) as:

> A state of wellbeing in which the individual realises his or her own abilities, can cope with the normal stresses of life, can work productively and fruitfully and is able to make a contribution to his or her community.

The key components of the WHO definition, as defined by Westerhof and Keyes (2010) are emotional well-being, psychological well-being and social well-being. A state of emotional well-being is a subjectively described feeling of happiness and satisfaction with life. Psychological well-being, as defined by Ryff and Keyes (1995) has six elements: self-acceptance, purpose in life, autonomy, positive relations with others, environmental mastery and personal growth. Social well-being is defined by Keyes as having five dimensions that, when met, indicate that an individual is functioning optimally in society (Westerhoff & Keyes, 2010). The five dimension are: social coherence, social acceptance, social actualisation, social contribution and social integration.

In contrast, the definition of a mental illness, within a clinical context (Stein et al., 2010), is a pattern of symptoms that manifest in an individual's mood, thought or cognition and are recognised behaviourally or psychologically (American Psychiatric Association (APA), 2012; Stein et al., 2010). The symptoms cause significant distress, disability or impairment in an important area of the individual's functioning (Stein et al. 2010). Mental illness is closely associated with an underlying psychobiological or neurological dysfunction and is not an expected response to common stressors or losses that form part of everyday life for most people (Stein et al. 2010).

Mental illness is not the absence of mental health, any more than mental health is the absence of mental illness (WHO, 2005). As previously stated, mental health and mental illness are considered to be two distinct continua, rather than a single continuum (Manderscheid et al., 2010; Westerhof & Keyes, 2010). Therefore, assessment must take into account, not only the correlates of mental illness, as recognised by diagnostic processes, but also the correlates of mental health, as recognised through person-centred, strengths-based assessment practices.

In coming to understand a mental illness, nursing assessment is based on understanding the whole person and how she or he is inextricably linked with the environment in a pattern of relationship. It is through examining the pattern of this relationship, as it occurs for an individual, that a nurse might understand the processes of health and illness in the context of the whole person (Newman, 2008). This is a relational worldview whereby we consider the person to be within an intricate web of social connections, with the person placed at the centre of his or her own individual web. Understanding and working with the social or environmental effects of mental illness within a person's lived experience is crucial in her or his journey of recovery. Once we have a comprehensive view of the person's relational world, we can assume many different perspectives of it; for example, how do the person's physiological, psychological and spiritual determinants of health play out across this view of his or her life?

Therapeutic communication within the assessment process

First and foremost, the key to an effective mental health assessment is the nurse's ability to develop a therapeutic relationship with the person and others within her or his supportive network, as early in the process as possible. This is important for developing rapport and trust.

Consumer narrative   John on therapeutic rapport

My first experience of giving my history was with a general medical practitioner (GP) and a medical student. Mum was waiting out in the car. The doctor didn't ask her to come in, I didn't think to ask her to come in and she didn't ask if she could come in, either. It probably would have been different if I had thought to ask her to come in. I felt very alone and it was a difficult experience. It wasn't until my first psychiatrist's appointment, with a registered nurse in the room, that I felt there was a bit of warmth in the assessment experience. I felt she was there for me. She was very good and she had a warm and a friendly face, and I felt that she was someone who was going to just be there [for me]. Whereas the psychiatrist, as wonderful as he was, had a medical perspective and medical requirements to be met, and he approached me from that frame. But one thing I needed in that situation was to develop a rapid therapeutic relationship. I needed it to help me feel at ease, to feel much more human, rather than just being an illness sitting in a chair, and also I needed it to feel safer talking about the stuff that was happening in my life. I always remember that nurse and the therapeutic relationship she developed with me at that difficult time.

As indicated by John's experience, developing trust early in the therapeutic relationship is necessary to guide the person towards feeling that safe and knowing that his or her privacy and confidentiality will be respected. The person has a right to expect to be treated with dignity, respect and cultural sensitivity, regardless of the circumstances of the current situation. The offer of a hot or cold drink, a pleasant environment and a non-judgemental and empathetic nurse, who is genuinely listening, will help to create trust and to ease the person's into opening up about her or his current situation. A complete assessment may need to be carried out over a series of interviews, and also with people the person nominates as important within his or her supportive network.

Once comfortable, the interview should commence with open questions concerning the person's present situation and experiences, followed by more specific questions to clarify ambiguities and confirm or refute initial impressions. Open, curious questions are important, such as: What brings you here today? What has been happening in your life? What are your main concerns? How may we help you? Talking with a competent, knowledgeable listener about the difficulties the person is experiencing provides the person with an opportunity to know himself or herself as never before (Peplau, 1994). Studies repeatedly provide evidence that being understood and listened to in a thoughtful and sensitive manner confirms an individual's sense of humanity and provides hope for the future (Jackson & O'Brien, 2009). Furthermore, the process of assessment is in itself a therapeutic intervention through which a person can begin to recognise patterns and relationships, which in turn can lead to changed attitudes and behaviour and progress towards new levels of health (Newman, 2008).

It is important to let the person 'tell her or his story', and therefore the onus is on the listener, the nurse, to take what the person is saying seriously. Listening is an essential part of being a nurse; listening to understand as opposed to listening to respond.

Listening to understand as opposed to listening to respond

When we listen to respond while the person is still actually speaking we may already be reacting to what has been said or we may be already thinking about our next question, and therefore we cannot truly 'hear' what the person is saying. When we listen to understand, we are present and available and are only listening to what the person is saying, not thinking about other things. Listening to understand requires a degree of self-awareness and self-discipline. Withholding our reactions to what is being said, hearing what is being said and then exploring the person's perspective with curious questioning, rather than launching into our own formulation, leads us to develop a more balanced and inclusive appraisal of the person's situation.

Here is an example that gives you the opportunity to reflect upon this listening strategy.

Malik says to the nurse:'I don't want to take my medication; I want to go home because I hate it here.'

Amune, the nurse, replies to Malik:'You know you should take your medication. You need to be here and it's not such a bad place.'

Malik walks away thinking:'You just don't understand.'

Lisa, another nurse, asks Malik to tell her about his concerns. By listening carefully to Malik, Lisa discovers that he is experiencing some well-known side-effects of his medication, that his mum and dad were due to visit him an hour ago and, furthermore, this is the first time he has been away from home. Lisa now knows that Malik is feeling very lonely, sad and anxious.

If a person becomes upset or distressed while you are listening to him or her, allow time for the person to calm down. Reflect upon any role you may have had in creating the distress. Try not to be distracted by other 'noise' in the environment. The person needs to feel that she or he has your full attention. Never divert your attention by checking your phone or other electronic device, particularly while the person is speaking to you. Do not be distracted by taking notes or reading past notes or other documents during the interview, and do not hide behind a checklist. If you must write, ask for the person's permission and let him or her know that you are taking notes to aide your memory and to accurately represent what she or he is telling you.

It is important not to feel under pressure to conduct a mental health assessment in a rush. You need to allow time to discover as much as the person is prepared to reveal, without having to hurry him or her along. Try not to use closed questions too early in the interview as this can give the impression of being task-focused.

Learn to be comfortable discussing sensitive topics, such as suicide, self-harm and harm to others, or potentially embarrassing topics, such as sexual history. This is a skill you can practise with your colleagues in the safe environment of peer or clinical supervision.

Reflective questions

Imagine that you are working with a consumer who is distressed at the time of your engagement with her. She is telling you that it is okay to undertake an assessment. The local working environment is under intense pressure and there are several competing demands being placed on your time. Asking personal questions about her situation is making you feel uncomfortable. Consider the following questions:

- What do you think you might be feeling or experiencing at this time?
- What do you think the consumer might be feeling or experiencing at this time?
- What steps can you take to respond to this situation? What options do you have? What might be the longer-term implications of the actions you take at this time?

It is important for the nurse to set professional boundaries, to respect privacy and confidentiality and to be non-judgemental. Do not take sides or collude with others with or against the person, and be particularly mindful of when your own beliefs, feelings, values and judgements are taking the lead in your assessment approach.

While conducting the assessment, holding out a sense of hope for the person and for her or his future is correlated with positive health outcomes, symptom reduction and development of a 'future orientation' (Harding, Zubin & Strauss, 1987; Kylmä et al., 2006; McGrath, 2006; Miller & Mason, 2011). Communicating sense of hope can support a person to take risks, and to get back up again and have another go when an attempt fails (Kelly & Gamble, 2005; Kylmä et al., 2006). 'Hope connects someone directly to the dreamed-of future' (Peterson & Seligman, 2004, p. 519). People who support others through believing in them and offering hope are supporting recovery (Ralph & Corrigan, 2005), and therefore this is an essential attitude for a clinician to hold (Moxham, Robson & Pegg, 2012).

The nursing assessment within a mental health context is based upon coming to know and understand the whole person, the current problem she or he is experiencing and, very importantly, the skills, competencies and strengths the person possesses that may significantly enhance the healing process and bring about a positive outcome (McCormack, 2007). Seeing the person you are assessing as an individual, within his or her own web of support, with hope and the strength and capacity to heal, and not to define the person as a set of symptoms, a disease or an illness is a principle that must underpin the model of assessment being used in practice (Kelly & Gamble, 2005).

The assessment process

As stated above, nursing assessment is based on understanding the whole person and how he or she is inextricably linked with the environment in a pattern of relationship. It is through examining the pattern of this relationship, as it occurs for an individual, that a nurse can understand the processes of health and illness in the context of the whole (Newman, 2008). The person's individual relational world can be viewed as an intricate web of connections, with the person at the centre.

Christine, a consumer of mental health services, has provided a description of her personal history (see page 96). While reading about Christine, you are encouraged to consider her as a person who is inextricably woven within her history, her experiences, her family and her responsibilities. An activity you could undertake as you read Christine's story is to plot her relational world as a freehand mapping exercise on a sheet of paper. What are Christine's family circumstances? What are the relationships like within that structure? Which relationships are supportive and which are challenging? What resources are already within her world? Which are challenges that could become future goals? Use different colours to denote strengths and challenges. What supports are available to help meet those challenges? Which areas are critical to improving health? Where are the longer-term challenges for Christine to be able to reach full recovery with dignity? The purpose of these exercises is to help you to think more broadly and deeply about the person in the context of her or his lived experience. In practice, working with the consumer's personal strengths and qualities would be a collaborative endeavour, with the consumer in the role of expert on his or her own experience and available support and resources. It is not our role to guess these or to determine them on behalf of the person and in her or his absence.

Guided by laws, evidence and policy, the process of assessment allows the nurse to clearly understand and document the reason the person is seeking help, the life context in which the problem exists, the person's history of mental health, any treatment she or he may receive for mental disorder and the desired outcomes. Through this, the nurse is able to identify any unmet needs, the supports that are in place to meet those needs and also strategies and supports that need to be developed. From this assessment, the person and nurse can work together to develop goals and commence a plan.

Consumer narrative   Christine's story part one

My family of origin: Is that I was number two in a family of five and I was the only girl. Mum had five of us in six years. My father was a very intelligent man and held a very high position but he was also an alcoholic, and as a father he was not very good. Something that I have only found out in recent years through my mum mentioning it is that my father went to a Christian school and he was assaulted there. Mum was a registered nurse and she often did night shift. In my family, which was very dysfunctional, there was intergenerational sexual, physical and emotional abuse. One brother committed suicide when he was 28 years old, another brother had a lung transplant and he's now died, and a third brother was diagnosed with bipolar disorder and he has a severely anorexic, 20-year-old daughter. Two of those brothers are also heroin addicts. I had a grandmother with an undisclosed mental illness and a cousin with bipolar, so there's obviously a genetic link there.

My childhood: My earliest memory was when I was four, of my father trying to kill my mother. I was trying to stop him. He was a very controlling man, and he used to make us polish boots. He used to wake me up at night time to iron his shirts if Mum wouldn't do it. I have no happy memories of him as a father figure. I struggled a lot and missed a lot of school. I couldn't concentrate. Sometimes they'd fight and Mum would actually leave for a few days and go to a motel, and she'd actually take me with her so I think she knew, deep down inside that he was abusing me, but it wasn't anything that she could have brought to the surface because of the situation she was in.

My adult years: I finished school and moved away from home, and then life became very different. I qualified as a general and paediatric nurse and then I did midwifery. Life was full with study and nursing.

My marriage: In 1981 I married a man after knowing him less than a year, and I used to think he was my soul mate. He was abnormally possessive and controlling. He ended up being physically abusive but normally didn't mark me. I have been married for nearly 32 years, and now I am in the process of separation and divorce. There were always problems in our marriage. My husband also suffered abuse as a child. He was on and off antidepressants. He used my illness as a form of control. Our sex life struggled, and I had an affair and I left him when our twins were really small, and that's when he confessed to me that he was a cross-dresser and that he needed me for his survival. It turned into a nightmare; cross-dressing was against my beliefs. Being a 'rescuer', I tried to save our marriage. We had lots of counselling, which my husband attended, but he didn't do anything the counsellor recommended. He would sometimes go out dressed as a woman and when, in 1986, he wanted to have sex dressed as a woman, I had my first breakdown and my first admission to hospital.

continued ›

My own family: I had my first child in 1983 and then I had twins in 1986; the boys all still live at home. My eldest son was born with cerebral oedema, and they said he'd be retarded but he's just completed his second university degree in law. One of the twins had a bad car accident as a passenger and his pregnant girlfriend died. He ended up with massive injuries – neck and spinal injuries. The other twin son got cancer and had the lower lobe of his left lung removed, and we've been told the cancer is likely to come back and also that his identical twin is likely to get it. The twin brother who had the car accident also got injured in a bike accident. I am also now a grandparent to my oldest son's child.

A person who is experiencing the symptoms of mental illness oftentimes will be under stress. This, in turn, can affect the person's sleep, appetite, physical fitness, relationships with important others, financial situation, faith, hope and dreams, and the person's relationship within her or his broader social setting. All too often, we regard activities of daily living to be the main problem, without fully appreciating that they are the result of larger problems embedded in life. The effects of stress are highly individual to each person; the extent of which is grasped during assessment. If the stress or condition has been long standing, the consequences may be compounded, particularly with regard to physical health and important supportive relationships. A comprehensive nursing assessment should support both the consumer and the nurse to gain a sense of the way in which current challenges are woven within the person's web of lived experience, and this emerging clarity may also contain the seeds of potential solutions. Acknowledging the personal experience and expertise of the individual, supporting his or her potential for recovery and assisting the person to achieve optimal quality of life are within the national Standards of Practice for Australian Mental Health Nurses (Australian College of Mental Health Nurses (ACMHN), 2010).

In adopting a person-centred approach to assessment, the nurse places the person in the central and most important position within her or his own individual health web. Health services play a part in providing the support needed to enable full recovery and sustain and improve health and well-being. Furthermore, the nurse works collaboratively to ensure the person has access to a multidisciplinary network to support current needs, which may include a community mental health nurse, general practitioner, psychiatrist, psychologist, social worker, occupational therapist, dietician, rehabilitation service and other allied health professionals as required. This supportive web of holistic care can facilitate the person's management of her or his own mental health within the context of daily life. However, it is important to note that family, carers and connection to the social world are the most important part of the web of support, and therefore the person's responsibilities within these relationships are an important part of assessment. Working in partnership with the individual affected by mental illness and significant others such as family, carers, support agencies and other health care providers are within the Standards of Practice for Australian Mental Health Nurses (ACMHN, 2010).

Mental status examination

Assessment processes include enquiring into specific aspects of a person's mental health condition, such as is evaluated through the mental state examination (MSE) and also various types of risk criteria such as potential to harm self, others or reputation. The MSE assesses the features and characteristics of each person's individual experience of a mental illness. No two people will have the same experience, and therefore the MSE provides a structured method for observing and describing an individual's current state of mind (APA, 2013). In particular, the MSE provides a framework for examining changes within the domains of appearance, attitude, behaviour, mood, affect, speech, thought process, thought content, perception, cognition, insight and judgement. Observations within these domains are combined with the person's subjective reports and biographical and historical information, to allow for an accurate opinion to be developed and a diagnosis to be formulated. This then contributes to planning for care and treatment within the person's journey of recovery.

The MSE is conducted and documented initially through a series of interviews by a person qualified and empowered to make psychiatric diagnoses, such as a psychiatrist. However, the MSE also forms an integral part of a nurse's daily encounter with a person receiving care. It needs to be much more than a 'tick and flick' exercise. It has the potential, in the hands of a skilled and competent nurse, to paint a composite picture of a person's mental state at the time of the assessment. Observations are made, questions are asked and subjective accounts are routinely collected and documented, to enable all members of the team delivering services to maintain awareness of the person's current state of mind and to respond to changes.

One common approach to conducting a MSE is described with the acronym BATOMI PJR. This is a minor adaption of the MSE, which we have used in clinical and educational settings:

Behaviour and appearance
Affect
Thought form and thought content
Orientation
Mood
Insight
Perception
Judgement
Risk.

Behaviour and appearance

The observation of behaviour is the non-verbal communication of the person being assessed: the person's attitude, behaviour, dress and grooming. By observing the person's behaviour it is possible to identify some specific characteristics of her or his underlying mental state. It is important to simply observe and document behaviour, and not to make judgements or interpretations, or to apply labels. Within the domain of behaviour and appearance, the following observations are made:

- Physical characteristics (height, weight, hair style and colour, body markings)
- Dress (neat, tidy and appropriate for climate; dishevelled or unkempt)
- Posture and body language (relaxed, rigid, tense, erect, closed)
- Facial expression (eye contact, fixed, passive, intense)
- Motor activity (slowed, immobile, restless, clumsy, tremors, wringing hands, pacing)
- Speech (tone, cadence, slow, rapid, loud, quiet, monosyllabic, pressure of speech, logical, coherent and relevant)
- Attitude to interview (engaged, reluctant, avoidant, hostile, suspicious).

Example of behaviour observation

Vid presents as a tall, slim man, appearing as his stated age of 58 years. He has a tattoo of a fish visible on his lower left forearm. He is wearing work clothes: black boots, blue work pants, a checked work shirt. The shirt and pants are heavily stained with a black substance. Vid is sitting very upright, in a rigid, immobile pose, with his arms crossed against his chest. He mostly gazes downwards towards his feet, making eye contact only sporadically with the assessing doctor and not at all with other staff in attendance. He answers questions with very few words, in a firm but quiet voice. His replies are coherent and logical.

In general, we all are tempted to make assumptions about people. This is not helpful. The nurse needs to withhold her or his assumptions until a full or composite overview of the person emerges.

Affect

The assessment of a person's affect refers to an objective assessment of the emotional expression that flows from the person. What is the type and intensity of the emotion behind his or her expression? Is it depression, elation, euphoria, anger, sadness, anxiety, fear, suspicion, resentment, apathy or lability? Additionally, the person may exhibit a range of emotions during the interview and this will result in a variation in certain facial expressions, tones of voice, uses of hands and body movements (gesticulating). When a person's affect is constricted, the range and intensity of expressed emotions are reduced. The range may be described as 'flat affect' (showing no change in facial expression), 'blunted affect' (facial expression is slow in responding), 'restricted affect' (only showing one type of emotion), 'incongruent affect' (facial expression does not match mood) or 'broad affect' (full range of emotional expressions).

Vid's face appeared anxious and slightly angry, and his range of facial expression was restricted to these emotions. Vid's affect was consistent with his stated mood of being anxious and tired.

Thought form and thought content

Thought form

Thought generally refers to any mental or intellectual activity involving an individual's subjective consciousness. It can refer either to the act of thinking or the resulting ideas or arrangements of ideas that are expressed.

Thought form or processes are the verbal record of *how* (as opposed to *what*) a person is thinking. Thoughts are usually logical and goal-directed. Some problems with thought form may be observed as an abundance of thoughts or a poverty of ideas. Thoughts may be vague or without substance. A person's thinking might be circumstantial (talks slowly and in detail about trivial or irrelevant topics), tangential (wanders and drifts, and may never return to the original topic, for example) or may be blocked (unable to move forward in thinking, may often move to another topic entirely, for example). Neologisms (made-up words or phrases), clang association (association by rhyming), flight of ideas (extremely rapid thinking), loose associations and incoherent thoughts may indicate that a person's thought form and processes are disturbed. These types of experience affect the ability to communicate in order to have needs recognised and met.

Vid's thoughts are expressed in a logical manner; however, he is speaking very minimally, which may indicate a poverty of ideas.

Thought content

Thought content is concerned with *what* a person may be thinking. Disturbances in thought content include delusions, preoccupations, obsessions, compulsions, phobias, plans, intentions and specific impulsive actions. In particular, thoughts of harm to self and harm to others must be assessed. It is also important to explore the person's level of hope for the future and her or his optimism as to whether things will improve. These aspects combine to allow the person's safety to be considered.

Thought content disturbances

Delusions are false, fixed beliefs that are not open to logical challenge. Therefore, do not try to change the person's beliefs with logic. Consider instead the implications for the person holding the beliefs and how the particular beliefs affect his or her daily life, and the associated potential challenges and risks.

Obsessions are recurrent thoughts that cause anxiety, and compulsions are the actions that are taken to relieve the anxiety. Since the thoughts are recurrent, so, too, are the actions intended to relieve them.

Thoughts of harm to self and others must be thoroughly explored in a very direct manner (Have you thought about suicide?). Discussing harm to self or others will not create a new suggestion or cause it to happen. Ask the person she or he is thinking. How would the person harm himself or herself (method)? Does the person have access to the method (means), and does the person have a plan for when she or he will carry it out (intent)?

The person's level of hope and optimism towards the future must also be assessed, as hopelessness is correlated with suicide risk (Davidson et al., 2009).

> Vid states that he knows his employers have been spying on him. They have bugged his home, his car and his mobile phone. His workplace's wi-fi system has been interrogating his phone for the industrial secrets his employers know he has. Vid is not going into work anymore and he only has this secret intelligence on his home computer. That is the only way he can protect them from his employers. He says his bathroom and kitchen are also bugged with listening devices. On being questioned, Vid states that he has never done anything to harm himself and he has no thoughts of doing so. He says that he has never hurt or assaulted anyone, and he has no criminal convictions.

Orientation

Orientation is usually assessed as a person's awareness; in particular, the person's awareness of who she or he is, where she or he is and the current time, day, month and year. Assessment of alterations to orientation and level of consciousness are important in considering whether a person may have sustained a physical trauma, such as a head injury, or has a physical illness.

> Vid is aware of the current day, month and year, although he is not sure of the date as he has not been paying attention. He is conscious and alert.

Mood

Mood is a person's emotional state, as conveyed by the person rather than what is observed (affect). Common adjectives used to describe mood include: depressed, despairing, irritable, anxious, angry, euphoric, empty, guilty, hopeless, frightened and perplexed. A person's mood may be labile, fluctuating or alternating between extremes.

> Vid states that he is tired from maintaining vigilance against those that are trying to get his secrets. He is anxious and also angry about their constant efforts against him.

Insight

A person having a level of awareness and understanding of his or her symptoms or condition, and the relevance of those symptoms to the person's current experience is often referred to as the person's degree of insight. For example, a person's level of insight may be described as: 'no insight', 'poor insight', 'limited insight' or 'good insight'. There are six criteria to consider when assessing a person's level of insight:

1 complete denial that anything is wrong;
2 slight awareness of being unwell and needing assistance; however, some level of denial is still apparent;
3 aware of being unwell; however, the problem is projected onto others, external factors or on physical factors;
4 awareness of being unwell, not able to identify a cause;
5 intellectual insight – acknowledgement of the condition and that symptoms or problems with social adjustment are due to the person's particular irrational feelings without applying this knowledge to future experiences; and
6 what is deemed as true emotional insight – the person is emotionally aware of his or her motives and feelings and those of significant others; this level of insight may lead to changes in the person's journey of recovery.

> Vid is convinced that he is being followed and that his house and possessions have been bugged. He has no awareness that these experiences might indicate a mental illness.
> How would you describe Vid's level of insight?

Perception

Perception (from the Latin *perceptio, percipio*) is the interpretation, identification and organisation of sensory information in order to represent and understand the environment. Disorders of perception may be experienced as false stimuli in any of the five senses: auditory, visual, gustatory, olfactory and somatic or tactile:

• auditory – hearing voices or sounds that do not exist in the environment but appear to be projections of inner thoughts and feelings;
• visual – seeing a person or object that does not exist in the environment;
• gustatory – tasting sensations that have no stimulus in reality;
• olfactory – smelling odours that are not present in the environment; and
• tactile or somatic – feeling strange sensations where no external objects stimulate such feelings.

> Vid states that he hears noises in his ceiling, and he thinks that the noises are the people hired by his employers to check the bugging devices in his house. They come mostly at night when they think he will be sleeping.

Judgement

Judgement is about decision-making, and refers to a person's capacity to make sound, reasoned and responsible decisions. Traditionally, the MSE included the use of standard hypothetical questions such as 'What would you do if you found a stamped, addressed envelope lying in the street?' However, contemporary practice is to enquire about how the person has responded or would respond to real-life challenges and contingencies. Assessment takes into account the individual's likely behaviour in terms of impulsivity, social cognition, self-awareness and planning ability.

> Vid has stopped attending work. He is not using his kitchen because it is bugged and he does not go into his bathroom very often.

Impaired judgement is not specific to any diagnosis but may be a prominent feature of illness affecting the frontal lobe of the brain. If a person's judgement is impaired due to a mental condition there might be implications for the person's safety or the safety of others.

Risk

Assessment of risk in the context of mental health is multifaceted and can include a person's capacity to harm himself or herself or others or to harm his or her own reputation or standing in the community. The person's level of insight into her or his current situation and the decisions the person is likely to make as a consequence must be considered in conjunction with the particular risk factors that are being assessed. Risk assessment and risk management form the platform for safe and effective care provided through competent nursing and the service's strategic approach (Royal College of Psychiatrists, 2008).

Risk assessment should be based upon the person's current mental state. The purpose of assessing risk is to determine the specific level of care to be provided, and to provide clear directions regarding therapeutic approach and the timing of the next review. The involvement of family, carers and other stakeholders in the overall risk assessment is necessary. In determining the level of risk and the associated therapeutic approach, it is important to uphold the person's rights, maintain respect for her or his autonomy and to allow the person the dignity of risk. This involves reasoned judgement, rather than an arbitrary application of a score-based assessment (Royal College of Psychiatrists, 2008). Some risk must be incorporated into the therapeutic process, and this is informed by the needs identified during assessment. Taking calculated risks is fundamental to recovery and to the development of resilience (Liersch-Sumskis, 2013); the Strengths-based Model of assessment is used within the risk assessment process to support recovery (Royal College of Psychiatrists, 2008). Although every care and precaution must be taken when the person's assessment indicates thoughts of suicide or harm to others, it is not acceptable to cast blanket restrictions that do not allow any dignity of risk within this type of care.

Studies have shown that predicting risk is an extremely difficult undertaking at an individual level (Royal College of Psychiatrists, 2008). Structured risk assessment tools are generally used to underpin risk management, and these activities are a required competence for nurses (ACMHN, 2010). However, risk assessment tools should not be used by people who have not been trained in their use. Studies have demonstrated that the person conducting the assessment is more important than the tool being used (Royal College of Psychiatrists, 2008). Nurses who are skilled at conducting holistic, culturally appropriate and non-judgemental risk assessments are ideally placed to balance the needs of the service and the needs of the person to experience some level of risk within her or his journey of recovery.

Strengths-based assessment

Assessment of an individual's mental health (as distinct from the correlates of a mental illness) must also be incorporated into the nursing assessment process to begin to identify the way forward. Various strengths-based models, such as the Tidal Model (Barker, 2002) and the Strengths Model (Rapp & Goscha, 2012) may be used to facilitate this within assessment. The underlying principle is that the nurse conducting the assessment needs to appraise the model being used and ensure that it contains components of a mental health assessment and does not characterise the person only in terms of illness, disability, deficit and dysfunction (Beecher, 2009; Rose et al., 2007). These latter characterisations do not support a hopeful view of the future based on the person's strengths, nor do they contain the seeds for recovery (Chadwick, 2009; Kylmä, et al., 2006; Repper & Perkins, 2003). Utilising an evidence base for practice (where evidence exists) and quality improvement processes, in order to provide the highest attainable standard of care is one of the Standards of Practice for Australian Mental Health Nurses (ACMHN, 2010).

A strengths-based assessment seeks to understand the person's life history: Where does the person come from? What important influences have shaped her or his personality, identity, race, culture, ethnicity, gender, spirituality and sexual orientation? What is her or his personal narrative? How does the person make sense of where he or she is in life? What are the person's values: what matters to her or him in life? What are the person's treatment preferences; what kind of help does the person want from mental health services and other sources? Enabling cultural safety, taking into account age, gender, spirituality, ethnicity and health values of people affected by mental health issues are among the Standards of Practice for Australian Mental Health Nurses (ACMHN, 2010).

Understanding is gained through engaging in a series of continuing and evolving conversations (McCormack, 2007). Within all notes and documentation, the storyteller's own words and metaphors are used (McCormack, 2007). This helps to prevent loss of the person's meaning through reinterpretation with technical, jargonistic or illness-laden language. All too often, during assessment a person is 'measured' in some way, with the result enclosed in clinical language and inaccessible to the understanding of the person, and not being used as a facilitation point for transformation of her or his own understanding and empowerment for self-directed improvement. The benefit of the strengths-based approach is that the solutions can be built into the assessment process in a language recognisable to the person. Furthermore, the person is treated as the expert on her or his own experiences, and the nurse is a collaborator who contributes his or her own knowledge and the skills, support and resources of health services.

Reflective questions

A colleague tells you that assessment of insight is a 'dubious concept' because such questions are 'really about finding out how much a consumer knows about and agrees with the psychiatric diagnosis she or he has been given'. This statement leaves you thinking more deeply about assessment in mental health and what the basis might be for this point of view. Working in small groups, answer the following questions:

- List the aims and objectives of undertaking a MSE.
- Why is therapeutic engagement a critical component of the MSE process?
- To what extent can a MSE be a useful guide to inform collaborative care?
- How might you respond to the statement that 'assessment of insight is a dubious concept'?

Consumer narrative Christine's story part two: Strengths-based assessment

I was allocated a male case manager who came and assessed the whole family individually. He engaged in communication and problem-solving training with us. He also did strengths assessment. It was the first time I had ever been asked what I was good at and what I wanted to do. That's just something that I have never been asked. I started to get a little bit of hope for my future. I thought that I'd never get back into the workforce; my husband said there was no way I could work and the doctors told him 10 years ago that I would never again work as a registered nurse but I received the help from the mental health team to actually do that. The strengths approach gave me confidence. When other people have hope and confidence in you it changes your perspective on life. I got to reflect on the abilities that I already had. In that 10-year period of being ill, and over all of the admissions to the mental health unit, I forgot the strengths that I already had. Through the strengths assessment I learned to believe in myself and I got the support to meet the goals that I decided upon. My goals initially were little things, like starting up a vegetable garden and going to the gym, but I also came to develop greater

continued ›

Consumer narrative continued ›

goals, like getting back to work to find an identity for myself. I know I have a severe illness and I become really unwell, but through the strengths treatment I've remained well, so that approach has worked phenomenally well for me. Medication and illness are now a small part of my life. Now, I work four days a week as a carer for clients with severe brain injuries, and I've applied to the Australian Health Practitioner Regulation Agency to become a registered nurse again. It's been a two-year process, and I've had to do a reconnect course, but I'm actually getting back into nursing and that's going to give me financial support. I have a long-term plan. I have value, I enjoy life, I'm responsible for my illness and I don't focus on my symptoms. I owe my life to the strengths model and to the nurses who didn't focus on my symptoms and who believed in me. Before that, I was just existing and not really living.

The Tidal Model

The Tidal Model was developed in England from a series of studies that explored the nature of the power relationship between nurses and people who have an enduring mental illness (Stevenson, Leamy & Barker, 2000). Mental illnesses are considered to be problems of living that exist within a human system, rather than being mysterious conditions a person has developed as an individual. The Tidal Model assumes a person's sense of self and world of experiences, including her or his experience of others, are inextricably tied to that person's life story and the various meanings generated within it. Hypothetical problems within this limit a person's ability to function effectively.

The Tidal Model does not seek to unravel the cause or course of the person's problems, but rather to chart the next steps in the life journey. Within this model, the assessment record is written entirely in the person's own voice, rather than being translated into a third-person account, using clinical language. Nurses work with the person to co-create a narrative account of the person's world of experience, including what the person needs and what needs to happen to meet that need (Barker, 2009).

The person's story, such as is imparted through the assessment process, is given primacy because this is the theatre of experience in which reflection and discussion result in a contemporaneous editing of the script. The caring process begins and ends here because all people express a need to develop (that is, create) a coherent account of what has happened and currently is happening to him or her. This account is most meaningful when framed in the person's own language, as drawn from her or his own history and sociocultural context. The story from the first holistic assessment becomes the opening chapter of the story of the current episode of care, and that story becomes a continuously developing narrative that flows through the episode of care (Barker, 2009).

Aboriginal mental health assessment

The person-centred, relational view of assessment that has been adopted within this chapter may be well suited to the needs of Aboriginal people who do not view illness as a split between mind and body, but rather take an holistic view of it being an experience rather than a symptom of an illness (Westerman, 2004).

In order to make a connection, it is important to be able to become familiar with the person's relatives, both past and present. Aboriginal people have a strong spiritual connection to their ancestors, based on the belief that in the beginning our ancestors were all connected to each other (Reid & Trompf, 1991). Self-disclosure about your own family and relations, providing you feel comfortable, is an effective way to engage in a conversation with Aboriginal clients. This process is seen as essential for an Aboriginal person to 'place' the clinician in a family/community context (Seru, 1994). It is important to be able to comfortably discuss relationships with land, country and genealogy (Westerman, 2004). To relate to a person at a deeper cultural level it is necessary for the clinician to understand differences in language, geographic boundaries and family groups of the communities in which they work (Westerman, 2010).

It is also important to recognise that Aboriginal people may view mental illness as being related to external forces and that, furthermore, having a mental illness may be associated with beliefs of having done something 'wrong' (Reid & Trompf, 1991). Using a liaison worker whenever available is essential in delivering culturally appropriate care, especially when commencing the therapeutic relationship and initiating an episode of care with Aboriginal people.

When working with Aboriginal people, there are examples of misdiagnosis due to the person being assessed outside her or his community or cultural context (Westerman, 2004). Hunter (2007), for example, noted that Aboriginal people assessed in places such as hospitals, prisons and detention centres are more distressed than they would be if the assessment were carried out in a culturally appropriate setting. Using several sources of information is likely to result in a more accurate diagnosis of mental health conditions in Aboriginal people. Collateral information, particularly when the nurse is from a different cultural background, is essential (Westerman, 2010).

The Westerman Aboriginal Symptom Checklist for young people aged 13 to 17 years (WASC-Y, Westerman, 2003) is the first culturally and scientifically validated psychological test developed specifically for use with Australian Aboriginal young people and is the first such measure for indigenous young people worldwide (Shields et al., 2002).

Assessment in the context of forensic psychiatry

Forensic psychiatry is the intersection between the law and mental health. Assessments in this context may emphasise specific aspects of a person's mental health state.

Evidence-based nursing practices for individuals experiencing a mental illness who have offended remain scarce; forensic mental health services are without effective assessment tools and interventions on which to base their treatment and rehabilitation programs (Abou-Sinna & Luebbers, 2012). The Camberwell Assessment of Need (CAN) (Phelan et al., 1995) and the Health of the Nation Outcome Scales (HoNOS) are two assessment tools that are well established and have been researched in the forensic setting (Abou-Sinna & Luebbers, 2012). HoNOS–secure (HoNOS–S) is the forensic version of HoNOS, which includes an additional seven-item security scale that assesses ongoing security needs.

While the HoNOS–S assesses similar underlying domains of need to the CANFOR–S (see below), it does not incorporate a broad range of criminogenic aspects that are related to general re-offending for these individuals. A forensic version of CAN, CAN–Forensic (CANFOR) (Thomas et al., 2003), has been developed to allow for an in-depth and integrated needs analysis of individuals with a mental condition who have offended.

A recent study into the use of these two instruments concluded that CANFOR–S is a forensic mental health needs assessment that assesses the criminogenic, mental health, and non-criminogenic needs relevant for the treatment needs of individuals experiencing mental illness who have offended.

It has been suggested that services would benefit from using assessments such as CANFOR–S, to measure outcomes among people who have a mental health condition who have offended (Abou-Sinna & Luebbers, 2012). In particular, nurses should consider the potential this kind of tool gives them to incorporate the person's perspective into her or his own treatment planning. This could be the bedrock of developing an effective therapeutic alliance between the person and the nurse.

Complete a CANFOR–S assessment for the case study of James

I first came in contact with James when he was 43 years old. He has had a diagnosis of paranoid schizophrenia since the age of 23. James is unmarried, lives alone and is currently unemployed. His parents are deceased and he has no living relatives. James first offended when he was accused of harassing a neighbour, whom he believed was plotting against him. At that time James was referred to me at the local mental health service for treatment under the Mental Health Act. James has had a number of court appearances since that time.

On this occasion, James believes a local café owner is poisoning his coffee, and physically assaults the café owner, believing that he was trying to kill him. The police are called during this assault, and James is arrested and taken into custody.

Following a mental health assessment while in custody, James is then referred by the magistrate's court to a forensic service for further assessment. James appears to be facing a number of psychological, social and clinical challenges. He appears to be distressed,

continued >

Complete a CANFOR–S assessment for the case study of James continued ›

and there are concerns related to his risk to others as he continued to believe he is being poisoned. James refuses to eat or drink. He isolates himself and refuses to associate with anyone. His accommodation is under threat as he has not been paying his rent. Physically James appears underweight, possibly dehydrated and has a dishevelled appearance.

James states that if people do not stop trying to poison him, he would 'do the job for them'. Historically James has refused treatment and is generally non-compliant with medication or other forms of therapeutic intervention. Each time I sit down to talk with James, he tells me that he does not believe that he has a mental illness, and wishes people would cease in their attempts to control and poison him.

Reflective questions

Using the items listed below, conduct an assessment of James and suggest recommendations for his ongoing care.

CANFOR: The Forensic CAN (CANFOR) is an assessment tool that highlights what can be significant challenges for people who have a mental illness and have offended. It has been developed for a variety of forensic mental health settings. It is based on the Camberwell Assessment of Need.

The short, one-page version of the assessment tool is in the form of a semi-structured interview and covers a range of psychological, social and clinical needs:

- Accommodation
- Food
- Looking after the living environment
- Self-care
- Daytime activities
- Physical health
- Psychotic symptoms
- Information about condition and treatment
- Psychological distress
- Safety to self
- Safety to others
- Alcohol
- Drugs
- Company
- Intimate relationships
- Sexual expression
- Child care

continued ›

Reflective questions continued >

- Basic education
- Telephone
- Transport
- Money
- Benefits
- Treatment.

Diagnosis of mental illness

Mental illness is currently diagnosed under two separate classification systems: one created by the World Health Organization (WHO), the International Classification of Diseases (ICD) (WHO, 1993) and the other developed by the APA, the Diagnostic and Statistical Manual of Mental Disorders (DSM) (APA, 2013). Both classification systems are regularly reviewed and updated. The APA has recently released the fifth edition of the DSM, and the WHO will release ICD version 11 in 2015 (APA, 2013; Reed, 2010; Stein et al., 2010).

The structured classification of symptoms, as represented in the above, is considered necessary for a common understanding of diseases and illnesses that can be shared, not only within communities, cities and countries, but also globally (WHO, 2008). Classification is also considered useful in identifying illnesses, providing education, designing and delivering treatment and for research and epidemiological purposes (Australian Government, 2012; Reed, 2010). The WHO's ICD diagnostic classification system is the global standard for health reporting and clinical applications (Reed 2010; WHO, 1993). In addition, the psychiatric professions in many countries use the APA's DSM (Ebert, 2008; Reed, 2010; Stein et al., 2010).

In the absence of pathophysiological certainty, psychiatric diagnoses are socially constructed (Robertson & Walter, 2007; Wolff, 2007; Young, 2009). Therefore, the diagnostic classification of mental illness has inherent problems, such as being based on values rather than facts (Robertson & Walter 2007; Stein et al. 2010). An example provided by Robertson and Walter (2007) is the diagnosis of acute delirium, which is a physical condition confirmable through tests, using validated measures. In comparison, a mental illness is diagnosed by considering patterns of behaviour (observed or not) that deviate from socially constructed norms. These structured classification criteria, which are essentially statements set against socially constructed norms, are regarded by some authors as unreliable (Garb, 2005; Reed, 2010; Robertson & Walter, 2007; Stein et al., 2010).

In the absence of definitive scientific evidence, the diagnosis of mental illness is made following a series of interviews by a person qualified and empowered to make psychiatric diagnoses, such as a psychiatrist. During the interview process, an extensive set of questions is asked, based on the previously discussed MSE. Opinions are formed, based on the combination of observations, questions and subjective responses within the domains of the MSE (APA, 2013). The findings of the assessment, together with collateral information from family members and friends when available, are matched with diagnostic criteria from the chosen diagnostic tool (DSM or ICD-10) and a diagnosis is given. It is important to understand that psychiatric classification for an individual has significant implications that reach well beyond the boundaries of a single diagnostic act.

Consumer narrative Christine's story part three: Diagnosis

I always felt guilty for having bipolar disorder, because of the effect it had on the kids and everyone around me, and honestly I felt that I had no value outside of the house, and no one expected me to recover from my diagnosed mental illness. They just expected me to get better, and there's a huge difference in that. Mum always introduced me as 'This is my daughter; she has bipolar', as if I was part of the disease. The kids always spoke to their friends about my bipolar, and that always made me feel less of a person. Mental illness isn't widely accepted. My eldest son did it to help people understand that bipolar is okay and that mental illness is okay, but I lost all confidence. I couldn't even make decisions anymore because I had no confidence. I had to get my son to help me to make decisions.

Consumer narrative   Anna's story: Diagnosis

My original diagnosis in 2000 was postnatal depression. I was put on antidepressants and I had to stop breast feeding. I didn't really recover properly from the depression, so then I was diagnosed with major depression with psychotic features. In 2004 I had a psychotic episode and I was admitted to hospital for two weeks, but they misdiagnosed me. They said I had Zoloft withdrawal, a psychotic episode and bipolar disorder type 2. I was put on anti-psychotic medication and then they diagnosed me with schizophreniform, which is basically a short-form version of schizophrenia that lasts between one and six months. After the six months was up I was still on both anti-psychotics and antidepressants. The psychiatrist didn't say to me 'You have schizophrenia', but I asked him whether he thought that my symptoms and the medication that I was on pointed to a diagnosis of schizophrenia, and he said yes. Then, in 2007, I had a manic episode and I was admitted to the hospital for six weeks. When I came out of hospital I had a really big depression, a big low, and so they put me on Epilim, a mood stabiliser, which didn't do much for me so the medication was changed over to lithium, which made me thirsty

continued ›

and made me urinate a lot. In 2008 I had to fill out a treating doctor's report so I could get a disability pension, and he put down that I had schizoaffective disorder, which basically means schizophrenia combined with a mood disorder, and the mood disorder was bipolar so that's been my diagnosis for the past five years. The changes to diagnosis have been frustrating but I've read up on each new diagnosis, usually in books from the library, to keep myself on top of the changes.

Chapter summary

This chapter has presented stories and information, supplemented with activities designed to deepen understanding of:

- the nature, scope and practice of assessment in mental health and mental illness across a range of situations;
- the ways in which various key concepts in mental health assessment are utilised in practice;
- how engagement is at the heart of therapeutic assessment, and possible barriers and enablers in this regard;
- the value of looking beyond taken-for-granted assumptions underpinning the therapeutic relationship; and
- the importance of respect, trust and dignity in mental health assessment and practice more generally.

Critical thinking/learning activities

1   Consider Christine's story. What interventions or services and supports might she need to consider to help work through her trauma, build resilience and live a more flourishing life?

2   Christine may need to access services or support from community, non-government and government settings, such as individual or group counselling, or a support group for survivors of abuse. What resources are available within the area in which you live for a person who has had Christine's experiences? What goals can you identify within Christine's story? How would you suggest Christine go about addressing any unmet goals?

3   What does the term 'assessment' mean in the field of mental health? How might various forms for assessment differ between various groups and across the lifespan? In mental health, assessment is a widely utilised concept. All government and non-government organisations will have a schedule of documentation and clinical/ organisational governance procedures. It is important to become familiar with a range of assessment techniques. Information can be found at the time of your clinical placement as well as from attending clinical seminars and symposiums. What type of assessment process would be appropriate for a person who has had Christine's experiences?

4   What do you think are the main reasons that Anna has received so many different diagnoses? Discuss what you think are the potential effects of this upon Anna, her family and her perception of herself and her place within society.

5   How do you think the nurse in John's experience developed therapeutic rapport with him so quickly? What would you do in the same situation? What might be some of the barriers you may encounter in doing so?

6   How might you identify and consider a person's strengths within the process of assessment? What methods might you use for doing this? What barriers might you encounter in taking a strengths-based view?

Learning extension

1 Review the list of terms used to undertake a MSE. Write a paragraph answering the following questions:
   - How and in what ways are these terms interrelated?
   - Would any of these terms be more or less acceptable to an Aboriginal person? Explain your answer.
2 Choose one of the assessment tools indicated above to assess Anna. Provide a one-paragraph summary of the MSE. Working in small groups, identify how the information arising from the MSE will inform nursing practice.

Further reading

Barker, P.J. (2004). *Assessment in Psychiatric and Mental Health Nursing: In search of the whole person.* Cheltenham, UK: Nelson Thornes.

O'Hagan, M. (2013). *Straight Answers to the Curley Questions in Mental Health.* Retrieved from www.maryohagan.com/Home.

Purdie, N., Dudgeon, P. & Walker, R. (eds) (2010). *Working Together: Aboriginal and Torres Strait Islander Mental Health and Wellbeing Principles and Practice.* Canberra: Department of Health and Ageing. Retrieved from http://apo.org.au/research/working-together-aboriginal-and-torres-strait-islander-mental-health-and-wellbeing-principl.

Shattell, M.M., Starr, S.S., Thomas, S.P. (2007). 'Take my hand, help me out': Mental health service recipients' experience of the therapeutic relationship. *International Journal of Mental Health Nursing, 16*: 274–84.

Wand, T. (2013). Positioning mental health nursing practice within a positive health paradigm, *International Journal of Mental Health Nursing, 22,* (2): 116–24.

Westerman, T. (2004). Engagement of Indigenous clients in mental health services: What role do cultural differences play? *Australian e-Journal for the Advancement of Mental Health, 3*(3): 88–94.

References

Abou-Sinna, R. & Luebbers, S. (2012). Validity of assessing people experiencing mental illness who have offended using the Camberwell assessment of need-forensic and health of the nation outcome scales-secure. *International Journal of Mental Health Nursing, 21*(5): 462–70.

American Psychiatric Association (APA) (2012). *DSM-5 Development.* Retrieved from www.dsm5.org/Pages/Default.aspx.

APA (2013). *Diagnostic and Statistical Manual of Mental Disorders: DSM-5.* Arlington, VA: Author.

Australian College of Mental Health Nurses (ACMHN) (2010). *Standards of Practice for Australian Mental Health Nurses: Setting the standard.* Canberra: Author.

Australian Government (2012). MHPOD: Classification of mental disorders. Retrieved 31 July 2012, from www.mhpod.gov.au/assets/sample_topics/Classification_of_Mental_Disorders.html.

Barker, P. (2002). The tidal model. *Journal of Psychosocial Nursing & Mental Health Services, 40*(7): 42.

Barker, P. (2009). *Psychiatric and Mental Health Nursing: The craft of caring.* London: Hodder Arnold.

Barry, P.D. (2002). *Mental Health and Mental Illness,* 7th edn. Philadelphia, PA: Lippincott.

Beecher, B. (2009). The medical model, mental health practitioners and individuals with schizophrenia and their families. *Journal of Social Work Practice, 23*(1): 9–20.

Chadwick, P. (2009). *Schizophrenia: The positive perspective*, 2nd edn. New York: Routledge.

Davidson, C. L., Wingate, L. R., Rasmussen, K. A. & Slish, M. L. (2009). Hope as a predictor of interpersonal suicide risk. *Suicide & Life-threatening Behavior, 39*(5): 499–507.

Ebert, M. H. (2008). *Current Diagnosis & Treatment: Psychiatry.* New York: McGraw-Hill Medical.

Garb, H. N. (2005). Clinical judgment and decision making. *Annual Review of Clinical Psychology, 1*(1): 67–89.

Harding, C. M., Zubin, J. & Strauss, J. S. (1987). Chronicity in schizophrenia: Fact, partial fact or artifact? *Hospital and Community Practice, 38*: 477–86.

Hunter, E. (2007). Disadvantage and discontent: A review of issues relevant to the mental health of rural and remote Indigenous Australians. *Australian Journal of Rural Health, 15*: 88–93.

Jackson, D. & O'Brien, L. (2009). The effective nurse. In R. Elder, K. Evans & D. Nizette, (eds), *Psychiatric and Mental Health Nursing*, 2nd edn (pp. 3–13). Sydney: Mosby Elsevier.

Kelly, M. & Gamble, C. (2005). Exploring the concept of recovery in schizophrenia. *Journal of Psychiatric and Mental Health Nursing, 12*(2): 245–51.

Keyes, C. (2005). Mental illness and/or mental health? Investigating axioms of the complete state model of health. *Journal of Consulting and Clinical Psychology, 73*(3): 539–48.

Kylmä, J., Juvakka, T., Nikkonen, M., Korhonen, T. & Isohanni, M. (2006). Hope and schizophrenia: An integrative review. *Journal of Psychiatric and Mental Health Nursing, 13*(6): 651–64.

Liersch-Sumskis, S. (2013). A Phenomenological Examination of the Meaning of Resilience as Described by People Who Experience Schizophrenia. Doctoral thesis, Wollongong University, Australia.

Manderscheid, R. W., Ryff, C. D., Freeman, E. J., McKnight-Eily, L. R., Dhingra, S. & Strine, T. W. (2010). Evolving definitions of mental illness and wellness. *Preventing Chronic Disease, 7*(1): A19.

McCormack, J. (2007). Recovery and strengths based practice. In Scottish Recovery Network (ed.), *SRN Discussion Series*, Report No. 6. Glasgow: Glasgow Association for Mental Health.

McGrath, J. (2006). Variations in the incidence of schizophrenia: Data versus dogma. *Schizophrenia Bulletin, 32*(1): 195–7.

Miller, R. & Mason, S. (2011). *Diagnosis: Schizophrenia: A comprehensive resource for consumers, families, and helping professionals.* New York: Columbia University Press.

Moxham, L., Robson, P. & Pegg, S. (2012). Mental health nursing. In A. Berman, S. J. Snyder, T. Levett-Jones, T. Dwyer, M. Hales, N. Harvey, Y. Luxford, L. Moxham, T. Park, B. Parker, K. Reid-Searl & D. Stanley (eds), *Fundamentals of Nursing*, 2nd edn (pp. 1220–46). Sydney: Pearson.

Newman, M. A. (2008). *Transforming Presence: The difference that nursing makes.* Philadelphia, PA: FA Davis.

Peplau, H. (1994). Psychiatric mental health nursing: Challenge and change. *Journal of Psychiatric and Mental Health Nursing, 1*: 3–7.

Peterson, C. & Seligman, M. (2004). *Character Strengths and Virtues: A handbook and classification.* Oxford: Oxford University Press.

Phelan, M., Hayward, P., Slade, M., Thornicroft, G., Dunn, G., Holloway, F. & McCrone, P. (1995). The Camberwell Assessment of Need – The validity and reliability of an instrument to assess the needs of people with severe mental illness. *British Journal of Psychiatry, 167*: 589–95.

Ralph, R. O. & Corrigan, P. W. (eds). (2005). *Recovery in Mental Illness: Broadening our understanding of wellness.* Washington, DC: American Psychological Association.

Rapp, C. A. & Goscha, R. J. (2012). *The Strengths Model: A recovery-oriented approach to mental health services*, 3rd edn. New York: Oxford University Press.

Reed, G. M. (2010). Toward ICD-11: Improving the clinical utility of WHO's International Classification of Mental Disorders. *Professional Psychology: Research and Practice, 41*(6): 457–64.

Reid, J. T. & Trompf, P. (1991). *The Health of Indigenous Australia.* Marrickville, NSW: Harcourt Brace Jovanovich.

Repper, J. & Perkins, R. (2003). *Social Inclusion and Recovery: A model for mental health practice.* London: Bailliere Tindall.

Robertson, M. & Walter, G. (2007). The ethics of psychiatric diagnosis. *Psychiatric Annals, 37*(12): 792.

Rose, D., Thornicroft, G., Pinfold, V. & Kassam, A. (2007). 250 labels used to stigmatise people with mental illness. *BMC Health Services Research, 7*(1): 7–97.

Royal College of Psychiatrists (2008). Rethinking risk to others in mental health services: Final report of a scoping group. *Psychiatric Bulletin, 32*(8): 32–37.

Ryff, C. D. & Keyes, C. L. (1995). The structure of psychological well-being revisited. *Journal of Personality and Social Psychology, 69*(4): 719–27.

Seru, G. (1994). Mental health issues for elders with a focus on grannies. *Aboriginal and Islander Health Worker Journal, 18*: 13–16.

Shields, M., Tremblay, M. S., Laviolette, M., Craig, C. L., Janssen, I. & Gorber, S. C. (2002). Fitness of Canadian adults: Results from the 2007–2009 Canadian health measures survey. *Health Reports*. Cat. 82–003. *21*(1): 1–15.

Stein, D. J., Phillips, K. A., Bolton, D., Fulford, K. W. M., Sadler, J. Z. & Kendler, K. S. (2010). What is a mental/ psychiatric disorder? From DSM-IV to DSM-V. *Psychological Medicine, 40*(11): 1759–65.

Stevenson, C., Leamy, M. & Barker, P. (2000). The philosophy of empowerment. *Mental Health Nursing, 20*(9): 8.

Thomas, S. D. M., Harty, M. A., Parrot, T. J., McCrone, P., Slade, M. & Thornicroft, G. (2003). *CANFOR: Camberwell Assessment of Need–forensic version.* London: Gaskell.

Westerhof, G. J. & Keyes, C. (2010). Mental illness and mental health: The Two Continua model across the lifespan. *Journal of Adult Development, 17*(2): 110–19.

Westerman, T. G. (2003). The Development of the Westerman Aboriginal Symptom Checklist for Youth: A measure to assess the moderating effects of cultural resilience with Aboriginal youth at risk of depression, anxiety and suicidal behaviours. Unpublished PhD thesis, Curtin University.

Westerman, T. (2004). Engagement of Indigenous clients in mental health services: What role do cultural differences play? *Australian e-Journal for the Advancement of Mental Health, 3*(3): 88–94.

Westerman, T. (2010). Engaging Australian Aboriginal youth in mental health services. *Australian Psychologist, 45*(3): 212–22.

Wolff, N. (2007). The social construction of the cost of mental illness. *Evidence & Policy: A Journal of Research, Debate and Practice, 3*(1); 67–78.

World Health Organization (WHO) (1993). *The ICD-10 Classification of Mental and Behavioural Disorders: Diagnostic criteria for research.* Geneva: Author.

WHO (2005). *Promoting Mental Health: Concepts, emerging evidence, practice.* Geneva: Author.

WHO (2008). Closing the gap in a generation: Health equity through action on the social determinants of health: Final report. In WHO (ed.) *Commission on Social Determinants of Health.* Geneva, Switzerland: Author.

Young, E. (2009). Memoirs: Rewriting the social construction of mental illness. *Narrative Inquiry, 19*(1): 52–68.

6

Legal and ethical aspects in mental health care

Helen P. Hamer, Anthony J. O'Brien and Debra Lampshire

Introduction 118
A legal and ethical framework for
  practice 118
Procedural justice and mental health
  nursing 126
Alternatives to compulsory treatment and
  the role of advance directives and crisis
  plans 129

Mental health legislation in the year
  2042 30
Chapter summary 133
Critical thinking/learning activities 133
Learning extension 133
Further reading 133
References 134

Learning objectives

At the completion of this chapter, you should be able to:

- Describe a legal and ethical framework for practice.
- Understand the effects of compulsion/coercion on people with mental illness and their families.
- Describe the tension between the therapeutic relationship and compulsory treatment.
- Understand a procedural justice framework to underpin human connectedness.
- Explain the role of the nurse in implementing mental health legislation.
- Incorporate alternative approaches to compulsory treatment, such as advance directives.

Introduction

This chapter explores the legal and ethical factors that inform mental health nursing, from multiple perspectives. The chapter proposes a legal and ethical framework that promotes human connectedness between the mental health nurse and people with mental illness and their families and *whānau*. The chapter includes theoretical and practical aspects of working within a legal framework, and provides a number of narratives to bring to life what it means to experience compulsory treatment. The chapter concludes by discussing proposed alternatives to compulsory treatment and a potential future legal framework that embraces a person's autonomy and human rights. New Zealand – and each Australian state and territory – has its own mental health legislation. Although there are differences between them, they share the essential features of providing for treatment without consent, criteria of danger to self and others, and certain procedural protections. Throughout this chapter we use the term 'mental health legislation' to refer to common aspects of the legislation in different jurisdictions.

> ***whānau***
> (Māori) extended family, family group; a familiar term of address to a number of people

A legal and ethical framework for practice

Mental health nurses encounter many challenges in caring for people with mental illness, such as the multifaceted explanations for the origins of mental distress and the requirement to uphold the people's well-being and safety though the use of mental health legislation. Such challenges can create moral and ethical dilemmas in practice.

Ethical framework

Ethics is described as a moral philosophy. Within nursing practice, ethics is concerned with the decision-making processes in which nurses engage, based on their reasoning about what is right and wrong (Bennett & Bennett, 2011). According to Beauchamp and Childress (2013), ethical decision-making requires the person to have the motivation and desire to understand what should be done in a given circumstance in order to perform the action required. The subsequent actions are thus based on the moral ideals of the person. Such ethical decision-making in nursing care is informed by the processes of reasoning, justification and argument (Beauchamp & Childress, 2013) in order to make a decision about the appropriate actions to take (Johnstone, 2009).

An ethical framework for nursing practice (Australian Nursing and Midwifery Council, 2008; Nursing Council of New Zealand, 2012) is based on four sound ethical principles: autonomy, beneficence, non-maleficence and justice (Beauchamp & Childress, 2013). Autonomy refers to the respect that is shown by nurses towards the people's decisions and choices. Beneficence requires the nurse to prevent evil or harm to people and non-maleficence obliges the nurse to avoid inflicting harm (Beauchamp & Childress, 2013; Bennett & Bennett, 2011). By following such ethical principles it can be argued that justice is reached by creating an encounter that supports fairness, equality and non-discrimination towards people with mental illness.

Example of an ethical dilemma in practice

The use of electroconvulsive therapy (ECT) remains one of the most controversial treatments in psychiatry, and poses an ethical dilemma for mental health nurses, the person with a mental illness and her or his family members (Bray, 2003). Many people who have experienced ECT find it helpful; others find it distressing, punitive and degrading (Bray, 2003; Weitz, 2013). ECT has permanent side-effects, such as memory loss or headaches, and has been regarded by some in the mental health service-user movement as a violation of a person's **human rights** (Weitz, 2013).

> **human rights**
> an expression of dignity, respect and equality; regardless of a person's religious, cultural or linguistic background, where the person lives or what the person thinks or believes, human rights are about being treated fairly, treating others fairly and having the ability to make real and genuine choices in our daily lives

The evidence and effectiveness for the use of ECT are also debateable (Read & Bentall, 2010). Since the administration of ECT is a medical procedure and requires the use of an anaesthetic, general rules of informed consent and preparation for a medical procedure apply. However, on occasions ECT may be administered in the case of an emergency and without the consent of the person. According to Bray (2003), the ethical dilemma nurses face is whether the therapeutic benefits of ECT outweigh some of the risks briefly listed here. Being able to voice the ethical dilemma with colleagues is important for the mental health nurse, who will be expected to care for and support the person throughout the process of deliberation and treatment. Bray further argues that there are alternative treatments to ECT; however, if the person consents to treatment with ECT after weighing up the risks and benefits, then there is no longer an ethical dilemma for the nurse (see Bray, 2003 for a full explanation of the role of the nurse in the procedure of ECT).

Reflective question

Read the article by Read and Bentall (2010) and then consider the key points you would cover in discussion with a family member who wishes to know the effectiveness of ECT.

Introduction to a legal framework

The **legal** framework for mental health nurses is underpinned by specific principles within the United Nations charter (United Nations High Commissioner for Human Rights (UNHCHR) 1991), which describes

> **legal**
> relating to the law

compulsory treatment
an initial period of assessment, at the end of which a legal determination is made about whether the person is to become subject to a legal order for further assessment and treatment, in an in-patient or community setting; while subject to compulsory treatment the person has a right to appeal her or his compulsory status, usually to a judge

the rights of people with mental illness who are subject to **compulsory treatment**. The charter declares that all people with mental illness have the right to voluntary treatment wherever possible. However, if involuntary treatment is required this must be authorised by a qualified mental health professional; a second medical opinion must be sought; and treatment must occur within an approved mental health facility. The four guiding ethical principles discussed earlier: autonomy, beneficence, non-maleficence and justice serve as guides to nursing practice in order to balance the tension between the rights of the individual to choose when and where she or he wishes to access health care and the responsibilities of the mental health nurse to safeguard the well-being of consumers when there are concerns about their capacity and competency to make such informed decisions (see Chapter 12 in this book for a detailed discussion of the definitions of competence and capacity). For example, Fishwick, Tait and O'Brien (2001) have argued that the responsibilities of nurses and their expected roles and duties enshrined within legislation will present conflicts between a paternalistic custodial role as a nurse and an ethical commitment to the person's autonomy.

If mental health nurses are required to maintain culturally competent human connectedness within a legal framework in order to preserve the partnership and collaboration with consumers, this will require the nurse to be cognisant of rights-based approaches to assessment and treatment, and to provide care within a least discriminatory way. Therefore, it is not our intention in this chapter to provide a practical, step-by-step guide to the various legislation throughout Australia and New Zealand. Rather, this chapter focuses on the social and political aspects of mental health law and the tensions that this may pose in the art and science of mental health nursing.

A background to mental health law

Mental health nursing as a specialty is unique in health care in providing a specific legislative framework for treatment without consent. Mental health legislation provides criteria for the compulsory treatment of consumers of mental health service and, in addition, sets out the rights of consumers, procedures to be followed in conducting assessments, and appeal and review processes. The criteria of legislation vary internationally and between jurisdictions. Almost every developed country has some form of mental health legislation.

The first mental health legislation was the English *Madhouses Act of 1774* (GB). This legislation was concerned with the regulation of private houses used for the detention and, in some cases, treatment, of people considered to be mentally ill. The main aim of the Madhouses Act was to prevent the abuses that were known to occur in private houses. Later, legislation specified the criteria and processes to be followed in making someone subject to compulsory assessment and treatment, a process referred to as 'committal'.

Mental health legislation typically provides for detention and treatment in hospital and for compulsory treatment in the community in the form of a community treatment order. Having a mental illness, even a severe mental illness, is not a sufficient criterion for someone to be made subject to detention and/or compulsory treatment. In addition to mental illness (in some cases referred to as 'mental disorder') the person must also present a risk to self or to others as a result of the mental illness. Risk may include risk of self-neglect, in the case of someone who is unable adequately to attend to activities of daily living.

For the self-neglect criterion to apply there would need to be a substantial threat to the person's health, not merely, for example, that he or she might lose weight or neglect personal hygiene. Inclusion of criteria of risk is sometimes referred to as the 'dangerousness standard' of mental health legislation, in contrast to the 'need for treatment standard' that applied in most countries until the latter half of the 21st century. The intention of the change to a dangerousness standard was to prevent detention in a hospital simply because health professionals believed the person needed treatment. Instead, only those who were considered as representing a significant degree of risk were thought to need compulsory hospital treatment. By moving the focus of treatment to the community, services were to be provided to the 'least restrictive alternative' standard.

Community treatment orders (CTO) are used to provide compulsory treatment in the community. Most commonly, the person will have been in hospital under compulsory care, and the CTO is a condition of her or his discharge from the hospital. CTOs are considered by those who use them as providing for the least restrictive treatment, with the idea being that treatment in the community, even under legislation, is less restrictive than treatment in a hospital setting. A person subject to a CTO is obliged by the order to accept treatment, which will usually consist of medication, some form of case management and periodic review. A case manager, often a mental health nurse, will provide contact in the form of home visits or attendance at a community clinic, and will broker other services such as employment, housing and income support, and therapeutic programs. A person who does not accept compulsory community based treatment may be returned to hospital, sometimes with the assistance of police.

Despite their widespread adoption internationally, there is limited evidence for the effectiveness of CTOs in achieving their main goal of reduced hospital admissions (Burns et al., 2013; Kisely et al., 2007). There is therefore concern to develop alternatives to compulsory treatment, such as joint crisis plans and **advance directives**.

> **advance directive**
> a legal document (such as a living will) signed by a living, competent person in order to provide guidance for medical and health care decisions in the event that the person becomes incompetent to make such decisions

Lamb, Weinberger and DeCuir (2002) noted that there are two common-law principles that provide the rationale for the police to take responsibility for persons with mental illness. These are their power and authority to protect the safety and welfare of the community, and their obligations to protect individuals with mental illness. However, as the first responders this places the police in a gate-keeping role. Police officers have to decide whether the person should enter the mental health system or the justice system. Many police officers have limited awareness and understanding about mental health conditions. Therefore, as first responders, their peace-keeping role can unwittingly increase the notion of risk and dangerousness of the distressed person, who may require compulsory assessment and treatment.

People who are voluntarily admitted to a mental health unit may be subjected to compulsory detention if, due to a deterioration in their mental health, a nurse believes that they now meet the criteria for compulsory treatment, and that compulsory treatment is necessary to contain a risk of harm to the person or to others. Mental health legislation, for example, Section 111 of the New Zealand legislation, usually provides powers for registered nurses to prevent someone from leaving an in-patient mental health unit or a general hospital environment if the registered nurse believes there is a significant risk within the terms of the legislation.

Mental health legislation sets out the rights of those subject to committal, and the processes available to support those rights and to seek review of their committed status. Rights include the right to information, access to a lawyer, to receive treatment, to receive visitors and other rights. In New Zealand, the Minister of Health appoints solicitors, formally known as district inspectors, to allow consumers subject to legislation to complain if they feel their rights have been breached, and about the standard of their care and treatment. A person may seek the opportunity to have her or his compulsory status reviewed by a judge who has the power to release the person from compulsory status.

Safeguards for the use of the Act include the Mental Health Review Tribunal in New Zealand (Diesfeld & McKenna, 2006) and Australia (Carney et al. 2011), which hears appeals about the treatment orders that mental health professionals have put in place and is able to confirm or revoke an order under the legislation. Each person who is subject to the legislation is supported by a legal representative (a solicitor), at no cost to the person.

Mental health legislation establishes specific statutory roles that in many cases are assumed by nurses. For example, in New South Wales an accredited person may sign a mental health certificate as part of the process of committal. The accredited person must be a health professional, and may be a nurse. In New Zealand, the role of duly authorised officer is instrumental in providing advice and arranging compulsory assessment, and that role is most commonly assumed by registered nurses. In addition to these roles, nurses may be involved in providing opinions to a court about a patient's compulsory status under mental health legislation. Legislated roles such as these present nurses with the dilemma that they have dual responsibilities: those created by legislation and those arising from their commitment as nurses to developing therapeutic relationships with consumers (O'Brien & Kar, 2012).

Mental health law and human rights

The human rights of people with mental illness in New Zealand and Australia have received increasing attention in the past two decades, more recently prompted in part by new obligations under the United Nations Convention on the Rights of Persons with Disabilities (UNCRPD) (UNHCHR, 2006; McSherry & Wilson, 2011). Enshrined in these instruments is the human right for individuals to not be subjected to medical treatment without full, free and informed consent (Bell, 2003; Quinn, 2011).

Like other citizens of Australia and New Zealand, people with mental illness have inalienable human rights (United Nations General Assembly, 1948). More recently, further guarantee of human rights for consumers have been enshrined within the UNCRPD. The document defines persons with disabilities as those who have long-term physical, mental, intellectual or sensory impairments that, in interaction with various barriers, may hinder their full and effective participation in society on an equal basis with others. The UNCRPD's purpose is to:

> Promote, protect and ensure the full and equal enjoyment of all human rights and fundamental freedoms by all persons with disabilities, and to promote respect for their inherent dignity (Article 1).

Though these declarations, principles and guidelines have no binding legal effect, they provide the moral force that provides practical guidance to governments to domesticate these within their statutes and protocols (The International Council on Human Rights Policy, 2006). In their review of Australian legislation, Callaghan and Ryan (2012) discussed how changes to the Victorian and Tasmanian legislation attempted to give effect to the UNCRPD by replacing the dangerousness standard with a competency standard.

The New Zealand *Mental Health (Compulsory Assessment and Treatment) Act 1992* (the Act) mandates the detention and compulsory treatment of people who are mentally ill in hospital or in the community. According to Bell (2003) the Act is designed to give force to the notion of the person's rights rather than perpetuating the paternalistic approach to treatment, and to promote the person's autonomy and provide the least restrictive intervention. However, the Act's definition of mental disorder (an abnormal state of mind) avoided diagnostic labels and instead focused on danger to self and others and the person's capacity for self-care (Bell, 2003). The Act obliges the state and its agents to provide health and social services to its citizens, as well as making a broad range of treatment options available. Legal safeguards are also in place in New Zealand, such as the input of the duly authorised officer (DAO), who provides expert information and advice on the mental health needs and services that may be required by people who are experiencing mental illness. Other safeguards are a review by a family court judge of a person's status under the Mental Health Act, legal representation by a solicitor and access to a review tribunal, as discussed earlier.

The law, reciprocity and recovery

Bell (2003) and Winick (2003) argued that the law governing the care of people who are mentally ill contains two principal powers. The first principle is that police powers protect society from those who are dangerous. The second principle relates to *parens patriae* (Latin for 'parent of the country') when the state delegates the power to the police to protect the best interests of citizens whose illness deprives them of the ability to make rational decisions.

There are many restrictions imposed on the rights and responsibilities of consumers who are subject to mental health legislation (Hamer, 2012). The legal principle of reciprocity (Hatfield & Antcliff, 2001; Richardson, 2003) is concerned with balancing the state's restriction on the liberty or autonomy of the citizen with its responsibility to provide an adequate treatment system. If the rights of consumers are to be curtailed, then the principle of reciprocity means there must also be benefit for consumers. Reciprocity is therefore the justification for the curtailment of a person's freedom. The notion of therapeutic jurisprudence (Winick, 2003) suggests that the law can be a therapeutic agent by advocating and reducing the curtailment of the civil liberty of people who are mentally ill when assessing them for compulsory treatment. However, given these legal precepts, the mental health legislation continues to have a profound influence on the liberty and rights of people who have a mental illness as autonomous citizens, and is a form of civil commitment in the absence of any crime (Winick, 2003).

The effects of involuntary treatment

Suzy Stevens (2003) gave a compelling account of her experience of involuntary containment and treatment. She suggested that psychiatry understood mental illness as a disease of the brain (Bracken & Thomas, 2001; Morgan, 2008) and completely separate from the human being. Suzy's initial and subsequent involuntary treatment in hospital, therefore, was more about suppressing her distress – by heavily medicating her – than bringing relief and calm to the turmoil she was experiencing at that time. Decisions about involuntary treatment led to irreparable breakdowns in her family relationships.

Examined in light of the ethical framework outlined earlier in this chapter, Suzy experienced significant limitations on her autonomy, and did not experience her care and treatment as beneficent. Her account also suggests that the ethical principle of non-maleficence was breached in her case, leading to her experience of care and treatment as harmful. A greater focus on human connectedness during Suzy's episode of care may have reduced her level of distress and led to better outcomes in terms of her family relationships.

Consumer narrative   Leigh's story

In my role as a district health board family advisor I would urge mental health nurses to maintain the human connectedness with the person and her or his loved ones during the legal process of compulsory assessment and treatment, and to help mitigate the effects on all concerned. As a family, *whānau* member I have at times felt in conflicted about whether to seek help for my loved one. Encouraging my family member to access help is always the first thing I do. However, when this does not happen, I have in the past been concerned enough to seek assistance on my family member's behalf. One experiences feelings of guilt about calling for assistance and then the person ends up under compulsion to enter the system. Sometimes the process takes on a life of its own, with the person

continued ›

Consumer narrative continued ›

being processed very quickly becoming involved with police and crisis staff. As a family *whānau* we have experienced trauma because of the process. When a family member ends up under compulsion to enter the system and is processed very quickly with police involvement and crisis staff, it is natural to wonder if you have done the right thing. Being involved in and witnessing your family member being taken away by the police is very distressing and potentially traumatic, especially for children. Often, the loved one being placed under the Act blames the family, as the system is too big to blame and then the family is alienated from the person they care about, left with feelings of guilt and regret which negatively affect their future relationship.

What the family member needs

I would like nursing staff to support and strengthen the relationship that the family *whānau* have with their family member. My relationship is not strengthened by being reduced to the role of 'the monitor' or 'the watcher' of my family member, or being asked to 'make sure they take their pills'. I would like some skills and knowledge to support my family member who is experiencing mental distress and not be afraid of the 'symptoms', so that together we can hopefully reduce the need for compulsory care under the Mental Health (CAT) Act. With the knowledge I have gained over the years, I no longer have fears about my family member hearing voices. I can talk about what is happening for my family member, normalise the situation and decide more accurately (with my family member) if there is a need to call for help. I would like nursing staff to encourage the use of advance directives that enable us as a family, *whānau* to discuss ahead of time what help and support is needed when things aren't going well. The system needs to also model the recovery process and support family, *whānau* to understand how they can do that, too.

Suzy Stevens (2003) described how the longer-term effects of being subjected to involuntary treatment dehumanised her when she 'became a statistic'. She had the label and stigma of psychiatric patient, and as she was removed from society she could no longer participate as she had no place within it. Suzy explained that people who are detained by law in a psychiatric hospital have very few rights (Mackenzie & Shirlaw, 2002). One cannot, for example, claim the right to refuse or change one's mind about the treatment on offer (Health and Disability Commission, 1996). Likewise, people with mental illness have restrictions placed on their right to vote, to enter into legal contracts or to leave the country. Suzy further explained that when compulsorily detained it is difficult for consumers to assert their rights, and thus they need the advocacy of others, including mental health nurses.

Compulsion and coercion through the use of the law represents an intrusion on the rights and liberties of an individual (Barnes & Bowl, 2001; Barnes, Bowl & Fisher, 1990; Bell, 2003; Sayce, 2000). It is a form of social control and regulation of the lifestyle of citizens (Bartlett, 2003; Bell, 2003). Hatfield and Antcliff (2001) contended that if governments promoted social policies that attended to economic inequalities and social exclusion of people with mental illness, rather than containing risk and rationing resources for mental health care, they may reduce the need for compulsory treatment. The following section outlines the concept of procedural justice, a framework that acknowledges the experience of coercion when consumers are subject to compulsory treatment, and which provides guidance for nurses in maintaining human connectedness when practicing within mental health legislation.

Procedural justice and mental health nursing

In keeping with the spirit of human connectedness within this book, people who face the requirement of compulsory treatment will, more than ever at this time, require mental health nurses to work within a legal and ethical framework that provides dignity and respect for people during the process of civil commitment. The requirement to work in partnership and to be an advocate for the person is also paramount during a time when the person and her or his family members are at their most vulnerable.

procedural justice
the legal decision-making processes that incorporate the principles of fairness, justice and distribution of resources

The concept of **procedural justice** (Lind, Kanfer & Earley, 1990; McKenna, Simpson & Coverdale, 2003) places an obligation on mental health nurses to include consumers in fair decision-making processes that incorporate the principles of fairness and justice. According to McKenna and O'Brien (in press) and McKenna and colleagues (2003), when mental health nurses work within a procedural justice framework, the decision-making process about commitment will minimise the value biases and the vested interests of the decision-makers, particularly nurses, and provide an opportunity for any erroneous decisions to be corrected.

When mental health nurses practice within a procedural justice framework, they model open dialogue (Seikkula & Olson, 2003) with consumers and their families, and foster the concept of human connectedness by adhering to the following principles:

Fairness: The person believes that the process of commitment is free from the biases and the self-interest of the nurse and other clinicians involved in the process, even when the person has no control over the decision itself.

Voice: The person is able to voice her or his opinions, choices and wishes about treatment options at that time, even though this may not influence the outcome of the process.

Validation: As above, the person experiences that his or her views and opinions are taken seriously by the nurse, facilitated by a collaborative discussion so the person's experience of distress is acknowledged and validated. Such frank discussion may not determine the outcome that the person desires, though. However, the therapeutic alliance is enhanced when the nurse bears witness to the person's often-traumatic experience of compulsory assessment and treatment, and fosters human connectedness.

Respect: The person feels that he or she has been treated in a respectful and dignified way.

Motivation: The nurse has conveyed that he or she is admitting the person into a hospital out of their concern for him or her.

Information: The person believes that she or he has had the opportunity to discuss all the relevant information with the nurse regarding the process of committal and is clear about the goals for this procedure. Providing information enhances the person's expectation of fair justice and participation, and that his or her voice has been heard.

Here, we turn to the idea of **insight** and its role in compulsory assessment and treatment. Hamilton and Roper (2006) and Diesfeld and McKenna (2006) have argued that though the term insight is used universally within psychiatry, and especially in processes of civil commitment, there is no consensus on a definition of the term. Despite this lack of concensus, insight forms a critical component of clinicians' assessment of the mental health of consumers. Lack of insight is frequently cited in the clinical reasoning that leads to a decision to use mental health legislation. The notion of insight can be 'troubling' (Hamilton & Roper, 2006, p. 416) when a person's explanation of her or his distress does not accord with the professionals' biomedical explanatory framework of illness. Hamilton and Roper (2006) argued that this often results in consumers being deemed as lacking insight, and that any further commentary or decision-making input that they would wish to have in regard to their care may be considered invalid or mistrusted. However, as the following example illustrates, attending to the individual's account of distress is experienced as validating and respectful.

> **insight**
> in psychiatry, the person's awareness and understanding of her or his own attitudes, feelings, behaviours, disturbing symptoms and self-understanding

Longden (2010) expressed how the attention to her story changed the relationship with her psychiatrist when she felt 'heard' and able to begin to give her own story or explanation for her mental distress:

> When the psychiatrist said 'I don't want to know what other people have told you about yourself, I want to know about you', it was the first time I had been given the chance to see myself as a life story, not as a genetically determined schizophrenic with aberrant brain chemicals and biological flaws and deficiencies that were beyond my power to heal. (p. 256)

In this case, if the psychiatrist had insisted that her or his own view of Eleanor's mental distress was the only correct view, Eleanor would have been assessed as lacking insight. In terms of the concept of procedural justice outlined above, Eleanor would have been denied a voice, would not have felt respected and would not have had her experience validated by the psychiatrist.

Reflective questions

- In pairs, discuss your understanding of the term 'insight'.
- Having read the stories of consumers' lived experiences in this chapter, how might these change your understanding of insight?

Evidence into practice

The use of the Act creates a collision between the mandate of the state to safeguard the great public and the autonomy of the individual. Restrictions on the person's autonomy will almost inevitably cause great alarm and distress for the individual. The parameters of the Mental Health Act dictate the responsibilities and role of mental health professionals toward the person; they then, in turn, determine the restrictions that are to be put in place. However, the individual's focus is on the effect of the restrictions and how this will impede her or his ability to function and live in the manner in which the person chooses for herself or himself. This tension will remain generally intact until the Act is lifted. It is not unusual for people with mental illness to feel significantly oppressed by service providers, which can lead to an adversarial relationship with the services and, in particular, the mental health clinicians. It seems a natural response that people will 'push back' when constraints are placed on their liberty and autonomy, particularly if they see the restrictions as unjustified. People then run the risk of being labelled as 'oppositional', 'non-compliant' or 'in-sightless', thereby reinforcing the notion that the person is unwell, incompetent and even untrustworthy. The person may perceive that he or she is being punished for being honest. Yet, by endeavouring to keep their integrity and stay true to their beliefs, people forfeit their freedom. This will add to the person's sense of persecution. It also raises the question: 'If the person acquiesces to the compulsory treatment and just tells clinicians what they want to hear, is this not an attack on their self-esteem and their honour?'

Mental health nurses need to be cognisant that our decisions and actions regarding compulsory treatment processes can help or hinder human connectedness, and not only with people with a mental illness; we are also required to maintain the human connectedness with their loved ones. In New Zealand, and in some parts of Australia, it is a requirement for mental health clinicians to consult with families during the legal process of making an application to place a person under compulsory treatment.

Murray (2013), provided an overview of how mental health nurses are able to support family members during this process. Murray contended that relationships form the cornerstone of recovery from mental illness and the often-traumatic effects that the process of being compulsorily detained has on both the person and her or his loved ones. She provides a useful acronym, RELATIONSHIP, that can be applied to mental health nurses' practice of procedural justice: **r**espect – build trust and rapport; **e**nhance – the family's ability to be with the loved one; **l**isten – in an empathic way; **a**ddress – the needs of children when a parent is compulsorily detained; **t**hink – about the implications for the person's relationship with a loved one when you make requests of the family; **i**nformation – about the process of the Mental Health Act and the service to be provided; **o**utcome tools – that track progress and improvement in the mental distress of the loved one (such as the HoNOS (Wing et al., 1998)); **n**ormalise – what is happening as the way the family views the situation can determine their response to the event; **s**trength – keep the door of communication open to help families to learn, grow and change; **h**elp – the family to hold hope; **i**nform – the family about available support services; and **p**rotect – families entrust nurses with their most precious and vulnerable family members, so it is important protect the relationship between the person with a mental illness and his or her family.

Consumer narrative Debra's story

It is hard to speak of the time when I am seated in that room with a group of strangers, all of whom seem to have an excessive amount influence on my future and how I will live my life, especially when they only know the vulnerable and confused me, not the capable, competent me. To be judged by any person is an uncomfortable and difficult position to be in, and when it is by people who appear to have no understanding or appreciation of your circumstances it appears quite unjust. To speak with any authority on another's life and know her or his history one must be witness to all facets of a person's life, surely, not just this snapshot, this moment in time when things are hard for me. I hardly know these people and, more importantly, they know almost nothing about me, so how can it be fair that they can exert such power over my existence? This cannot be right; it most certainly can't be an honest assessment of me. They speak around me as if I don't exist. It all seems so predetermined. I don't understand why I'm here and no one seems to be listening to me, no one has told me what to expect and what to do. I feel betrayed and assaulted by those very people who profess to help me. If these are the very people who can condemn me, they can also free me. How do I navigate that relationship knowing I have no choice but to do so? What will this mean for my present and for my future?

Alternatives to compulsory treatment and the role of advance directives and crisis plans

As explained at the beginning of this chapter, most countries have some form of mental health legislation that covers both in-patient and community care. Because mental health legislation overrides the usually accepted principle of autonomy in health care, there is a concern to limit the use of mental health legislation and to develop alternative responses to the needs of consumers experiencing acute episodes of distress. Two alternatives that have been attempted are joint crisis plans and advance directives. Both of these alternatives aim to decide in advance how mental health services can best respond to an acute episode and, in particular, they aim to provide a response that respects the wishes of the individual.

Joint crisis plans are clinical plans negotiated between individual consumers and their clinical teams (Henderson et al., 2004). Typically, the joint crisis plan will document an person's early warning signs of mental health deterioration and specify responses such as the consumer initiating contact if he or she feels a crisis is imminent, options such as intensive support at home, respite care or voluntary hospital admission, medication and other measures. The process of negotiating a joint crisis plan helps consumers to express their preferences, increases understanding between consumers and clinicians, and leads to consumers feeling more involved in their care. Joint crisis plans are also aimed at reducing the use of compulsory treatment. An initial study of joint crisis plans (Henderson et al., 2004) showed that holders of such plans were half as likely to be admitted to hospital under compulsion, although a more recent, randomised controlled trial did not demonstrate the same effect (Thornicroft et al., 2013). A reason for this difference is that it may be easier to implement joint crisis plans in small health districts where more intensive coaching of staff leads to the joint crisis plan being more effectively implemented.

Advance directives are similar to joint crisis plans, with the difference being that an individual consumer can develop an advance directive without consulting her or his mental health team (Atkinson, 2007). Advance directives cover many of the same aspects as joint crisis plans, but can also cover anything of concern to the person, including care of children or pets, care of the person's home, financial matters and other issues. In relation to compulsory treatment, advance directives are aimed at avoiding the use of compulsion and promoting consensus between clinicians and consumers about care and treatment.

The New Zealand Health and Disability Commission (n.d.) has promoted the option of advance directives as a mechanism for consumers to express their treatment preferences for future mental health care. Advance directives are commonly used in health care and are usually completed by people who have long-term illnesses and who anticipate that they may experience a deterioration in health. An advance directive allows the person to set out his or her preferences for treatment during an episode of illness when he or she may be unable to decide or communicate these. Advance directives, in part, protect consumers' right to choice of treatment; however, they are not legally binding, and can be overridden if the person is subject to the Act.

Mental health legislation in the year 2042

In this concluding section of the chapter we ask the reader to suspend judgement and consider the future of mental health law if the principles of least-restrictive approaches to mental health care were to be firmly embedded within the legislation, mental health delivery and nursing practice. In the following we have chosen to summarise the innovative ideas of Mary O' Hagan, a consumer activist who has offered many visionary approaches to mental health care within New Zealand and Australia (see www.mary@maryohagan.com).

In the first instance, we are reminded that mental health legislation is underpinned by the principles of harm to self and harm to others. Mary argues that the harm to self principle is unfair in that it does not apply to people who have physical illnesses; for example, they are free to refuse treatment. Likewise, with regard to the harm to others principle, within a criminal justice context a person cannot be deprived of his or her liberty unless the person has committed a crime (Wexler & Winick, 1996). Therefore, Mary suggests that people who are vulnerable and at risk because of mental illness are required to have advanced advocacy and support rather than deprivation of their liberty.

Because the media continues to perpetuate the perceived dangerousness of people with mental illness (Angermeyer & Matschinger, 2003; Angermeyer, Matschinger & Corrigan, 2004; McKenna, Thom & Simpson, 2007), members of the public expect mental health professionals to safeguard them from the mentally ill (Hazelton, 1999; Rose, 1998). This stance presents an ethical dilemma for mental health nurses in that they are required to balance their responsibility to both the public and the person with a mental illness with the least restrictions on people's liberty and autonomy.

According to Mary, even though the risk of harm to self and others can result in death, this is likely to happen only in extreme circumstances, and need not be a driver of the mental health systems in Australia and New Zealand, which are dominated by risk management, often at the expense of the therapeutic relationship (Hamer, 2012; Hamer, Finlayson & Warren, forthcoming; Hazelton, 1999; Sawyer, 2005). Ideally, the state must provide advocacy and supportive interventions that are least restrictive for people experiencing mental illness.

It has been acknowledged above that current mental health laws are discriminatory. Mary O'Hagan offers a visionary set of mental health laws in an effort to honour the rights of those who experience mental illness. Mary suggests that future legislation will embody the principles of a 'Care without Coercion' law and a 'Health Consumer Treatment Act', which will support decision making that recognises the best interests of the person and his or her family, places least restrictions on the person's autonomy and sustains the person's equal access to the rights accorded to other citizens. Such principles will minimise the harm to people with mental illness and their loved ones through advanced support by state health services to guard against abuse and exploitation of this vulnerable group.

Further advance directives will provide for the treatment wishes of people with continuing and recurring mental illnesses. Mary O'Hagan suggests that the in-patient or CTO would be superseded by a 'right to treatment order' (RTO), which will require mental health services to provide specified treatment, support and advocacy for people with cognitive challenges to make their own decisions.

Further, Mary proposes that a Health Consumer Treatment Act (HCT Act) will regulate treatment without consent for all people experiencing mental illness. For example, she recommends a single capacity test that assesses the person's ability to communicate her or his wishes, facilitated by professional assessors. However, this will be overridden in the case of a medical emergency. Assessing capacity puts to one side the measure of the person's incapacity and focuses on the person's capacity to express his or her wishes (see Chapter 12 for a fuller definition of competency and capacity).

Here, we remind the reader of the importance of advance directives. Mary's idea that the law needs to focus on adequate treatment, rather than containment, means that within a new HCT Act the person or her or his loved ones can apply to the court for an RTO rather than a CTO. This option echoes the legal principle of reciprocity, concerned with the balance of the state's restriction on the liberty or autonomy of people and, in return, its responsibility to provide an adequate treatment system (Hatfield & Antcliff, 2001; Richardson, 2003).

In conclusion, Mary O'Hagan proposes that such legislation will change the care of people with mental illness; for example, all hospitals will be replaced by community based crisis houses and in-home options for treatment and care. Open access to suicide prevention houses will be established, and forensic services will be absorbed into a humanistic criminal justice system.

It is incumbent on all health professionals, primarily psychiatrists, to be thoroughly familiar with the mental health legislation including the relevant statutory criteria and case law related to civil mental health matters (Neilson, 2005). Similarly, mental health nurses must also have sufficient knowledge of mental health law to effectively work within the law and hold respectful regard for their responsibilities toward the people they serve, their families and members of society.

We urge nurses working with consumers subject to mental health legislation to familiarise themselves with the ethical framework outlined above, and with the concept of procedural justice. While these measures alone will not resolve all professional and ethical issues arising from the use of compulsion in mental health care, we believe that if they are applied with concern for maintaining human connectedness in clinical practice, they will assist nurses in providing humanistic interpersonal care, and will promote respectful care for consumers.

Chapter summary

This chapter has presented stories, information and activities designed to deepen understanding of:
- a legal and ethical framework for mental health nursing practice;
- the effects of compulsion/coercion on people and their loved ones;
- the role of procedural justice in nursing practice to underpin human connectedness;
- the tensions between the therapeutic relationship and compulsory treatment;
- the role of the nurse in the legal processes and procedures of compulsory assessment and treatment; and
- the alternative approaches to compulsory treatment and legislation.

Critical thinking/learning activities

1 Review the acronym RELATIONSHIPS. Are these principles currently being modelled in clinical practice by other mental health nurses, or by you?
2 Consider the aspects of the procedural justice framework; does it seem easy to implement this framework into your current practice? If not, discuss what may hinder you from doing so.
3 Consider the process of developing an advance directive; if you became physically or mentally unwell, discuss what wishes you would record for your care.
4 Imagine a world with new mental health legislation as described by Mary O'Hagan. How might this affect your current understanding of the role of the mental health nurse?
5 Discuss the advantages and disadvantages of having alternative treatment facilities such as community based crisis houses, in-home options for treatment and care, and suicide prevention houses.

Learning extension

Mary O'Hagan's description of potential future mental health legislation is strongly linked to a human and citizenship rights-based platform. In small groups, discuss how other marginalised groups, such as people living with a disability, have claimed their right to fair and just health care.

Further reading

Fishwick, M., **Tait, B.** & **O'Brien, A.J.** (2001). Unearthing the conflicts between carer and custodian: Implications of participation in Section 16 hearings under the *Mental Health (Compulsory Assessment and Treatment) Act (1992)*. *Australian and New Zealand Journal of Mental Health Nursing*, 10(3): 187–94.
This paper discusses the tensions and conflicts mental health nurses may be confronted with when a person is subjected to compulsory assessment and treatment.
Galon, P.A. & **Wineman, N.M.** (2010). Coercion and procedural justice in psychiatric care: State of the science and implications for nursing. *Archives of Psychiatric Nursing*, 24(5): 307–16.
This paper gives an overview of procedural justice.

Hamilton, B. & **Roper, C.** (2006). Troubling 'insight': Power and possibilities in mental health care. *Journal of Psychiatric and Mental Health Nursing, 13*(4): 416–22.

This paper offers both the mental health nurse's and consumer's view of insight.

Seikkula, J. & **Olson, M. E.** (2003). The open dialogue approach to acute psychosis: Its poetics and micropolitics. *Family Process, 42*(3): 403–18.

This paper is based on a family systems approach, and provides an inclusive process of dialogue with consumers, their loved ones and mental health clinicians.

Stevens, S. (2003). Where is the asylum? In K. Diesfeld & I. R. Freckelton (eds), *Involuntary Detention and Therapeutic Jurisprudence: International perspectives on civil commitment* (pp. 95–112). Aldershot, UK: Ashgate.

This chapter is a first-person account of the effects of compulsory assessment and treatment.

References

Angermeyer, M. C. & **Matschinger, H.** (2003). The stigma of mental illness: Effects of labelling on public attitudes towards people with mental disorder. *Acta Psychiatrica Scandinavica, 108*(4): 304–9.

Angermeyer, M. C., **Matschinger, H.** & **Corrigan, P.** (2004). Familiarity with mental illness and social distance from people with schizophrenia and major depression: Testing a model using data from a representative population survey. *Schizophrenia Research, 69*: 175–82.

Atkinson J. (2007). *Advance directives in mental health. Theory, practice and ethics.* London: Jessica Kingsley Publishers.

Australian Nursing and Midwifery Council (2008). Code of Ethics for Nurses in Australia. Retrieved from &www.nursingmidwiferyboard.gov.au/Search.aspx?q=code%20of%20ethics.

Barnes, M. & **Bowl, R.** (2001). *Taking over the Asylum: Empowerment and mental health.* Basingstoke, UK: Palgrave.

Barnes, M., **Bowl, R.** & **Fisher, M.** (1990). *Sectioned: Social services and the 1983 mental health act.* London: Routledge.

Bartlett, P. (2003). Capacity and confinement: When is detention not detention? In K. Diesfeld & I. R. Freckelton (eds), *Involuntary Detention and Therapeutic Jurisprudence: International perspectives on civil commitment* (pp. 339–58). Aldershot, UK: Ashgate.

Beauchamp, T. L. & **Childress, J. F.** (2013). *Principles of Biomedical Ethics*, 7th edn. New York: Oxford University Press.

Bell, S. (2003). Rights issues in compulsory community treatment. In K. Diesfeld & I. R. Freckelton (eds), *Involuntary Detention and Therapeutic Jurisprudence: International perspectives on civil commitment* (pp. 485–501). Aldershot, UK: Ashgate.

Bennett, B. & **Bennett, A.** (2011). Law, ethics and mental health nursing. In K.-L. Edward, I. Munro, A. Robins & A. Welch (eds), *Mental Health Nursing: Dimensions of praxis* (pp. 88–120). South Melbourne: Oxford University Press.

Bracken, P. & **Thomas, P.** (2001). Postpsychiatry: A new direction for mental health. *British Medical Journal, 322*(7288): 724–7.

Bray, J. (2003). The nurse's role in the administration of ECT. In P. Barker (ed.), *Psychiatric and Mental Health Nursing: The craft of caring* (pp. 466–75). New York: Arnold.

Burns, T., **Rugkasa, J.**, **Molodynski, A.**, **Dawson, J.**, **Yeeles, K.**, **Vazquez-Montes, M.** … & **Priebe, S.** (2013). Community treatment orders for patients with psychosis (OCTET): A randomised control trial. *Lancet, 381*(9878): 1627–33.

Callaghan, S. & **Ryan, C. J.** (2012). Rising to the human rights challenge in compulsory treatment – new approaches to mental health law in Australia. *Australian and New Zealand Journal of Psychiatry, 46*(7): 611–20.

Carney, T., **Tait, D.**, **Vernon, A.**, **Perry, J.** & **Beaupert, F. A.** (2011). *Australian Mental Health Tribunals: Space for fairness, freedom, protection & treatment? Sydney Law School Research Paper.* Retrieved from http://papers.ssrn.com/sol3/papers.cfm?abstract_id=1969713.

Diesfeld, K. & **McKenna, B. G.** (2006a). *Insight and Other Puzzles: Undefined terms in the New Zealand Mental Health Review Tribunal. Summary report.* Wellington: Mental Health Commission.

Diesfeld, K. & McKenna, B. G. (2006b). The therapeutic intent of the New Zealand mental health review tribunal. *Psychiatry, Psychology and Law, 13*(1): 100–9.

Diesfeld, K. & Sjöström, S. (2007). Interpretive flexibility: Why doesn't insight incite controversy in mental health law? *Behavioral Sciences and the Law,* 25(1): 85–101.

Fishwick, M., Tait, B. & O'Brien, A. J. (2001). Unearthing the conflicts between carer and custodian: Implications of participation in Section 16 hearings under the *Mental Health (Compulsory Assessment and Treatment) Act* (1992). *Australian and New Zealand Journal of Mental Health Nursing, 10*(3): 187–94.

Galon, P. A., & Wineman, N. M. (2010). Coercion and procedural justice in psychiatric care: State of the science and implications for nursing. *Archives of Psychiatric Nursing, 24*(5), 307–316.

Hamer, H. P. (2012). Inside the City Walls: Mental Health Service Users' Journeys Towards Full Citizenship. Unpublished PhD thesis, University of Auckland.

Hamer, H. P., Finlayson, M. & Warren, H. (forthcoming). Insiders or outsiders? Mental health service users' journeys towards full citizenship. *International Journal of Mental Health Nursing.*

Hamilton, B. & Roper, C. (2006). Troubling 'insight': Power and possibilities in mental health care. *Journal of Psychiatric and Mental Health Nursing, 13*(4): 416–422.

Hatfield, B. & Antcliff, V. (2001). Detention under the Mental Health Act: Balancing rights, risks and needs for services. *Journal of Social Welfare and Family Law, 23*(2): 135–53.

Hazelton, M. (1999). Psychiatric personnel, risk management and the new institutionalism. *Nursing Inquiry,* 6(4): 224–30.

Health and Disability Commission (n.d.). *Advance directives in mental health care and treatment.* Retrieved from www.hdc.org.nz/publications/resources-to-order/leaflets-and-posters-for-download/advance-directives-in-mental-health-care-and-treatment-(leaflet).

Health and Disability Commission (1996). *The Health and Disability Commissioner (Code of Health and Disability Services Consumers' Rights) Regulations 1996.* Retrieved from www.legislation.govt.nz/regulation/public/1996/0078/latest/DLM209080.html.

Henderson, C., Flood, C., Leese, M., Thornicroft, G., Sutherby, K. & Smukler, G. (2004). Effect of joint crisis plans on use of compulsory treatment in psychiatry: Single blind randomised controlled trial. *British Medical Journal, 329*(7458): 136.

Johnstone, M.-J. (2009). *Bioethics: A nursing perspective,* 5th edn. Sydney: Churchill Livingstone.

Kisely, S., Campbell, L. A., Scott, A., Preston, N. J., & Xiao, J. (2007). Randomized and non-randomized evidence for the effect of compulsory community and involuntary out-patient treatment on health service use: Systematic review and meta-analysis. *Psychological Medicine, 37*(1): 3–14.

Lamb, H. R., Weinberger, L. E. & DeCuir, W. J. Jr. (2002). The police and mental health. *Psychiatric Services, 53*(10): 1266–71.

Lind, E. A., Kanfer, R. & Earley, P. C. (1990). Voice, control, and procedural justice: Instrumental and noninstrumental concerns in fairness judgments. *Journal of Personality & Social Psychology, 59*(5): 952–9.

Longden, E. (2010). Making sense of voices: A personal story of recovery. *Psychosis: Psychological, Social & Integrative Approaches, 2*(3): 255–9.

Mackenzie, S. & Shirlaw, N. (2002). *Mental Health and the Law: A legal resource for people who experience mental illness.* Wellington: Wellington Community Law Centre/Educational Resources.

McKenna, B. G. & O'Brien, A. J. (in press). Mental health nursing and the Mental Health Act. In J. Dawson & K. Gledhill (eds), *New Zealand Mental Health Act.* Wellington: Victoria University Press.

McKenna, B., Thom, K., & Simpson, A. I. F. (2007). Media coverage of homicide involving mentally disordered offenders: A matched comparison study. *International Journal of Forensic Mental Health, 6*(1): 57–63.

McKenna, B. G., Simpson, A. I. F. & Coverdale, J. H. (2003). Patients' perceptions of coercion on admission to forensic psychiatric hospital: A comparison study. *International Journal of Law and Psychiatry, 26*(4): 355–72.

McSherry, B. & Wilson, K. (2011). Detention and treatment down under: Human rights and mental health laws in Australia and New Zealand. *Medical Law Review, 19*(4): 548–80.

Morgan, A. (2008). *Being Human: Reflections on mental distress in society.* Ross-On-Wye, UK: PCCS Books.

Murray, L. (2013). Ko te whānau te kī mo te oranga o te tangata: The family is the key to the wellbeing of the person. *Handover, 23*(23): 12–13. Retrieved from www.tepou.co.nz/library/tepou/handover-issue-23-autumn-2013.

Neilson, G. (2005). The role of mental health legislation. *Canadian Journal of Psychiatry, 50*(11): S1.

Nursing Council of New Zealand (2012). *Code of Conduct for Nurses*. Retrieved from http://nursingcouncil. org.nz.

O'Brien, **A.J.** & **Kar**, **A.** (2012). The role of second health professionals under New Zealand mental health legislation. *Journal of Psychiatric and Mental Health Nursing, 13*(3): 356–63.

Quinn, **M.** (2011). *Mental Health and Human Rights in Victoria*. Retrieved from http://rightnow.org.au/ topics/disability/mental-health-and-human-rights-in-victoria/.

Read, **J.** & **Bentall**, **R.P.** (2010). The effectiveness of electroconvulsive therapy: A literature review. *Epidemiology and Psychiatric Sciences, 19*(4): 333–47.

Richardson, **G.** (2003). Involuntary treatment: Searching for principles. In K. Diesfeld & I.R. Freckelton (eds), *Involuntary Detention and Therapeutic Jurisprudence: International perspectives on civil commitment* (pp. 55–73). Aldershot, UK: Ashgate.

Rose, **N.** (1998). Governing risky individuals: The role of psychiatry in new regimes of control. *Psychiatry, Psychology and Law, 5*(2): 177–95.

Sawyer, **A.-M.** (2005). From therapy to administration: Deinstitutionalisation and the ascendancy of psychiatric 'risk-thinking'. *Health Sociology Review, 14*(3): 283–96.

Sayce, **L.** (2000). *From Psychiatric Patient to Citizen: Overcoming discrimination and social exclusion*. Basingstoke, UK: MacMillan Press.

Seikkula, **J.** & **Olson**, **M.E.** (2003). The open dialogue approach to acute psychosis: Its poetics and micropolitics. *Family Process, 42*(3): 403–18.

Stevens, **S.** (2003). Where is the asylum? In K. Diesfeld & I.R. Freckelton (eds), *Involuntary Detention and Therapeutic Jurisprudence: International perspectives on civil commitment* (pp. 95–112). Aldershot, UK: Ashgate.

The International Council on Human Rights Policy (2006). *Human Rights Standards: Learning from experience*. Retrieved from www.ichrp.org/files/reports/31/120b_report_en.pdf.

Thornicroft, **G.**, **Farrelly**, **S.**, **Szmukler**, **G.**, **Birchwood**, **M.**, **Waheed**, **W.**, **Flach**, **C.** … & **Marshall**, **M.** (2013). Clinical outcomes of joint crisis plans to reduce compulsory treatment for people with psychosis: A randomised control trial. *The Lancet, 381*(9878): 1634–41.

United Nations General Assembly (1948). Universal Declaration of Human Rights. Retrieved from www.un.org/ en/documents/udhr/index.shtml.

United Nations High Commissioner for Human Rights (UNHCHR) (1991). *United Nations Principles of Care and the Improvement of Mental Health Care*. Geneva: Author.

UNHCHR (2006). *Convention on the Rights of Persons with Disabilities and Optional Protocol*. Geneva: Author. Retrieved from www.un.org/disabilities/documents/convention/convoptprot-e.pdf.

Weitz, **D.** (2013). Electroshock: Torture as 'treatment'. *Mad Matters: A critical reader in Canadian mad studies* (pp. 158–69). Toronto: Canadian Scholars' Press.

Wexler, **D.B.** & **Winick**, **B.J.** (eds) (1996). *Law in a Therapeutic Key: Developments in therapeutic jurisprudence*. Durham, NC: Carolina Academic Press.

Wing, **J.K.**, **Beevor**, **A.S.**, **Curtis**, **R.H.**, **Park**, **S.B.**, **Hadden**, **S.** & **Burns**, **A.** (1998). Health of the Nation Outcome Scales (HoNOS). Research and development. *British Journal of Psychiatry, 172*, 11–18.

Winick, **B.J.** (2003). A therapeutic jurisprudence model for civil commitment. In K. Diesfeld & I.R. Freckelton (eds), *Involuntary Detention and Therapeutic Jurisprudence: International perspectives on civil commitment* (pp. 2–54). Aldershot, UK: Ashgate.

7

Mental health and substance use

Rhonda L. Wilson

Introduction 138

Harm minimisation 138

Overview of substance-use problems 139

An overview of drugs and the effects
they have on people 140

Reasons people use drugs and alcohol 145

An holistic framework for understanding
people who use drugs and those who
misuse drugs 146

Mental illness and substance-use problems
in combination with each other 158

Mental health and drug and alcohol models
of care 158

Chapter summary 162

Critical thinking/learning activities 162

Learning extension 162

Acknowledgement 162

Further reading 163

References 163

Learning objectives

At the completion of this chapter, you should be able to:

- Recognise the effects of legal and illegal drugs which, when misused, can adversely affect mental health and well-being.
- Consider the ways in which person-centred care can promote the recovery of people with combined drug, alcohol and mental health problems.
- Identify holistic care opportunities related to professional care of mental illness and drug and alcohol problems.
- Recognise the physical and mental health care needs of people affected by drug misuse.
- Consider how harm minimisation can be implemented to improve mental health outcomes for individuals and communities.

Introduction

This chapter introduces the intersections between mental health care and drug and alcohol care. It addresses the implications for holistic health care needs related to dual drug and alcohol use, and concurrent mental illness. It tells the contemporary, real-life story of a person who developed an episode of psychosis following consumption of premixed alcohol and caffeine drinks. The chapter also describes change models applied to substance use and recovery, such as motivational interviewing and stages of change readiness. Both common and less common drugs and their misuse affect the physical, social, cognitive and mental health dimensions of people with mental illness. Reflective exercises guide readers to consider how they will be able to promote mental health and well-being and minimise drug-related harm to individuals and communities in a practice context.

Harm minimisation

Australian and New Zealand drug policies have been underpinned by a **harm minimisation** philosophy, which has a 'three pillars' approach to implementation: supply reduction, demand reduction and harm reduction. This collaborative approach includes stakeholder partnerships across government agencies, including those responsible for health, education and law enforcement (Department of Health and Ageing, 2011; Ritter, King & Hamilton, 2013). Supply reduction is largely a role for policymakers, legislators and justice systems, while reducing demand and reducing harm to individuals, groups and communities are a focus for health and education service providers. Health services aim to provide enough information to assist people to make healthy lifestyle choices and thereby deter the harmful uptake of drug and alcohol use, and/or to help people reduce or cease the use of harmful drugs and alcohol if this has occurred.

> **harm minimisation**
> a multi-agency drug policy approach, aimed at addressing supply reduction, demand reduction and harm reduction

Reflective questions

Alcohol and tobacco are drugs that are available for purchase in Australia and New Zealand under legally regulated conditions of sale and consumption. Take some time to consider the pros and cons of legalisation and regulation of supply.

- What are the health and social influences and the consequences of alcohol and cigarette smoking in your community?
- Have our laws and regulations achieved a balanced approach to management of these two legal drugs?
- List some changes you would like to see in the future, and explain why.

Overview of substance-use problems

The use of **drugs** can be considered as a problem or 'non-problem', based on the health, social, behavioural and cognitive outcomes related to that use. There are three main groups of drugs that are used or misused for non-therapeutic purposes, described in Table 7.1. It should be noted that there is a range of subjective variability related to the experiences people may have with drugs within these categories (Ritter et al., 2013). For instance, alcohol is a depressant but, when used in small quantities, some people experience behavioural stimulation promoting a sense of social disinhibition, which may be considered a desirable outcome by the person consuming the alcohol (Ritter et al., 2013). In addition to these broad categories, it is important to consider poly drug use, which may include the use of drugs across categories, thereby further complicating the effects of the drug. The setting or context in which the drug is taken along, with the mood in which the drug is consumed, are both important considerations (Zinberg, 1984). Thus, if alcohol is consumed in a context in which the mood is low, and the person is alone, the alcohol effects will most likely reinforce a state of depression. However, if the alcohol is consumed when the person's mood is happy, and in a social and celebratory setting, the alcohol effects more likely will stimulate the drinker's behaviour. An assessment of the drug type, along with the context and mood, will be required in order to understand the dynamics related to an individual's drug experiences.

drugs
in the context of this chapter, the use of legal or illegal substances that have a psychoactive effect on the central nervous system and are taken for the purpose of achieving pleasurable or normative personal experiences

Table 7.1 Drug categories

Depressants	Drugs that cause the central nervous system to be inhibited or depressed. Symptoms include decreased respirations and heart rate.	Examples: alcohol, benzodiazepine (e.g. Valium), opioids (such as heroin, pethadine, morphine, methadone, endone, oxycontin) and cannabis
Stimulants	Drugs that cause an increase in central nervous system activity and arousal. Symptoms include increased heart rate, respirations and blood pressure; increased temperature, especially with amphetamine-based drugs; and some increase in agitation and aggression.	Examples: Methylenedioxymetham-phetamine (known as MDMA, or ecstasy), amphetamines, methamphetamine (known as 'ice'), cocaine, caffeine, nicotine and synthetic, cocaine-like 'bath salts'
Hallucinogens	Drugs that alter the central nervous system so that perceptions, thinking or cognition, feelings or emotions and sense of time or place are distorted. Symptoms include the sometimes-frightening experiences of delusions and paranoia.	Examples: LSD (acid), mescaline (peyote cactus), psilocybin (magic mushrooms), cannabis, kronic/spice (synthetic cannabis) and daytura (stramonium leaf)

An overview of drugs and the effects they have on people

Alcohol

Alcohol is a depressant drug, and it acts to slow heart and respiratory rates. Alcohol is often associated with mood-related conditions, and especially so in people who experience depression (Attenborough, 2010). Alcohol is a legal drug that is the most likely of all drugs to be misused in Australia, and it is sometimes misused by people who attempt to regulate their distress by modifying both low and elevated moods (Attenborough, 2010; Australian Institute of Health and Welfare, 2011). Alcohol is frequently associated with death by suicide (Attenborough, 2010). Suicide is the most significant problem caused by alcohol misuse in Aboriginal men and represents the most common cause of death for this group, while alcohol misuse related to suicide is the fourth-most common cause for deaths among Aboriginal women in Australia (Wilkes et al., 2010). Longer-term, risky alcohol consumption is particularly harmful, with implications for decline in physical and mental health (for example, liver failure and cirrhosis; gastrointestinal haemorrhage and ulceration; depression; alcohol-related dementia). Withdrawal from alcohol dependency should be monitored and managed carefully because abrupt alcohol withdrawal can trigger seizures resulting in death. A carefully managed, gradual withdrawal is required to support a person who has planned to reduce or cease his or her use of alcohol (Mental Health and Drug and Alcohol Office (MHDAO), 2008). In addition, social and psychological support will be needed to provide holistic support for a comprehensive withdrawal (MHDAO, 2008).

Low-risk alcohol consumption consists of no more than two standard drinks per day, and should include some alcohol-free days each week (NHMRC, 2009). A standard drink is equivalent to 10 grams of alcohol. The percentage by volume of alcohol in any drink will differ depending on the type of beverage consumed; for example, in a standard drink of beer, the percentage of alcohol by volume is the same – 10 grams – as in a drink of liquor/spirits (Department of Health and Ageing, 2013). Alcohol is metabolised by the liver, and for a healthy adult it typically takes approximately one hour for the liver to process one standard drink. No more than four standard drinks should be consumed in one sitting, as the risk of alcohol-related injury increases considerably for that episode (NHMRC, 2009; Edward & Alderman, 2013).

binge drinking
drinking alcohol with the intention of drinking of becoming drunk

Binge drinking is described as drinking alcohol with the intention of drinking to become drunk. Young people are more likely to binge drink, with 20 per cent of young people reporting this behaviour (Australian Institute of Health and Welfare, 2011).

Caffeine

Caffeine is a stimulant found in products like tea, coffee, chocolate and cola soft drinks. Increasingly, it is found in premixed alcoholic and non-alcoholic energy drinks. In small doses, caffeine has effects that include increased heart rate, energy and stimulation. This is a pleasant sensation for many people; however, even at low doses withdrawal can result in discomfort such as headaches and agitation. At higher doses and in combination with other drugs, caffeine can contribute to the experiences such as those that Mark reports in his story (see page 150). And, as Mark's story demonstrates, not all people will be aware that they are consuming both alcohol and caffeine in premixed alcoholic beverages.

Cannabis

Cannabis (delta-9 tetra hydro-cannabinol (or THC)) is a drug that is often associated with both depression and psychosis. Attempts to understand causal relationships between the use of cannabis and the experience of these mental health problems have been the subject of much research; however, empirical evidence of a causal relationships in either direction – that is, that cannabis causes psychosis, or that psychosis predisposes people to decisions to consume cannabis – remains elusive, despite the efforts of many researchers (Dubertret et al., 2006; Ferdinand et al., 2005; Fergerson, Horwood & Ridder, 2005; Green, Young & Kavanagh, 2005; Mental Health Council of Australia, 2006; Ritter et al., 2013; Solowij & Michie, 2007).

Cannabis is most commonly consumed by smoking the dried leaves or heads of the cannabis plant, either as a paper-rolled cigarette – sometimes combined with tobacco – or with the use of a water pipe ('bong'). It is also consumed in baked products such as 'hash cookies'. Inhalation provides a fast effect, and for this reason it is most likely to be smoked.

Synthetic drugs

Some synthetic copies of cannabis and other drugs have become prominent in recent times. They are frequently marketed as 'herbal cigarettes', or as incense, in an attempt to connect with customers who are curious and looking for a legal and safe alternative to illegal drugs such as cannabis, amphetamines and cocaine. It is difficult for regulators to keep up with the rapid pace in which these types of drugs are varied and manufactured, and so legislation through therapeutic goods administration and regulation of their sale lag behind in listing new products as illegal substances (Barratt, Cakic & Lenton, 2013). Synthetic cannabinoids are sprayed onto inert plant matter, which is then smoked using the methods typical of cannabis inhalation. Some common names for these substances are 'kronic' and 'spice' (Ritter et al., 2013). These substances should not be considered safe, or a lesser risk, than other known drugs, because it is impossible to accurately know their ingredients and concentration. In the case of kronic, there are known cases of debilitating psychosis and other mental and physical health problems that have been triggered by the use of these drugs (Barratt et al., 2013). Synthetic drugs are best avoided because so little is known about them, and the adverse consequences are thought to be significant. Furthermore, people who use synthetic drugs tend not to seek help (Barratt et al., 2013).

Amphetamines

Amphetamines (sometimes referred to as 'speed') were discovered about 100 years ago, and have been used in a clinical context for much of that time (Heal et al., 2013). However, misuse of amphetamines in its various forms is problematic. Amphetamines act to stimulate the central nervous system. They are consumed in various forms, such as oral tablet or wafer, inhaled nasally, or injected intravenously. People misuse amphetamines in search of pleasurable, alert and energetic effects. This experience usually lasts for several hours, while with continued heavy misuse paranoid, perceptual, cognitive and delusional problems can occur. The resulting behaviours and sensations can be frightening, and they can place individuals in risky circumstances (for example, thinking they are safe to drive at high speeds). The physiological risks include increases to blood pressure, heart rate, respirations and body temperature, with increased body temperature placing individuals at high risk of serious and life-threatening neurological damage, in particular. Amphetamine-style drugs are sometimes considered 'party' drugs (for example, MDMA/ecstasy), and in a party setting where it is hot, there is poor air circulation and cooling, perhaps some dancing and alcohol consumption, the risk of dehydration and elevation in temperature is high.

Methamphetamine

Methamphetamine (sometimes known as 'ice' or 'crystal') is one type of amphetamine that has become popular among people who use stimulant drugs. However, it has some particularly challenging side-effects, which include anger and aggression in combination with psychosis, and these have complicated the care of many people presenting to accident and emergency departments in recent years (Degenhardt, Roxburgh & McKetin, 2007).

Cocaine

Cocaine is a stimulant drug that is usually injected or inhaled, and has many of the same problems and effects as amphetamine drugs. However, the immediate euphoric effects and arousal that is experienced following consumption of cocaine is short-lived and dissipates within a short time – around half an hour. Despite the reduced sensations, the brain continues to be affected, and often with racing thoughts, irritability, depression and insomnia. People sometimes attempt to modify these symptoms with further doses of cocaine, but while the brain remains saturated with the drug, the pleasurable effects are minimal, and a downward neuro-chemical and behavioural spiral unfolds.

Opioids

Opioids are used therapeutically to manage strong pain in the form of injectable (intravenous or intramuscular) morphine and pethadine, or endone and oxycondine in tablet form for pain such as cancer-related pain. Opioids are important clinical medications for the management of both acute and chronic physical pain. However, they are also drugs that are often misused, in the illegal form of heroin in particular. Fentanyl is a potent synthetic opioid that is an effective analgesic, but illegal diversion and use of this drug, when combined with other depressant drugs, has seen a recent increase in deaths among younger men who have a history of using injectable drugs (Roxburgh et al., 2013).

Heroin is usually injected intravenously and has an immediate euphoric affect; however, less commonly it is smoked, which also has a very quick affect. A sensation of relaxation and calm follows use of this drug and this can last several hours. Heroin is a depressant drug and its side-effects include respiratory depression, reduced heart rate and low blood pressure. Combining heroin with other depressant drugs such as alcohol can amplify the physiological responses, and this can lead to unconsciousness and death.

Tolerance builds exponentially with continued misuse of opioids, including heroin which means that people require more of the drug to achieve the desirable effects; however, over time the pleasurable effects are reduced and depression develops. People feel compelled to continue to use this drug to achieve a normal effect, and thus a dependency develops. It is very difficult to break this cycle once it has developed, and the social consequences are complicated because the escalating rates and amounts of use are extremely expensive to maintain, and frequently people become involved in crime, selling their goods, or providing services to others (for example, sexual services) to pay for their supply of drugs. This circumstance is detrimental to the basic requirements of a healthy life, such as the procurement of quality food, housing, clothing, health care and training. The health, social and economic risks are significant for individuals who misuse heroin, and include the risk of infectious diseases such as HIV/AIDS and hepatitis C if needles, syringes or other drug-using paraphernalia are shared between injecting drug users to reduce costs or enhance convenience.

Benzodiazapines

Benzodiazapines (some common trade names include Diazepam/Valium, Temazepam, Lorazepam and Rohypnol) are among a group of drugs that are legal to use but require a medical prescription to obtain. They can be misused and are sometimes obtained illegally on the black market. They are used in a therapeutic form to address the short-term distress of people experiencing anxiety or stress, and, sometimes, to assist in enhancing sleep. Benzodiazepines are only effective for short-term treatment of acute conditions; however, once they are introduced for longer-term use, or misuse, they are extremely difficult to withdraw from. The side-effects are very uncomfortable and include depression, anxiety, panic attacks, psychosis, hallucinations, insomnia and nightmares. People who choose to withdraw from benzodiazepines usually need a great deal of clinical support, which might include cognitive behavioural therapy, motivational interviewing and change management to achieve withdrawal or reduction in their drug use.

Benzodiazepines are extremely effective depressive drugs, and they will dampen the mood; this sometimes makes people think that they are lacking any feeling or emotion at all. To counteract this, some people combine benzodiazapines with other drugs, such as alcohol, to enhance a sense of sociability and confidence. However, the risks associated with this include a bolstered sense of being indestructible, and it is in this condition that coordination is impaired, and sense of self-confidence is high, when risks are taken that can have consequences compromising the safety of the person misusing the drugs, other people and/or property.

Nicotine

Nicotine is found in tobacco cigarettes. It is a drug that is associated with harm, both to physical and mental health. Nicotine stimulates dopamine neuro-chemical responses and promotes a sense of calm and well-being; however, during withdrawal, anxiety, stress and depression are likely to be experienced (Edward & Alderman, 2013). People with mental illness are twice as likely as the general population to smoke cigarettes (Lawrence, Mitrou & Zubrick, 2009). Smoking increases the risk of respiratory and cardiac diseases, and these are major contributors to the total burden of disease for Australia and New Zealand. Nicotine influences the metabolism of caffeine and some medications for mental illness; any reduction or cessation of smoking may also reduce the effective dosage rate of some medications, thereby reducing the effects of high doses and related side-effects (Edward & Alderman, 2013).

Solvents

Solvents are volatile substances. They either vaporise or evaporate when they come in contact with air. People who inhale or sniff these substances are at immediate risk of neurological and/or cardiac and/or respiratory risk, which can include irreparable damage to the brain and cardiac systems. There is no way to assess which episode of use will cause irreversible damage, and the risk is exceedingly high. Solvents are found in products such as aerosol cans, glues, petrol and other fuels, nail polish and correction fluids. People who inhale these solvents experience an immediate effect of the gaseous toxins, which enter the blood stream and central nervous system extremely quickly, followed by a momentary sensation of euphoria that dissipates quickly. Regular use increases tolerance, and this promotes the use of increased doses and increased frequency of use to achieve the desired outcomes, which in turn amplifies the risks. Solvents are relatively cheap to purchase and they can be easily obtained from a range of common household products, and this availability has an influence on use and access.

Communities in central Australia have identified a particular problem with a high number of young people inhaling petrol, and government, community and retail stakeholders are working together to explore ways to minimise the risks to the population in regard to petrol sniffing. One intervention has reduced the availability of opal petrol fuel and has increased availability of petrol modified to remove harmful volatile solvents and thereby minimise supply of a substance known to cause harm to people (Schwartzkoff et al., 2008).

Paracetemol

Paracetemol and other over-the-counter medications are sometimes used in suicide attempts, or as a method of self-harm. Some people who overdose on products such as paracetemol report that they do so in an attempt to ease emotional discomfort, and sometimes with a view that they would like to 'go to sleep and not have to wake up'. Frequently, people are not aware of the serious consequences of paracetemol toxicity. Paracetemol toxicity can cause life-threatening liver failure and sometimes requires admission to a critical care unit in a hospital so that liver function can be carefully monitored (Daly et al., 2008). Nausea, vomiting and abdominal pain (right upper-quadrant) may signify excessive use of paracetamol. If a person is receiving care in a critical care unit, then consideration should be given to the physical environment, in which there may be many accessible and lethal means of suicide available. Close monitoring in regard to mental health safety and ongoing mental health assessment in conjunction with building a therapeutic rapport are equally as important as the management for prevention of liver failure.

Understanding the time delay between the taking of excess paracetamol and admission to health care will influence the selection of treatment protocols. If within one hour, an orally administered, activated charcoal may be a sufficient response. Up to eight hours following ingestion and based on the extent of liver function, obtained through a blood test, a decision needs to be made about the level of toxicity and whether intravenous infusion of N-acetylcysteine may need to be commenced, measured against the paracetamol toxicity nomograph tool (Daly et al., 2008). If ingestion is known to be longer than eight hours prior to receiving health care, then an N-acetylcysteine infusion is likely to be commenced immediately, and liver function monitoring commenced (Daly et al., 2008). If other drugs such as alcohol are also present, this adds further clinical complexity and risk, especially as alcohol is metabolised largely in the liver (Daly et al., 2008). It may be difficult to ascertain a clear history of ingestion of tablets and alcohol if the person is intoxicated, sedated or cognitively compromised. There are no pleasurable effects following use of paracetamol. A vulnerability for repeating overdose of paracetamol has been identified at four weeks following the initial episode, and therefore mental health follow-up is warranted during this period to the reduce risk (Ayonrinde et al., 2005). The safe use of paracetamol is described by New South Wales health polices and clinical guidelines (NSW Health, 2009).

Reasons people use drugs and alcohol

There are some common explanations for drug use. For some people, the pleasure and reward sensations derived from drug use influences and reinforces their drug use or misuse (Heal et al., 2013). For others, drug use creates a normative environment in which people consider they can think, behave or socialise effectively (Ritter et al., 2013). Still others might choose to use drugs (e.g. steroids, peptides) to enhance their performance; for example, in sports. The use of drugs to enhance performance is beyond the scope of this chapter. Readers who are interested to know more about this topic should explore the Australian Sports Anti-Doping Authority's website (www.asada.gov.au) to learn more.

Reflective questions

- Do you, or does anyone close to you drink wine, beer or other types of alcohol? Why? Reflect on when either you, or others you know well, drink alcohol. How does it make you, or them, feel? Is there any pleasure associated with alcohol consumption? Does it help you/them to 'fit in' with others in a social context? Could you/they manage without alcohol? Does it matter?
- Write a short, reflective paragraph about your experiences with alcohol. How have your experiences shaped your views and beliefs about alcohol consumption, and how will this influence your health care of others?

An holistic framework for understanding people who use drugs and those who misuse drugs

Mental health professionals are often in the position to provide care for people who have both a mental illness and a drug and/or alcohol problem, and the combination of these problems can result in increasingly complex situations for people. Both mental illness and drug and alcohol problems often need to be managed simultaneously to produce a good health outcome for people. This is difficult to achieve for a range of reasons, not the least of which is that some health services designate these problems to different streams of care, or service providers, and therefore the coordination and transition of meaningful, comprehensive health care is difficult to achieve for people with a dual diagnosis. Health care professionals should consider how they might achieve a seamless and coordinated approach to the care of people with mental illness and drug and alcohol problems, and they should work towards an holistic model of care, despite the challenges of service delivery structures and classification systems.

Holistic care models value an approach that is person-centred and recognises that people and their health and well-being are affected by a variety of life circumstances. Health and well-being cannot be fully understood without taking into consider the *biological, psychological, social, cultural, spiritual, developmental and ecological* elements of human life experiences. Nurses should take active leadership roles in further developing meaningful, combined mental health and drug and alcohol care. Nursing models of care are central to minimising the harm and promoting health related to these types of problems. A nursing framework is pivotal to understanding how to deliver holistic care to people who have combined mental illness and drug and alcohol problems. Central to nursing is the concept that health and well-being, health promotion and recovery are critical for individuals, families and communities.

Biological influences on the experiences of mental health and substance use

A broad understanding of the biological explanations of brain functioning is important if we are to understand the mental health and drug and alcohol implications and if we are to reduce the burden of related health problems in our society. The brain contains around 100 billion neurons (brain cells), each with multiple dendrites that receive incoming information and an axon that sends information outwards; together these neurons, dendrites and axon culminate in about 1000 synapses for each neuron. That translates into about 100 trillion connections within the brain. The synaptic gap between neurons is where messages transfer along the nervous system to achieve actions. Simply stated, the synapses are activated by electrical impulses and neuro-chemicals, and these trigger the transfer of messages along the neural pathways (Blows, 2011).

Some neuro-chemicals of particular interest to the study of drug and alcohol dependence and mental illness include serotonin (because it influences a sense of contentment), dopamine (because it influences motivation levels) and adrenaline (because of its capacity to trigger stimulation and alertness) (Blows, 2011). These neuro-chemicals are also described as neuro-transmitters. When triggered, a neuro-transmitter (which is shaped like a key) travels across the synaptic gap to locate a neuro-receptor (shaped like a keyhole to match the key), and a chemical message is transferred along a neural pathway. For example, to achieve the sensation of contentment, sufficient levels of serotonin need to be available to adequately saturate the synaptic gap, and at the same time there needs to be an equally sufficient quantity of serotonin receptors ready to receive the transmission of the serotonin. Too few, too many or unequal supplies of receptor and transmitter chemicals, and a vulnerability exists for mental illness or drug and alcohol problems to develop (Blows, 2011). This physiological process goes some way to explaining the influence chemicals have on our mood and cognitive functions.

Chocolate and its biological effects on the brain

Any drugs (and sometimes foods) that alter the chemical balance in our brains will have consequences for our mood and cognition (Cornah & Van De Weyer, n.d.; Van De Weyer, 2005). Chocolate consumption provides a useful way to describe this process. Most people have some experience of eating chocolate and can attest to a temporary enhancement of their mood after consumption! Chocolate gives us a boost continued ›

Chocolate and its biological effects on the brain continued ›

of a neuro-chemical called noradrenalin. Noradrenalin boosts our sense of pleasure in, and enthusiasm for, life and it has an immediate effect. The brain is stimulated and begins to down-regulate in an effort to get back to a state of homeostasis. With the flood of chocolate or noradrenalin, the brain receptors start to close down to noradrenalin until the excess can be metabolised, which in turn prompts the person consuming the chocolate to increase her or his intake (that is, the person eats more chocolate) in order to achieve a release of noradrenalin that the brain now sense it is missing. This results in an imbalance, with more neuro-transmitters and fewer neuro-receptors. To stop this cycle, the brain needs to use up the oversupply of neuro-chemicals and return to homeostasis, but to do so the person needs to stop eating chocolate. Thus, a period of depressed mood will follow, before homeostasis can be achieved again. It is a vicious cycle in some respects but it is this general process that, in part, describes some of the science behind the craving sensations that can be experienced in relation to chocolate, and the general idea can be extrapolated towards an understanding of the neuro-dynamics related to other drugs. Despite this, people usually repeat the experience of eating chocolate. This analogy mirrors experiences of other drugs by some people.

Cognitive brain activities, such as learning and memory, are triggered by the repetitive firing of synapses (Blows, 2011; Geake, 2009). The more frequently a synaptic pathway is accessed for cognitive activity the more that pathway is thickened and reinforced, and the easier it is to retrieve the information or memory that is needed; thus the phrase 'neurons that fire together, wire together' (Bennett, 2008a; Blows, 2011; Geake, 2009). People need to have cognitive functionality that is adaptive so that logical decisions can be formulated, problems solved and appropriate behaviours selected (Geake, 2009). Where thinking is slowed, or delays in cognitive processing occur, capacity for risk is accentuated. For example, cannabis is known to interrupt cognitive functioning, and this is problematic in a practical setting in which perceptual skill is required and decisions need to be made quickly and accurately, such as when driving a motor vehicle.

Long-term use of drugs such as cannabis alters the wiring structure and firing capacity of neural pathways, and this can result in perceptual changes that can in part explain some of the symptoms of mental illnesses such as psychosis (Blows, 2011). However, there is evidence to suggest that the brain has some limited capacity to recover and learn new pathways in a process known as plasticity, and it can best do this if cannabis is eliminated from the neuro-chemical environment (Early Psychosis Writing Group, 2010).

Psychological influences on the experiences of mental health and substance use

Psychological explanations for drug use and misuse also contribute to an holistic understanding of this topic. Exploring patterns of behaviours displayed by people who use drugs, and the cause and effect relationships in connection to human behaviours and experiences, is relevant to the general mental health and well-being of people. A psychological perspective of holistic mental health care seeks to describe and classify behaviours and to look for normal and abnormal parameters for a range of behaviours and experiences. Understanding why people use drugs will help to identify ways in which drug misuse can be reduced. Some people choose to use drugs because they experience satisfying sensations of pleasure in doing so, and generally pleasurable experiences are ones that people choose to replicate in the future (Ritter et al., 2013). Thus, interventions that acknowledge the satisfying experiences of pleasure related to experience of drug use, can assist people to identify new and safe ways in which to experience satisfying life experiences and reduce their drug use, will in turn promote mental health and reduce the risk of harm.

Some people use drugs because they consider that it will assist them by bolstering their confidence in stressful situations (Ritter et al., 2013). Their experiences form a basis from which they have learned to cope in response to stress or anticipated stress, and this then is the underlying mechanism that reinforces future behaviours. Drug use represents a very limited repertoire from which to draw coping skills, and unless others skills are developed, and as tolerance to drugs increases, the only avenue available to solve stress-related problems is to increase drug use. As drug use increases, so, too, does the risk of harm associated with drug misuse, and perhaps, drug dependence. This escalating spiral is a very uncomfortable human experience, and interventions that aim to build a healthy range of coping strategies related to stress management will alleviate the distress that accumulates for people and will also reduce the harm associated with their continued harmful drug use. It is of particular importance to recognise the human distress that accompanies harmful drug use, and for mental health care delivery to work towards supporting a person towards recovery.

For some people, the experience of psychological trauma or adversity precipitates vulnerability in regard to the uptake and use of drugs or alcohol. For example, complex mental health and drug alcohol problems sometimes develop as a result of an experience of child sexual abuse, or other childhood abuses. It is not the aim of this chapter to explore the consequences of abusive circumstances in any depth, but rather to note that frequently the combination of mental illness and drug and alcohol problems are linked to early life trauma.

Social influences on the experiences of mental illness and substance use

Social interactions are powerful components of human experience. Social connectedness is a critical aspect of a developed sense of self-esteem and confidence. Social interactions also carry a degree of vulnerability, as relationships between people can be sensitive to change, and sometimes flexibility and adaption are difficult to achieve when perspectives or circumstances differ. Some social anxiety is useful because it helps to self-moderate behaviour; however, when anxiety becomes disabling or distressing people often explore ways to deal with this tension. Some choose to isolate themselves from certain social settings, while others choose to utilise drugs to assist in overcoming, or dampening, a sense of anxiety. Alcohol is often used and misused in this way, to achieve a normalising and sociable affect in Australian and New Zealand communities. In rural settings, the local public bar (pub) might be a location for social meetings (and in some communities might be the only avenue for social exchange), thus the setting, and the context, are both linked to the consumption of alcohol. This is by no means problematic for all people; however, for a vulnerable few, the combination of social setting, context and alcohol can pose some risks, and these risks need to be considered in terms of the health and well-being (and the minimisation of harm) for individuals and their communities. Mark's story provides an example of social setting and context in relation to alcohol consumption.

Consumer narrative — Mark's story part one: Social setting and context

Having a few days of leave from work, I went into the city to catch up with a couple of mates I went to university with about 10 years ago.

It was nearing midnight when I arrived at the club. The music was loud and it was very warm. I usually drink vodka and soda with fresh lime. I went to order one and was told they did not serve anything in a glass after midnight. The bar staff said they had a similar drink, but would need to decant it into a plastic cup. I assumed all was fine and didn't think to ask what it was.

Cultural influences on experiences of mental illness and substance use

People are inherently cultural creatures (Kellert, 2012). We are influenced by the culture in which we are immersed in our day-to-day lives. Culture influences our attitudes and our practices with regard to drugs and alcohol. The following examples highlight the diversity of culture and drug or alcohol interactions.

Kava is an active ingredient in the root of a pepper plant (*piper methysticum*). It is used in Pacific Islander communities and in the northern parts of Australia as a part of cultural ceremonies and social interactions. The effects of kava include sedation and relaxation and, on occasion, psychosis in some individuals (Ritter et al., 2013). The use of kava is intertwined with ceremony and culture, and therefore the social value of this drug is relevant to note. However, there are detrimental consequences in relation to frequent consumption of kava that need to be considered carefully. Legislation exists to minimise the health, social and economic harms associated with use of kava (Northern Territory Government of Australia, 2011).

Another example is the prevalence of cigarette smoking among Aboriginal and Torres Strait Islander people, which occurs at a much higher incidence than non-Indigenous people. By way of contrast, the interventions offered in Australia to promote smoking cessation are predominantly targeted towards non-Indigenous people. It has been identified that the cultural basis of interventions such as those offered by Quitline may need to be developed in order to better target health promotion and prevention campaigns that align with Aboriginal and Torres Strait Islander cultures so that healthy outcomes are improved for this section of the community (Cosh et al., 2013).

Spiritual/meaning-making influences on experiences of mental illness and substance use

Making meaning from life experiences and circumstances is very important for people. We strive to understand how and why our experiences influence our views of the world, and these experiences have a depth of personal influence that develops our character. Our ability to find some experiences deeply satisfying or meaningful, and to develop a hopefulness for the future, are important aspects of a rich personal inner life, and for some people these experiences have a religious dimension. However, for all people it could be considered that these matters are deeply spiritual. In the real-life story of Mark, which is interwoven in this chapter, Mark expresses something of what it is like to reflect on his life circumstances and to make sense of what happened to him.

Developmental influences on experiences of mental illness and substance use

We know that long-term and risky use of drugs such as alcohol and cannabis adversely affect cognitive brain function (MHDAO, 2009; Mental Health Council of Australia, 2006), and this is especially relevant when we consider that the human brain does not complete its developmental growth phrase until about the age of 22 years (Blows, 2011). Cognitive flexibility is important so that people can learn and remember information, and can then select appropriate information to solve problems and make decisions. This process is used in every developmental stage of life; however, the brain structure that has not completed developmental maturation is vulnerable to damage occurring during the developmental phase (Bennett, 2008b; Blows, 2011). Alcohol and drug use pose risks to the developing brain and can compromise, or slow, both the availability of neurochemicals and the synaptic actions.

Ecological influences on experiences of mental illness and substance use

Family systems and social systems place significant influences on the people within those groups (Kellert, 2012). It is necessary for people to have an environment that fosters thriving and surviving, otherwise mental health will be compromised. Drug and alcohol exposure and misuse can represent a toxic environment, and unless these influences can be minimised, vulnerabilities and risks to mental health will occur.

So – what is it like experience a drug-related mental illness? Mark's story gives us a real-life example to learn from, and to recognise aspects for both the client and the clinician that influence a respectful and holistic recovery journey.

Consumer narrative

Mark's story part two: Recognising that something is not quite right and trying to get some help

A few hours later I left the club. I recall catching a taxi to a suburb about 10 minutes away from the city. I then purchased a ticket to go on a train to an outlying suburb, about 30 minutes further out of town. When I left the train I felt an urge that I needed help. I felt incredibly drunk and was in a very unfamiliar location.

I made my way out of the train station and towards the sound of music. I recall seeing a payphone and decided to call a taxi to take me to the nearest hospital. When I arrived at the hospital, I made my way to the triage nurse. She looked at me and said I looked fine. I tried to explain that I didn't feel right, but I didn't know what was wrong with me and I couldn't really explain why I felt something was wrong with me. I said I thought my drink had been spiked. She was about to dismiss me for a second time, then decided to allow me to lie down on an emergency room bed. I couldn't articulate what was wrong with me, but I just knew I didn't feel right. I noticed a group of police officers talking to her after I was allowed onto the bed.

It is a very confusing and unsettling situation for people who experience perceptual and cognitive changes as a consequence of drug or alcohol use, especially if they have not experienced these types of situations before. In the next part of Mark's story he gives a vivid account of his experiences of perceptual changes and paranoid thought processes.

Consumer narrative

Mark's story part three: The accident and emergency department experience during an acute episode of drug and alcohol-induced psychosis

I recall my thoughts starting to become more paranoid. This was because no doctor had seen me and I felt I was not being taken seriously. I recall the sounds of the nurses' voices becoming distorted. They were some 20 metres away but I could hear, crystal clear, what they were saying; or at least, what I think was them. Time didn't really seem to have any boundaries.

One of the nurses approached and tried to make me admit what I had taken to make me feel the way I was. I tried to explain my evening, but she was adamant that I must have taken something; that it was normal to feel the way I did. I tried to explain that I have never consumed any drugs in my life, not even a cigarette. Her questioning kept making me feel more paranoid.

The doctor came over to see me. He asked if I would like to have some tests done to see what is causing me to feel the way I was. I consented and was escorted

continued ›

to a toilet, where I gave a urine sample. I recall returning with it and hesitating to hand it over, fearing that if my drink was spiked and drugs were detected, what would happen to my reputation? Would the police be involved?

The next period became very intense. I started to feel my body tense up and my thoughts become more paranoid. At the time, they just appeared to be what I thought was reality. The examination light overhead turned into a lie detector. It was used by the nurse and police (who I thought were in the bed next to me) to read my thoughts. They would talk or ask questions, and whatever my first thought or opinion was, would be used to determine whether I was telling the truth. If I lied, a particular sound would be heard. If I told the truth a different sound would be heard. The curtains were drawn around my cubicle so I could not see anyone. All I could focus on was this object above my bed.

The voices and questions started off from the nursing and medical staff. Sometimes, I could hear the voices of the police, who I thought were investigating me. As time went by, I thought I was being set up for something I had not done, so I had to prove them wrong. I worked out that if I used my mental powers to disarm the lie detector they would not be able to read my thoughts. I felt violated by the interrogation of the hospital staff. I became less trusting of anyone who made an approach to me. I thought they were on the 'other side'.

I learned at times to overcome the power of the machine by focusing on saying 'I love my mum and dad'. Both my parents had passed away – one in 2002 and the other in 2010. I can never recall ever saying to them in my life that I loved them, but somehow, if I focused on my love for them, it stopped the machine from reading my thoughts. This went on for what felt like hours.

The questions became more personal and the intensity of the experience increased ten-fold. The voices changed from the medical staff to people from my past, some former students I have taught, current and former colleagues and my extended family. They asked many personal questions, for which only I would have known the answers. Many of the questions were mistakes or oversights I had made in my life. Not remembering to mark a particular question in the detail that I should have, relying on third-hand information about a particular incident are examples. Normally small issues, but with this 'machine' everyone was asking questions.

The voices increased even more in intensity. Rather than the machine having one person speak, all of a sudden more voices appeared and people were in groups, asking questions. At one stage, there were at least four groups asking questions at the same time, often with competing responses from me. If I heard one question, but thought a response for a different question, it meant I was lying and a sound would indicate that.

I never actually saw any of the people. I could recall very clearly their questions and their voices, but I never saw them. At one stage, I remember thinking it would have been impossible to fly everyone there in time to ask the questions. This sense of reason quickly disappeared as the onslaught of questions continued.

continued ›

Consumer narrative continued ›

> There came a point, when I realised I was about to go to gaol. I don't know why I thought that, but it was at this point I felt incredibly fatigued and unable to fight the power of all these questions. I recall believing that a bedside court hearing for bail was being conducted. Again, all of this was behind the curtains. I didn't actually see anything.

Mark goes on to tell us how he began to lose hope and he felt tired and worn out, and was no longer able to communicate effectively. Eventually, he was subjected to the relevant section of the Mental Health Act and was required to be transported to an involuntary mental health unit because he was experiencing a psychotic episode. Read on to gain some insights into his experiences.

Consumer narrative
Mark's story part four: Ideas about dying, losing hope and safety

I thought about just being dead. I knew somehow I couldn't kill myself – I was in a hospital – but if I willed myself to die, that would make this all end. I felt a need to admit defeat as I could no longer keep up. I just lost focus on trying to fight them, and just let them ask the questions. I lost a sense of wanting to prove I was not lying in my thoughts.

There came a point when a doctor, a psychiatrist, came to ask me some questions. I had incredible difficulty focusing on his questions, as I could hear all of these sounds taking place and all these questions being asked of me from all these voices. I would try my hardest to focus on him, but I just couldn't answer sometimes because I was looking at him, but hearing all these other questions. I couldn't keep up.

There came a point when I just remember falling asleep. I was so fatigued and I couldn't put up with this anymore.

I woke and the voices had stopped. I was unsure what had happened. Had they left, had they got what they wanted? It was surreal. I didn't know what was happening, but the voices and the sounds had stopped.

The psychiatrist explained that I was being 'scheduled' and that I had elevated levels of alcohol and caffeine in my system. He explained that I had a psychosis and that I needed to get help. I knew what he was saying, but the question in my mind was, 'How'?

The people Mark met along the way each had an influence on his recovery experience. Some (but not all) of the health services staff members were able to convey respect, care and helpfulness, and where this was achieved, Mark felt supported. The unfamiliar environment and people in an involuntary mental health unit, combined with a sense of personal embarrassment and uncertainty, is both a confronting and uncomfortable personal experience. Mark shares some of this discomfort.

Consumer narrative

**Mark's story part five:
Fear and the experiences of being cared for as an involuntary client in an acute bed-based mental health setting**

I was prepared for transport. Security staff came to my bed and assisted me out of the emergency room and into a patient transport vehicle. I recall feeling very embarrassed, as by this stage I thought I looked a wreck. I recall getting into the transport vehicle and being told they were taking me to Inverness. I became concerned as I had driven to Sydney, and what would happen to my car? The nurse, who was with me, became concerned and tried to explain that I had no choice. I understood that, but why Inverness? The hospital there is much smaller. I was settling into what I thought was a six-hour drive. Within about 10 minutes, I arrived at this facility and was told we had arrived. I was hesitant to question why it took so little time. I thought my sense of time was still distorted. Upon walking out of the van, I discovered that Inverness was actually the name of facility, not the name of the country hospital I had thought I was being transferred to. I was relieved.

Once inside, I met the nurse in charge. He was rather large, but very polite. He started a conversation about what I did for work, where I lived etc. He seemed friendly. When I explained to him these details, he looked at me as though he didn't believe me. My belongings – wallet keys etc. were handed over and I was escorted to a room. I walked through the doors. I could hear screams, voices and noises. I hesitated for a moment, questioning in my own mind if they were real or not. I walked past one room where a large, bearish man was banging and screaming on the door. I could see faeces down the glass panel.

I was shown to my room and my door was opened. I was told that if I heard voices or needed anyone, to press a button in my room. I was assured that only staff could get into my room. I was given some paperwork to read over – my rights and what would happen during this process.

I lay on the bed and could hear the screams and yelling through the air-conditioning ducts. I knew they were real and I looked for logical explanations. I was still trying to understand what I had just been through. I was cautious not to rely on my thoughts because I couldn't be sure that this was not just another trick being played on me.

Mental health care services are offered in somewhat public settings, and often people receiving care are in close social proximity with each other. Safety is a high priority, and clinicians are responsible for regularly monitoring the safety of the people they are helping. Consideration also needs to be given to the privacy and reputation of people within such a setting. In Mark's excerpt below he describes how he found the care environment to be challenging.

Consumer narrative

**Mark's story part six:
The experience of person-centred and respectful care**

Morning came. I was asked to shower. I went into a cubical, where there were cameras. I'm a rather private person, so knowing that I needed a shower but had to shower with others watching made me rather uncomfortable. After the shower, it was time to make my way to breakfast. It was at this point I could see the other people I had heard earlier. I felt they were strange. I sensed they were heavily medicated. We sat to eat breakfast with plastic knives and forks. The staff members were nice and friendly, and did whatever they could to ensure I felt comfortable at breakfast.

After breakfast I watched the news on TV. The other people were pacing around the rooms. One gentleman was exceptional with poetry. Staff would give him a topic or word and he would recite or give a poem that lasted hours. His language was sophisticated and he appeared to be very knowledgeable. I recall another person who called herself Miss Monica. She had difficulty keeping her clothes on and would spit at other people. Several times she was excluded to a separate area. Time and time again, staff treated her with respect.

Consumer narrative

**Mark's story part seven:
The importance of therapeutic rapport**

At 11.00 a.m. I was due for a meeting with a team of psychiatrists who would make the assessment about whether I needed to be scheduled for 72 hours or if I could be released. There were two. One, a younger lady who took notes and did not speak, and an older lady, who asked all the questions. I felt this older lady was particularly rude. She was the only person who I can recall who didn't show any respect. She attempted to lecture me about drinking and putting myself in a vulnerable state. She said I should be ashamed of myself. What was I thinking? No matter how I attempted to reason with her, she would not accept my position. I was fearful that if I challenged her too much, she would be offended and would schedule me for longer. I didn't want to stay. I needed to play her game. Rather than verbally denigrate her and her 'professional conduct', I just copped it on the chin.

I was released. I was allowed out the back door. I thanked the staff and congratulated them on a good job. They had shown compassion to the patients and I felt assured they cared for them. There was never any treatment of those vulnerable people that made me feel uncomfortable.

It is important that the interprofessional connections between clinicians and ancillary staff occur respectfully and seamlessly. Building a therapeutic rapport with people enhances communication and supports recovery. Mark was able to identify clinicians with whom he could develop a rapport, and other clinicians with whom there were significant barriers. In the next section of Mark's story he relays how he felt and coped with the various types of communication he was exposed to during his stay in hospital. On reflection, Mark started the process of making meaning of his life experiences. He shares some of the conclusions that he has drawn about his experiences, and what this will mean for his future.

Consumer narrative   Mark's story part eight: Meaning making and recovery

I spent the next few days with family, trying to overcome and piece together what really had happened. I was trying to figure out how I could move forward. This was a time of deep personal reflection. This event had changed my life.

I made the decision to sell many of my personal assets in the months that followed this experience. I left the job I was in and returned to teaching. I felt comfortable that this experience was an act of God. I obviously had many unresolved matters in my life that I needed to finalise or set to order, and the time was right. I felt a sense of inner peace.

Today, I get worried sometimes when I hear sounds or have strange thoughts. I have to check to make sure they are not foreign thoughts. I never want to experience this again.

So, what was in my system to cause this episode? I had been drinking an alcohol beverage that was heavily laden with caffeine and alcohol. Each single serve (250 millilitres) contained 1.9 standard drinks and significant amounts of caffeine. I'm a non-coffee drinker (including a non-energy drink consumer), so caffeine in my system, no matter how much, is significant. I've only ever had about two coffees in my life, and prior to this experience my last coffee was in 2006, and then I stayed awake for 12 hours after consuming the single cup of coffee (at about 5.00 p.m). I had consumed in the space of three hours the equivalent to 28 standard alcoholic drinks and the equivalent of approximately 30 cups of coffee. That's what they believed caused the episode. My blood tests returned no other traces of drugs.

How could this happen to a well-educated, 30-year-old professional who has spent much of his life working with young people and warning them of these types of problems? How could I have allowed this to happen? Being naïve. Had I just questioned the staff about the alcoholic beverage at the club, this could have been avoided. Had the sweetness of the drink not masked the strong alcohol and caffeine content, this could have been avoided. Had the club served the alcohol beverage in its original packaging, this may have been avoided.

Was this an act of God? I'm not sure. I carry my faith with me and I hold strongly to the power of the experience. It has made me more humble and wise. It has taught me, that even the most innocent people can have such experiences, all because of one foolish mistake.

I have to live with this experience for the rest of my life. The memories and voices have faded over time, but the conviction of the experience is still very strong in my mind.

Mental illness and substance-use problems in combination with each other

Mark's story demonstrates some characteristics of the mental health problems that can occur with drug and alcohol use. This real-life event also demonstrates how easily and rapidly such problems can develop, how frightening the experiences can be and how important it is for health professionals from all disciplines to work together in a collaborative and respectful manner. Drug and alcohol use have implications for the mental health and well-being of people, and the inverse is true, too; personal experiences of mental health and well-being can influence the type, extent and experiences of drug and alcohol. It can been seen from Mark's story that judgement, blame, invoking embarrassment and reinforcing stigma are not useful positions for the people being helped or the health professionals responsible for helping, and that these positions serve to promote discomfort rather than recovery. A more helpful approach is one that is respectful of the person and is both polite and caring, and that these characteristics promote hope for the future. Mark's story is a very powerful one; he is a well-educated young man and someone who is able to reflect on his own experiences and convey the meaning of those experiences to others very clearly. But not all people are as skilled as Mark in this regard. Many people may not be able to describe their feelings and experiences in such a clear way.

Reflective questions

- Think about what it would be like to be in Mark's shoes. How do you think it might feel? What if you thought no one believed you? How would you act? What would you choose to say, or not say?

Mental health and drug and alcohol models of care

Traditionally, mental health services and drug and alcohol services have operated as 'silos' of care; occasionally, health services have been able to integrate care so that people with both mental illness and substance use problems can receive simultaneous care. Withdrawal experiences from drugs and alcohol can be very uncomfortable for many people, and many people will benefit from the support of interprofessional mental health and drug and alcohol support during this time. Most public health services have clinical guidelines to promote recovery experiences (MHDAO, 2008).

Motivational interviewing

Motivational interviewing may be a useful strategy to start a conversation with a person with a drug and alcohol problem (Miller & Rollnick, 2002). The aim of motivational interviewing is to engage people towards a future in which they are less ambivalent and more engaged and motivated to work towards the changes they will need to make in their lives to minimise the risk of drug-related harm. Initiating and instilling hope for the future is also a useful mental health intervention, and so the same model is useful across both clinical problems.

Stages of the change

Understanding the dynamics related to the **readiness to change** is a useful framework for drug and alcohol care, and can also apply to mental health care. Distinct phases are evident, and they are: precontemplation (no recognition that a change in behaviour is warranted), contemplation (recognition of a need to change, marked with some ambivalence), preparation (engaged in planning for a sustainable life change), action (change behaviour has commenced, including cessation or reduction in drug or alcohol use), maintenance (the desired change has become embedded in a lifestyle for a substantial period of time) and exit/relapse (an exit from the cycle occurs where no relapse has occurred for a long period of time, or a trigger event occurs and the person returns to the original behaviour) (Prochaska, DiClemente & Norcross, 1992). A skilled clinician is able to apply an understanding of these phases and to assist and motivate people towards phases of action to reduce the harmful effects of drugs and alcohol, to promote health and well-being in a maintenance phase and to assist people to recognise triggers that may result in relapse, with a view to intervention so as to prevent relapse. This process may need to be followed a number of times before an exit is achieved; however, there are health gains when periods of action and maintenance become longer, and relapses become shorter.

> **readiness to change**
> a multi-dimensional state concerned with a change in health behaviour; readiness to change is marked by both cognitive and behavioural phases, including precontemplation, contemplation, preparation, action, maintenance and exit/relapse. In later stages of readiness to change, people are actively doing things to change or maintain the changes they have been able to make

Solution-focused therapy

Solution-focused therapy is a person-centred approach towards helping people with drug and alcohol problems and with mental illness, which explores personal strengths, resources for coping and a vision for a healthy future (Wand, 2010). The clinician aims to help the person to explore and elaborate on what is going well at the moment (rather than confining the discussion to a traditional problem focus), and to help or guide the person to identify for herself or himself what it is that she or he is currently doing to survive, and what the person might like to be different in the future, so that the person is able to refocus and improve her or his health and well-being in a supported context (Wand, 2010). Change is seen as a normal dynamic in everyday life and an activity that most people will have a history of success in negotiating in their lives. Adapting to change is something that all people have to do frequently, and so this current problem is an opportunity to do adapt normally. The clinician guides the person towards recovery, helps the person find a way to imagine a future without drug and/or alcohol problems, and to explore ways to create small achievable goals, rather than setting unrealistic, big goals at an early phase. As people see that small things can be changed, and are able to reflect on their success, they are able to take further, constructive steps to achieving more positive changes in their lives. Solution-focused interventions include structuring a scaling process so that people learn to evaluate change within their lives (for example, on a scale of 0 to 10 rate 'I feel I can make X change in my life'). In this way, outcomes can be recognised and complimented, while new motivation for future changes can be encouraged and nurtured (Wand, 2010). Solution-focused interventions are positively framed and they align usefully with other interventions such as motivational interviewing, change readiness, cognitive behavioural therapy, and withdrawal planning and interventions.

What needs to change in the future?

Remember Mark's story? He has some ideas about improvements that could be made so that others are less likely to experience the distress he did.

Consumer narrative | Mark's story part nine: Reflections and recommendations for change

I wouldn't change the nurses working at the coal-face. Perhaps I was fortunate with the nurses I encountered at the facility, but their care and compassion was very deep and I felt safe with them nearby. I felt human and that I had rights. I felt they were making the best decisions for me.

The experience with the psychiatrist in the facility is one I never want repeated. She thought she had all the answers. I felt that she was annoyed that I didn't have traces of other drugs in my system. I didn't feel a sense of compassion or warmth from her. I felt she was very focused on the power she had in decision-making. Several times, she made reference to her authority to make the decision to extend my stay.

Alcohol venues need to be more responsible. While their policy may have stopped me being 'glassed', it may have contributed to me experiencing this episode. I can never be sure if I would have read the label – I would like to think I would have. At the very least, I would have made an informed decision if I had the chance to read the label. I feel a sense of being personally violated because I could not.

My work, colleagues and extended network were very supportive. I thought they would think I was mad, but they didn't. The support was overwhelming and that was reassuring.

It is interesting that Mark identified that he felt safe, human and that his rights were maintained, and that he could sense the care and compassion of the nurses. These qualities are not tangible; they are not interventions that can be administered from the medication trolley. You cannot get compassion from the treatment room, as you might a dressing; you cannot measure it as if were a vital sign such as blood pressure, but these characteristics are the invisible hallmarks of excellent nursing care. Safety, care and compassion are noticeable, both in their presence and in their absence, they do require some emotional intelligence and investment by nurses and they are especially vital skills needed for the expert delivery of care towards people with mental illness and/or substance-use problems.

Chapter summary

This chapter has presented stories, information and activities designed to deepen understanding of:

- harm-minimisation strategies that underpin quality mental health outcomes for individuals and communities;
- how legal and illegal drugs, when misused, can adversely affect mental health and well-being;
- person-centred care that promotes the recovery of people with combined drug, alcohol and mental illness;
- holistic care related to mental health and drug and alcohol care as an interprofessional responsibility and a framework that enhances respectful, recovery focused relationships with people; and
- how the physical and mental health of people are affected adversely by drug misuse.

Critical thinking/learning activities

1 List some ways in which the brain is affected by drug use.
2 List some ways in which you as a new graduate health practitioner could support a person in his or her decision to reduce or cease consumption of drugs.
3 List the holistic domains that might apply to the care of a person with drug or alcohol problems.
4 What are some of the physical and mental care needs of a person who has ingested excessive quantities of paracetamol?
5 In what ways do harm-minimisation policies affect mental health outcomes for individuals and communities?

Learning extension

Samson and Delilah (directed by Warwick Thornton in 2009) is a film that portrays the experience of a young couple in central Australia who are affected by solvent sniffing. View a trailer by the film's director to find out more about this informative film and to explore some of the complex drug, mental health and social issues that relate to solvent misuse.

Acknowledgement

Thanks to Mark for sharing his story and for his contribution to this chapter in providing a real-life account of the mental health problems related to alcohol and caffeine use.

Further reading

Alcohol and Other Drugs Council of Australia: www.adca.org.au
Australian Government National Drug Strategy: www.nationaldrugstrategy.gov.au
Mental Health Foundation, UK: www.mentalhealth.org.uk/publications/feeding-minds
This is a link to the report: *Feeding Minds. The impact of food on mental health*, published in 2006. The companion report *Changing Diets, Changing Minds* is also available on the website.
Victorian Alcohol and Drug Association: www.comorbidity.org.au/sites/www.comorbidity.org.au/files/ AOD%20and%20MH%20prompt%20card%20information.pdf.
This link is to free alcohol and drug prompt cards designed to assist new practitioners and students to remember some key clinical characteristics of drug and alcohol misuse. Consider printing these cards for quick reference in the clinical setting.

References

Attenborough, J. (2010). Alcohol and mood disorders. In P. Phillips, O. McKeown & T. Sandford (eds), *Dual Diagnosis. Practice in context.* (pp. 76–88). Oxford, UK: Wiley-Blackwell.

Australian Institute of Health and Welfare (2011). 2010 National Drug Strategy Household Survey Report. *Drug Statistics Series no.25. Cat. no. PHE 145.* Canberra: Author.

Ayonrinde, O.T., Phelps, G.J., Hurley, J.C. & Ayonrinde, O.A. (2005). Paracetamol overdose and hepatotoxicity at a regional Australian hospital: A 4-year experience. *Internal Medicine Journal,* 35: 655–60.

Barratt, M.J., Cakic, V. & Lenton, S. (2013). Patterns of synthetic cannabinoid use in Australia. *Drug and Alcohol Review, 32*: 141–6.

Bennett, M.R. (2008a). Dual constraints on synapse formation and regression in schizophrenia: Neuregulin, Neuroligin, dysbindin, DISC1, MuSK and agrin. *Australian and New Zealand Journal of Psychiatry, 42*: 662–77.

Bennett, M.R. (2008b). Stress and anxiety in schizophrenia and depression: Glucocorticoids, corticotrophin-releasing hormone and synapse regression. *Australian and New Zealand Journal of Psychiatry, 42*: 995–1002.

Blows, W.T. (2011). *The Biological Basis for Mental Health Nursing*, 2nd edn. New York: Routlege.

Cornah, D. & Van De Weyer, C. (n.d.). *Feeding Minds. The impact of food on mental health.* London: Mental Health Foundation. Retrieved from www.mentalhealth.org.uk/content/assets/PDF/publications/Feeding-Minds.pdf?view=Standard.

Cosh, S., Maksimovic, A.L., Ettridge, K., Copley, D. & Bowden, J. (2013). Aboriginal and Torres Strait Islander utilisation of the Quitline service for smoking cessation in South Australia. *Australian Journal of Primary Health, 19*: 113–18.

Daly, F., Fountain, J.S., Murray, L., Graudins, A. & Buckley, N.A. (2008). Guidelines for the management of paracetomol poisoning in Australia and New Zealand – explanation and elaboration. A consensus statement from clinical toxicologists consulting to the Australasian poisons information centres. *Medical Journal of Australia, 188*: 296–301.

Degenhardt, L., Roxburgh, A. & McKetin, R. (2007). Hospital seperations for cannabis- and methamphetamine-related psychotic episodes in Australia. *Medical Journal of Australia, 186*(7): 342–5.

Department of Health and Ageing (2011). *National Drug Strategy 2010–2015.* (D0224). Retrieved from www.nationaldrugstrategy.gov.au/internet/drugstrategy/publishing.nsf/Content/nds20102015.

Department of Health and Ageing (2013). *Standard Drinks Guide.* Retrieved from www.health.gov.au/ internet/alcohol/publishing.nsf/Content/drinksguide-cnt.

Dubertret, C., Bidard, I., Ades, J. & Gorwood, P. (2006). Lifetime positive symptoms in patients with schizophrenia and cannabis abuse are partialy explained by comorbid addiction. *Schizophrenia Research,* 86: 284–90.

Early Psychosis Writing Group (2010). *Australian Clinical Guidelines for Early Psychosis*, 2nd edn. Melbourne: ORYGEN Youth Health.

Edward, K. & Alderman, C. (2013). *Psychopharmocology: Practice and contexts*. South Melbourne: Oxford University Press.

Ferdinand, R. F., Sondeijker, F., van der Ende, J., Selten, J.-P. & Huizink, A. (2005). Cannabis use predicts future psychotic symptoms, and vice versa. *Society for the Study of Addiction.*, *100*: 612–18.

Fergerson, D. M., Horwood, L. J. & Ridder, E. M. (2005). Tests of causal linkages between cannabis use and psychotic symptoms. *Society for the Study of Addiction*, *100*: 354–66.

Geake, J. G. (2009). *The Brain at School. Educational neuroscience in the classroom*. Berkshire: Open University Press.

Green, B., Young, R. & Kavanagh, D. (2005). Cannabis use and misuse prevalence among people with psychosis. *British Journal of Psychiatry*, *187*: 306–13.

Heal, D. J., Smith, S. L., Gosden, J. & Nutt, D. J. (2013). Amphetamine, past and present – a pharmacological and clinical perspective. *Journal of Psychopharmacology*, online first, doi: 10.1177/0269881113482532

Kellert, S. (2012). *Birthright. People and nature in the modern world*. New Haven: Yale University Press.

Lawrence, D., Mitrou, F. & Zubrick, S. (2009). Smoking and mental illness: Results from population surveys in Australia and the United States. *BMC Public Health*, *9*(1): 285.

Mental Health and Drug and Alcohol Office (MHDAO) (2008). *Drug and Alcohol Withdrawal: Clinical practice guidelines – NSW*. (GL2008_011). Sydney: NSW Health.

MHDAO (2009). *NSW Clinical Guidelines for the Care of Persons with Comorbid Mental Illness and Substance Use Disorders in Acute Care Settings*. Sydney: NSW Health.

Mental Health Council of Australia (2006). *Where There's Smoke … Cannabis and Mental Health*. Melbourne: ORYGEN Youth Mental Health Service.

Miller, W. R. & Rollnick, S. (2002). *Motivational Interviewing. Preparing people for change*, 2nd edn. New York: The Guilford Press.

National Health and Medical Research Council (NHMRC) (2009). *Australian Guidelines to Reduce Health Risks from Drinking Alcohol*. Canberra: Australian Government.

Northern Territory Government of Australia (2011). *Kava Management Act*. Darwin: Author.

NSW Health (2009). *Paracetamol Use*. Clinical Policy PD2009_009). Sydney: Department of Health, NSW. Retrieved from www0.health.nsw.gov.au/policies/pd/2009/pdf/PD2009_009.pdf.

Prochaska, J. O., DiClemente, C. C. & Norcross, J. C. (1992). In search of how people change: Applications to addictive behaviours. *American Psychologist*, *47*(9): 1102–14.

Ritter, A., King, T. & Hamilton, M. (eds). (2013). *Drug Use in Australian Society*. South Melbourne: Oxford University Press.

Roxburgh, A., Burns, L., Drummer, O. H., Pilgram, J., Farrell, M., & Degenhardt, L. (2013). Trends in fentanyl prescriptions and fentanyl-related mortality in Australia. *Drug and Alcohol Review*, *32*, 269–275.

Schwartzkoff, J., Wilczynski, A., Reed-Gilbert, K. & Jones, L. (2008). *Review of the First Phase of the Petrol Sniffing Strategy*. Canberra: Department of Families, Housing, Community Services and Indigenous Affairs.

Solowij, N. & Michie, P. T. (2007). Cannabis and cognitive dysfunction: Parallels with endophenotypes of schizophrenia. *Journal Psychiatry Neuroscience*, *32*(1): 30–52.

Van De Weyer C. (2005). *Changing Diets, Changing Minds: How food affects mental well being and behaviour*. London: Sustain: The alliance for better food and farming. Retrieved from www.mentalhealth.org.uk/content/assets/PDF/publications/changing_diets.pdf?view=Standard.

Wand, T. (2010). Mental health nursing from a solution focused perspective. *International Journal of Mental Health Nursing*, *19*: 210–19.

Wilkes, E., Gray, D., Saggers, S., Casey, W. & Stearne, A. (2010). Substance misuse and mental health among Aboriginal Australians. In N. Purdie, P. Dudgeon & R. Walker (eds), *Working Together: Aboriginal and Torres Strait Islander mental health and wellbeing principles and practice*. (pp. 117–33). Canberra: Australian Government, Department of Health and Ageing.

Zinberg, N. (1984). *Drug, Set and Setting: The basis for controlled intoxicant use*. New Haven: Yale University Press.

8

Nutrition, physical health and behavioural change

Denise McGarry

Introduction 166
Prevalence 167
Comorbidity 168
Common physical illnesses and
      conditions 174
Interventions 187

Chapter summary 191
Critical thinking/learning activities 191
Learning extension 191
Further reading 192
References 192

Learning objectives

At the completion of this chapter, you should be able to:

- Understand mental health care as incorporating physical health.
- Understanding the commonly experienced physical health problems of people who experience mental illness.
- Incorporate preventative strategies and monitoring approaches into future practice.
- Recognise physical health care as a human right for people with mental illness.
- Approach physical health care as a collaborative endeavour undertaken with the person with a mental illness, her or his carers and other members of the health team.

Introduction

significant mental illness
also referred to as serious or severe mental illness, SMI ordinarily refers to psychotic illness including schizophrenia and affective conditions, but may also include anxiety conditions

prevalence
the proportion of a population that experiences a certain condition

comorbidity
a concomitant but unrelated pathological or disease condition

Experiencing a mental illness has long been recognised as being associated with a range of physical illnesses that shorten life or impose limitations on physical health. Although the causes of this association are uncertain, it is absolutely clear that the experience of **significant mental illness** (SMI) in both Australia and New Zealand will be associated with a shorter life (Australian Bureau of Statistics (ABS), 2008). Indeed, schizophrenia, one of the major medical diagnoses among SMIs, has been described for some time as a 'life-shortening disease' (Allebeck, 1989).

This chapter explores the characteristic problems encountered in physical health by people with mental illness. The **prevalence** of physical ill health is identified. The causes that can be recognised are generally considered to be problems arising from lifestyle, also known as non-communicable diseases, and from treatments for mental illnesses.

The chapter will address the more commonly experienced physical illnesses (also known as **comorbidities**), looking at the prevalence and specific characteristics of such physical illnesses among those with mental illness.

The final part of the chapter will look at interventions that are useful in preventing, if possible, and limiting the effects of these comorbidities. These issues are fundamentally of a human rights nature. Physical health care is often overlooked in the presence of SMI or given a lesser priority. The right to physical health care is independent of a person's mental health status, as addressed in the United Nations Convention on the Rights of Persons with Disabilities (Office of the Commissioner for Human Rights, 2007). Article 25 specifies that 'persons with disabilities have the right to the enjoyment of the highest attainable standard of health without discrimination on the basis of disability'. Reference in this context is made to government policy directing the approaches of some (usually public) mental health services (Mental Health and Drug and Alcohol Office (MHDAO), 2009).

Reflective questions

Consider your prior knowledge of the physical health status of people with mental illness.
- Were you aware that it was so different from the physical health of the general Australian and New Zealand populations? Is this well understood in the wider society? What factors may limit this understanding of the poor physical health experienced by those with mental illnesses? List a few points in response to these questions.

Prevalence

Determining the characteristics of premature death among those with mental illness is difficult. Dilemmas exist about whether to include or exclude death due to suicide (Glozier, 2012). Ordinarily this is done. Another difficulty is to determine whether someone whose death is examined also had a coexisting mental illness. Consequently, many reports of premature death are derived from those who experience schizophrenia rather than other medical diagnoses of mental illness.

People with mental illness have a life expectancy in Australia of 15–20 years less than the general population (ABS, 2008, 2012). It is well known that Australian Indigenous communities experience significantly greater mortality and greater physical disease occurrence overall than the general Australian population (Parker, 2010; Vos et al., 2009). Examination of mental health in Australian Aboriginal and Torres Strait Islander communities has been incidental in other studies, making definitive understanding incomplete (Jorm et al., 2012). Review of available studies does confirm there is greater prevalence of mental illness in Indigenous communities and that this is evident from a young age (Jorm et al., 2012). Analysis of the physical health of Indigenous Australians who experience mental illness is not readily available.

The reduction in lifespan of those with mental illness is also experienced in other countries. For example, a Finnish study (Tiihonen et al., 2009) reported a life expectancy of 22.5 years fewer than the general population in 2006. Figures reported from the United Kingdom suggest a life expectancy of 16–25 years less than that of the general population (Blythe & White, 2012; Department of Health, 2011). Literature from the United States reports death among people with mental illness as 25–30 years earlier than the general population (Newcomer, 2007).

The national Australian study People Living with Psychotic Illness 2010 (Morgan et al., 2011) was primarily concerned with gathering detained information on the lives of people with psychotic illness who received publicly funded, specialised mental health services. The survey's methodology involved a random sample of 1825 people, most whom had a diagnosis of schizophrenia, being interviewed. Topics covered included socio-economic and demographic characteristics, activities of daily life, social participation family contact, physical conditions, nutrition and exercise. Scales were also included to determine the affects of psychotic illness on overall functioning, quality of life, smoking, alcohol and drug use, cognitive functioning and perceived need for mental health and other support services. Figure 8.1 is based on participant reports from the study. It describes physical health morbidity, as diagnosed or assessed by their doctors at any time in the past and covering a wide range of conditions. Rates for all conditions except cancers were higher in people with psychosis, compared to the general population (Morgan et al., 2011).

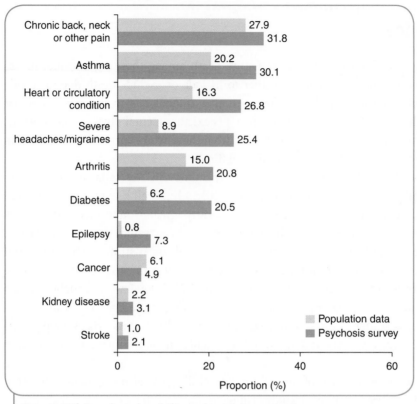

Figure 8.1 Lifetime physical morbidity, and population comparison

Comorbidity

Te Rau Hinengaro: The New Zealand Mental Health Survey (Oakley et al., 2006) noted the higher prevalence of several chronic physical conditions among New Zealanders with mental illness. These conditions are the same as those experienced in Australia, namely cardiovascular diseases, metabolic syndrome, type 2 diabetes, obesity, smoking and high blood pressure. Conversely, the authors also observed that those experiencing chronic physical conditions had a higher prevalence of mental illness. The range of physical health conditions experienced by people with mental illness is far broader than these chronic health conditions; sexual health, oral health, dysphagia, incontinence, nutritional intake and cancer were also considered.

The phenomenon of **diagnostic overshadowing** (Jones, Howard & Thornicroft, 2008) is also relevant in understanding the difficulty in accessing physical health care experienced by people with mental illness. This was first proposed as occurring among people with an intellectual disability, and recognised the tendency for physical ailments to be ascribed to the individual's cognitive

diagnostic overshadowing
the tendency for comorbid conditions to be ascribed to the individual's initial presenting problem

disability (Reiss, Levitan & Szyszko, 1982). It is, however, observed as happening to other people who experience an enduring health (or other) condition such as mental illness. It is postulated that this occurs because of three possible factors: the severity of the other condition and its symptoms, any cognitive or communication impediments that the person may also experience and the experience of the attending clinicians (Jopp & Keys, 2001). However, the phenomenon is not fully understood.

Listening to those who live with physical ill-health as well as a mental illness signals the urgency for mental health care that also incorporates physical health. Steph's story highlights this experience from a consumer's perspective.

Consumer narrative   Steph's story

Drugs become angels or demons. We need to stay on them at all costs, or get off them at all costs. We look only at the risks, or we're too frightened to look at the risks at all. There is no compromise: it's black and white, all or nothing (Hall, 2012).

I have been delivering consumer-led education in communities and workplaces, drawing on my lived experience of mental illness, for over seven years. Though I am still involved in delivering education with a focus on signs and symptoms in some contexts, the more time I have devoted to thinking about mental illness over the years, the more I have found it helpful to use words like 'crisis' or 'experiences' in place of diagnostic terms. Spending time rethinking and re-authoring my experiences has opened up more complex conversations and reflective processes, and has better prepared me to deal with new life challenges as they arise. I would like to acknowledge the role of other consumer educators in this enriching process and to encourage mental health workers of all disciplines to approach their work with creativity and philosophical flexibility, and to explore consumers' experiences in language that is meaningful for each individual.

In my mid-20s I went through a stressful two-year period, which culminated in a dramatic crisis and landed me a 'psychosis' diagnosis. I live with ongoing vulnerabilities to psychosis and need to make frequent tactical decisions in managing my mental well-being and professional and personal life.

The journey that I would like to outline is actually my pathway to diagnosis of diabetes type 2, given that people receiving treatment for psychosis, particularly those prescribed second-generation, atypical anti-psychotic medications, are at much higher risk than the rest of the population of developing metabolic complications and type 2 diabetes.

In the first national Australian survey regarding psychotic illness conducted in 1997–8 (Jablensky et al., 1999), 37.1 per cent of respondents were using second-generation, anti-psychotic medication. However, by the second national Australian survey (Morgan et al., 2011), the rates had risen dramatically and 78.4 per cent of respondents were using second-generation, anti-psychotic medication.

continued ›

The second survey found that 20.5 per cent of respondents had diabetes type 2 (a rate of three times the general population), many more had metabolic syndrome, and weight gain was the third most problematic side-effect reported from the consumers' perspective.

My personal story provides some context for understanding the lack of disclosure and effective service response to these emerging issues.

In 1998 I was prescribed anti-psychotic medication and stayed on it for several years. At the time I was told I was lucky to be being prescribed this medication as it had fewer side-effects than previous anti-psychotic medications. No health professional in those early years ever advised that these medications could cause weight gain, and I had never heard of a medication causing weight gain. I did not have contact with other people on similar treatment, so I had no idea why I seemed hungrier and my weight was going up steadily.

I put on a total of 40 kilograms in the first two-and-a-half years of treatment. On top of all my other challenges, it did terrible things to my sense of self-esteem and identity. No health professional had ever undertaken any metabolic screening or started a conversation about my weight.

Later, I had several years off medication and my weight stayed exactly the same. I even reported to my general medical practitioner (GP) at the time that it seemed strange that my weight felt 'stuck' despite my good diet, but no tests were ordered at the time.

Eventually, I began to meet other people who had also put on 20, 30 or 40 kilograms of weight while taking anti-psychotic medication, and someone I met had benefited from being supported by an endocrinologist and using the diabetes drug Metformin.

I saw a different GP and asked to be referred to that endocrinologist. The GP seemed annoyed but reluctantly referred me, and the endocrinologist turned me away, saying he/she could not help with 'just anti-psychotic weight gain'. The endocrinologist simply asked my GP to run standard metabolic monitoring (which at that point did finally show metabolic abnormalities).

At around this time I was again having mental health treatment and my weight increased by another 20 kilograms while taking second-generation anti-psychotic medication.

I then took things into my own hands. I changed GPs. I looked on the Dietitians Association of Australia's website to see if anyone specialised in mental health. There were only two dietitians with an interest in mental health, and I went and saw one of them. This dietitian's practice mainly supported people living with diagnoses such as anorexia and bulimia, but I felt that I had good psychiatric support in place and was comfortable explaining my mental health challenges. I felt we could pool our knowledge. The dietitian knew how to work respectfully in a multidisciplinary way, and we explored the best way to approach losing 60 kilograms while still dealing with reasonably frequent mental health challenges. I saw her as I might see a psychologist, and we spent 45 minutes of each session talking about ongoing challenges and goal setting. She was studying

continued ›

counselling on top of her qualifications in dietetics. Having some dedicated support and a hopeful relationship was crucial in me developing the self-belief that losing 60 kilograms was possible.

I believe strongly in the role of the mental health workforce, especially nursing, to take up some of this work. There were sometimes psychological barriers, such as having had vulnerable sexual experiences while in crisis. Losing weight brought up feelings of being unsafe if I was attractive. I have heard trauma survivors talk about traumatic feelings resurfacing as they lost weight. We don't need an army of people coming in to order us around with regard to our lifestyles without appreciating some of the complexities of our psychological and life challenges.

I begged this dietitian to write a book for people with experiences of treatment with anti-psychotic medication. We have unique challenges, including learning how to deal with the strong feelings of hunger should we choose to take medication. I used to feel so hungry at lunchtime that if I didn't eat a decent-sized lunch, I would have trouble concentrating at work in the afternoon. I would love to see more research done on hunger and how people have learned to cope with this. I lost 23 kilograms in seven months once I was correctly diagnosed as having metabolic problems, prescribed Metformin and accessed the regular support of this dietitian.

At that point in time I could afford a dietitian as I was working full-time. However, financial problems are often a very real part of many of our lives. I was actually living with relatives, because once I paid for my private psychiatrist, my private psychologist, my gym, my dietitian, my health fund and my medications, I did not have enough money left over to pay rent in Sydney.

I have often joked that I had more people in my 'entourage' at that point than a movie star. I have found that has been an effective metaphor for workers engaged in multidisciplinary work, and I am actively involved in advocacy at the moment, trying to articulate the need for dietitians and exercise physiologists to be included in standard mental health care teams, and for physical health initiatives to be embedded in mental health practice as core business.

Things changed again. My dietitian moved interstate. Then I returned to study and couldn't afford private care. Then my career got busier. My time at the gym was depleted and I had some hassles tolerating Metformin while travelling and training so much. I eventually did find myself an endocrinologist who would work with me, but this practitioner diagnosed that I had slipped into the diabetes zone for not having lost the weight quickly enough.

There is a history of lack of disclosure from drug companies on this issue, so a lot could have been done earlier to support people like me to make informed decisions about medication, and a lot of work and advocacy could have been done to put in place appropriate supports for those people who find second-generation anti-psychotic

continued ›

medication helpful in overcoming distressing experiences. There definitely needs to be better links between GPs, endocrinologists and psychiatrists. Psychiatrists should be routinely monitoring for metabolic risks as they do for lithium levels.

I am excited to see that the National Mental Health Commission acknowledged the state of physical health care of mental health consumers as 'a national disgrace' (Glozier, 2012), and my hope is that members of the mental health workforce will develop a passion for this area of health care. From my perspective it is one of the most important dimensions to the future of mental health work and an area of interest in which people can make a huge difference.

One of the issues that most concerns me is the amount of coerced medication use. Should society be able to force someone to take a medication with this known life-shortening, side-effect profile? The United Nations Convention on the Rights of Persons with Disabilities (Office of the Commissioner for Human Rights, 2007), which Australia ratified in 2008, provides a justification for mental health consumers to make all decisions that affect their mental or physical health. Given that Australia has retained a coercive medication regime in psychiatry, what is being done to inform consumers about the risks to which they are being exposed? For example, Clozapine and Olanzapine have been identified as being particularly likely to cause weight gain, yet they are frequently prescribed on community treatment orders and in hospital settings. Are all consumers being routinely offered screening and support in relation to these risks?

Even though I have rarely been coerced into taking medication, I still can attest to the fact that there is also a lot of softer coercion in terms of community attitudes about risk and dangerousness, with TV and newspaper reports creating stereotypes about people who are 'not taking their medication'. This all influences my friends and family, and creates an additional layer of anxiety around the times when I am attempting to cope with less or no medication.

I have successfully come off two types of medications with no emergence of the experiences for which they were prescribed. In each case, I was the one who made the suggestion that I come off this medication, and I managed the process with support of my medical practitioners. There are a number of side-effects that I gladly no longer experience, including sexual dysfunction. Recent research shows that nurses consider talking about sexuality as 'not my job' (Quinn, Happell & Welch, 2012), which leaves me wondering who is talking about sensitive issues like sexuality and weight gain caused by medication.

I would like to see a greater clinical emphasis on recognising that reducing or coming off anti-psychotic medication makes it easier to manage weight and metabolic risks. That it is a form of positive risk-taking. In fact, I am actively pursuing self-management strategies such as taking up meditation to reduce the amount of times I reach for anti-psychotic medication. I am also making long-term career choices to reduce

continued ›

Consumer narrative continued ›

my use of anti-psychotic medication because I notice that I use them more during periods when I travel a lot for work.

I believe we have to firmly let go of the words 'compliance' or 'adherence': 'Findings have revealed that non-adherence may not always reflect psychopathology or a lack of insight, but rather a personal choice directed toward engaging in activities that provide meaning and purpose' (Roe & Swarbrick, 2007, p. 39).

We need to move to a recovery-oriented focus whereby medication is considered to be one possible tool (among many) that consumers may choose to support their self-chosen recovery goals. Dr Patricia Deegan, a leader in the consumer/survivor movement and psychologist by training, has done leading work over the years on decision-making in psychiatry. Her work and that of others were drawn on in advisory paper by the Devon Partnership Trust & Recovery & Independent Living Professional Experts Group (Maddock & Hallam, 2010).

There are big philosophical questions to consider about the ways in which the Australian mental health system responds to 'psychosis' or crisis experiences. Can we better prevent psychosis by attending to the high levels of trauma experienced by people accessing mental health services? Is our highly medicalised response helping people lead the lives they want to lead? What can other frameworks offer? For example, the International Hearing Voices Network (see www.intervoiceonline.org) starts with an acceptance of the voice-hearing experience by accepting people's accounts of hearing voices without stigmatising or marginalising them, and the Finnish Open Dialogue method has attracted attention for its low use of anti-psychotic medication and good employment and disability outcomes. Specifically, the open dialogue approach saw many with symptoms have few hospital days and return to their studies or a full-time job. What sort of nursing and psychiatric practice will emerge from proper attendance to both physical and mental health risks?

Reflective questions

Think about Steph's story.

- How was her physical health care was integrated during mental health interventions? Did she experience any barriers to accessing physical health care?
- How may her physical health have been best maintained during her mental health care?
- Whose responsibility is it to ensure Steph, or any other person in her situation, has her physical health needs addressed?

Common physical illnesses and conditions

Metabolic syndrome

The metabolic syndrome (MetS) is a cluster of factors that significantly increase the risk of developing and dying from cardiovascular disease. These risk factors include insulin resistance, hypertension, central obesity and dyslipidaemia. Newcomer (2007) attributed the premature age at death in people experiencing mental illness to an increased prevalence of the metabolic syndrome and its components, which are risk factors for cardiovascular diseases and type 2 diabetes. This has to be assessed against general populations in which rates of cardio-metabolic syndrome have increased (Moodie et al., 2013). But evidence strongly suggests that the prevalence of metabolic syndrome is much greater among people with mental illness (Newcomer, 2007). It has been found that 32 per cent of men and 51 per cent of women with schizophrenia meet criteria for metabolic syndrome (John et al., 2009); the prevalence is higher in women than in men (Narasimhan & Raynor, 2010). Overweight and obesity, hyperglycaemia, dyslipidaemia, and hypertension are all risk factors of this syndrome that have higher prevalence among people with mental illness (Lambert, 2011). In the study described above (Morgan et al., 2011), three-quarters (79 per cent) of participants gave blood for metabolic analysis. These participants were assessed for key metabolic risk factors outlined in Table 8.1. An alarmingly high proportion of participants (81.1 per cent) met at-risk criteria for abdominal obesity. Half had at-risk levels of high-density lipoproteins (49.7 per cent), blood pressure (48.8 per cent) or triglycerides (48 per cent), and more than one-quarter had elevated plasma glucose, which is frequently associated with diabetes.

The reasons metabolic syndrome rates are high are complex and contested. Social factors such as poverty decreasing access to medical services are recognised contributors. So, too, is the use of psychotropic medications (van Winkel, De Hert & Wampers, 2008). Understanding of these factors may help consumers of mental health services make

Table 8.1 Metabolic syndrome and cardio-metabolic measures

	Proportion (%)
Met criteria for metabolic syndrome[*]	49.9
Met 'at-risk' criteria for individual cardio-metabolic measures:	
Abdominal obesity	82.1
High-density lipoproteins[†]	49.7
Blood pressure	48.8
Triglycerides[†]	48.0
Plasma glucose[†]	28.6

[*]International Diabetes Federation metabolic syndrome consensus criterion 13 applied to those with no missing data.
[†]Fasting.

Source: Morgan et al., 2011.

informed decisions about their treatment options. However, reversal of increased risk is not simple for those experiencing mental illness, as it is not for the general population. Factors may be screened for and recognised. Reversing or countering such factors as overweight, obesity, hyperlipidaemia and hyperglycaemia are stubborn issues. There are no simple responses (Lambert & Newcomer, 2009).

Hyperglycaemia and diabetes

Diabetes prevalence has increased rapidly in the developed world over the past several decades. The International Diabetes Federation reported that 'the number of people around the world suffering from diabetes has skyrocketed in the last two decades, from 30 million to 230 million' (World Federation for Mental Health, 2010, p. 12). The association of depression with diabetes has been recognised for some time. The World Federation for Mental Health reported that 25 per cent of people with diabetes would experience depression, and that the risk of developing depression and the prevalence of depression was twice that of the general population (World Federation for Mental Health, 2010). Further, that the risk of mortality in people with diabetes was increased by 30 per cent when they also experienced depression (World Federation for Mental Health, 2010).

The occurrence of diabetes among people with mental illness has been observed for a long time. Maudsley, the famous British psychiatrist, observed in 1897 that 'diabetes is a disease which often shows itself in families in which insanity prevails' (cited in Koran, 2004, p. s65). While the rate of diabetes among the general population is thought to be around 5 per cent (Busche & Holt, 2004), the prevalence among those with schizophrenia is 15 per cent (Holt & Peveler, 2005).

The understanding of why diabetes has greater prevalence among people with SMI is not clear. The best explanations point to the recurrent association with family histories, low physical activity, poor diet, smoking and the metabolic effects of some anti-psychotic medications (Gough & Peveler, 2004).

An additional concern observed about diabetes in the general population is an extreme delay in diagnosis. Explanations of this delay are not clear, but the delay is estimated at up to 12 years (Department of Health, 2001). Moreover, this delay in recognition, diagnosis and treatment has a number of serious health effects. Eye damage and blindness, kidney impairment that may result in renal failure and nerve damage are all potential consequences. This is also the case for people with SMI who develop diabetes. Data about delays in diagnosis for people with mental illness is not known, but one could speculate that the delay is greater than for the general population. If this is the case, the consequences on health could be serious.

Hyperlipidaemia

Monitoring of lipids is low among those experiencing SMI, despite longstanding position statements by relevant professional bodies (Royal Australian and New Zealand College of Psychiatrists, 2005). Further, the efficacy of statins, the usual pharmacological treatment for hyperlipidaemia, has rarely been studied among people who are also being treated for mental illness. This raises concerns that there may be effects other than those intended.

Cardiovascular disease (hypertension, cardiac arrhythmias)

Cardiovascular disease rates as noted are higher among people experiencing mental illness than the general population. This is not solely as a sequalae to hyperlipidaemia, but arises from the higher prevalence of hypertension and cardiac arrhythmias as well. Table 8.2 summarises data collected by Morgan and colleagues (2011) in Australia pertaining to consumers living with psychotic illness, most commonly schizophrenia. Almost one-third of those who were assessed met the criteria for absolute risk of a cardiovascular event in five years, with 7.2 per cent of the total at medium risk and 24.0 per cent at high risk. Although lifestyle factors such as reduced activity levels, obesity, poor diet and limited medical screening are implicated, medications used to treat mental illness are known to contribute. Drugs such as tricyclic antidepressants and some anti-psychotics are understood to change cardiac function. Clozapine requires monitoring to respond to iatrogenic cardiac effects, including myocarditis (Raedler, 2010).

Table 8.2 Absolute five-year risk of cardiovascular disease

	Proportion (%)		
	18–34 years*	35–64 years	Persons
Low risk	87.2	56.3	68.8
Medium risk	0.0	12.0	7.2
High risk	12.8	31.7	24.0

*Framingham risk equation 15–16 applied to those with no missing data. The Framingham risk equation is not normally used with people under 35 years of age. However, 12.8 per cent in the younger age group met risk criteria. In all cases, this was due to pre-existing cardiovascular disease or other high-risk medical conditions.

Source: Morgan et al., 2011.

Obesity

Rates of overweight and obesity have risen markedly over the past 20 years in the developed world and elsewhere (Sassi et al., 2009). The 2007–8 National Health Survey of Australians reported that 62 per cent of Australians were either overweight or obese (Australian Institute of Health and Welfare, 2009). So it should come as no surprise that levels among those with mental illness are also high. All the reasons suggested as significant for the rises in obesity in the general population – a food-rich environment, reduced levels of incidental physical activity and increased consumption of calorific-rich foods – also hold true for those with mental illness. However, there are additional factors that make the challenge of maintaining a healthy **BMI** (body mass index) more difficult.

BMI
(body mass index) an index of weight-for-height that is commonly used to classify underweight, overweight and obesity in adults

In Figure 8.2, which presents data from the Morgan and colleagues (2011) study, the level of physical activity that participants had undertaken in the seven days prior to interview was measured using the International Physical Activity Questionnaire (Craig et al., 2003). One-third (33.5 per cent) of participants was classified as sedentary; that is, inactive or with very low levels of activity, while the other two-thirds were classified as having a low level of activity.

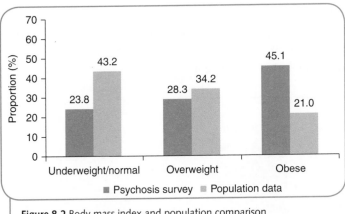

Figure 8.2 Body mass index and population comparison

The reduced income – indeed poverty – of many people with mental illness, especially of a SMI nature, presents the first hurdle. Relatively speaking, prepared foods are often a cheaper as well as more convenient food choice. These foods are often high in calories, and also a range of other ingredients detrimental to good health, such as saturated fats, low fibre and high sodium levels.

Poverty or significantly reduced income also increases the individual's chances of weight gain by yet another means. The capacity to pay for exercise opportunities, whether through gym membership or sporting club registration is severely limited, if not lost. A common response to activity needs provided to the general population is often denied to those with SMI before any application of stigma that may reduce social inclusion in such venues.

Psychotropic medications also play a role. Many are sedative. Measures of basal metabolic rates for people taking Clozapine are very low, further enhancing weight-gain trajectories. People experience lethargy when taking many of the anti-psychotics, such as Olanzapine (McEvoy et al., 2007).

There is also an association between anti-psychotic medications and weight gain. Young people experiencing a first episode of psychosis are particularly vulnerable to rapid weight gain. This is can lead to development of cardio-metabolic changes (Foley & Morley, 2011). The observation has been made that increased appetite is also experienced in association with anti-psychotic medication use (Basson et al., 2001).

Psychotropic drugs are suspected of interfering with the sensation of satiety. This in-built physiological feedback mechanism does not react to signal that the person has consumed sufficient food or calories. Some people have been known to complain of constant hunger that severely impedes self-restraint and moderation in feeding. Histamine neuro-transmitters are suspected to be instrumental in these atypical (second-generation), anti-psychotic-induced weight gain effects (Deng, Weston-Green & Huang, 2010). Consider Steph's comments regarding this problem.

Finally, the nature of many SMIs in themselves can reduce an individual's motivation to participate actively in life – including healthy rates of daily exercise. The study of people living with psychotic illness (Morgan et al., 2011, see Figure 8.3) found that those in the older group aged 35–64 years were more likely to be in the sedentary category when compared with the younger age group of 18–34 years. The most commonly reported barriers to being physically active were lack of motivation (36.4 per cent), tiredness (19.2 per cent) and pain or discomfort (15.2 per cent).

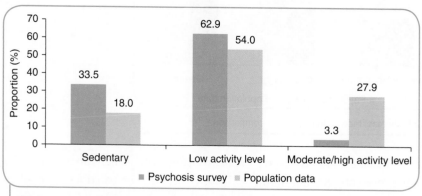

Figure 8.3 Level of physical activity in the past week and population comparison

Nutritional patterns

Independent of the effects of psychotropic drugs, the nutritional patterns of people with mental illness are poor and do not meet healthy eating guidelines (National Health and Medical Research Council (NHMRC), 2013). In a study of 159 people who had been diagnosed with schizophrenia, Simonelli-Muñoz and colleagues (2012) reported that 51 per cent of people reported that their meal times took less than 15 minutes, 40.8 per cent did not eat fresh food daily and 63.1 per cent did not eat fish. These poor dietary habits were associated with increases in BMI and waist circumference – a prime indicator of adipose fat patterns, the development of obesity and metabolic syndrome.

Cancers

The prevalence of cancers among people with mental illness shows contradictory patterns. On the one hand, some cancers appear more frequently while others are less frequently experienced. This apparently confusing pattern has been explained by a closer analysis of individual cancers, suggesting that some cancers that may be expected to be a common cause of mortality, such as lung cancer, are not represented as expected because people with SMI have died earlier from other causes such as cardiovascular diseases. Lung cancer typically occurs at a later age than death from cardiovascular disease, providing a possible explanation for its lower representation, and given the high levels of smoking among people with SMI (Robson & Gray, 2007).

Digestive and breast cancers, however, are well recognised as having higher rates of mortality (Robson & Gray, 2007; Schoos & Cohen, 2003). Several possible explanations are offered for this situation in relation to breast cancers. Among these includes lower participation by people with mental illness in screening activities – routine self-examination, examination by GPs and breast scans. Some anti-psychotic medications are known to increase prolactin levels, and this is suspected to increase prevalence and mortality. In addition to reduced screening participation, increased prevalence of digestive cancers among people with mental illness is associated with poor diet and increased alcohol consumption.

Hepatitis and HIV/AIDS

Most of studies on the prevalence of HIV/AIDS among people with SMI have been undertaken in the United States (Rosenberg, Goodman & Osher, 2001; Sewell, 1996). These studies have reported rates of between 3 and 7 per cent. A person with schizophrenia is 1.8 times more likely to contract HIV/AIDS than the general population, whereas people with a diagnosis of a depressive illness are 3.8 times more likely to contract HIV/AIDS (Blank et al., 2002).

Behaviours that particularly expose people with mental illness to increased risk of HIV/AIDS include failure to use condoms routinely – perhaps influenced by poor knowledge (Arrufo et al., 1990), planning skills or access to condoms (Kalichman et al., 1994). Alcohol and drug use, including injectable drug use, are also implicated (Cournos, McKinnon & Sullivan, 2005).

Data on survival rates for people with mental illness living with HIV/AIDS are not readily available. Since the adoption of anti-retroviral treatment has had significant effects on survival rates in the general population, it is of interest to know whether this treatment is offering the same benefit to those with SMI. However, it is suspected that effective delivery of this treatment for HIV/AIDS may be complicated by diagnostic overshadowing.

Sexual dysfunction

Sexual difficulties and dysfunction are common among those with mental illness. People whose mental illnesses are enduring experience sexual difficulties, both in establishing sexual relationships and also in high rates of relationship breakdown (Berner, Hagen & Kriston, 2007; Fortier et al., 2003). Stigma and self-image also contribute to such difficulties (Davison & Huntington, 2010; Volman & Landeen, 2007).

The prevalence of high-risk sexual behaviours among people with mental illness are difficult to determine, but there is some evidence that sexually transmissible infections are more common that in the general community (Dyer & McGuiness, 2008).

Sexual disinhibition experienced by some people with bipolar illness increases risks for relationship breakdown and for sexually transmissible infection (McCandless &

Sladen, 2003; Rosenberg et al., 2005). Sexual exploitation and abuse are more commonly experienced by people with mental illness than in the general population; estimates are that 68 per cent of women and 40 per cent of men experience sexual exploitation or abuse (Elliott, Mok, & Briere, 2004), in contrast to 22 per cent and 3.8 per cent, respectively, in the general population (Goodwin & Happell, 2007).

An additional factor contributing to sexual difficulties among people with mental illness are the side-effects of anti-psychotic medications (Khawaja, 2005). This is reported as a factor among some people who discontinue their anti-psychotic medications (Deegan, 2001). Sexual dysfunction has been reported as commonly experienced by men taking olanzapine, risperidone, quetiapine or haloperidol, with substantial effects on their quality of life (Olfson et al., 2005). Sexual dysfunction has been reported as also experienced by between 30 and 60 per cent of people treated with selective serotonin re-uptake inhibitors (SSRIs). SSRIs appear to be the class of antidepressants that most commonly causes sexual dysfunction; however, all classes of antidepressant medications have these adverse effects (Gregorian et al., 2002).

Reflective questions

- Did Steph describe sexual difficulties?
- How did she address these?
- How would you talk about sexuality with people who have a mental illness?

Smoking

Morgan and colleagues (2011) found that rates of smoking among people with SMI were significantly higher than in the general population (see Figure 8.4). The proportion of smoking was higher in males, with 71.1 per cent reporting that they were current smokers at the time of interview, compared to 58.8 per cent of females. Participants in the study smoked on average 21 cigarettes per day. Elsewhere, smoking rates among people with SMI have been reported to be between 58 and 88 per cent, and up to three times the rate of the general population (de Leon et al., 2002; Hughes et al., 1986). Furthermore, the amount of smoking behaviour is at the higher level, with a majority of people with SMI smoking more than 25 cigarettes a day (Kelly & McCreadie, 2000).

The reasons for such high rates of smoking are multifactorial and have been extensively researched. Neuro-biological, psychological and sociological factors together make it additionally difficult for people with mental illness to alter this behaviour. The attitudes of health professionals working with people accessing mental health services have been resigned to high levels of smoking. Some staff of mental health services have expressed the belief that smoking is a human right and one of a small number of pleasures available to those with SMI. They expressed confusion about actively promoting smoking cessation among people with mental illness (McNeill, 2001). This retarded the attempts by some people with mental illness to give up smoking; studies have shown that many people with mental illness were keen to be offered support to give up smoking (Addington et al., 1998).

Inhaling nicotine has the effect of controlling some of the experiences of psychoses, including negative symptoms, cognitive deficits and side-effects of anti-psychotic medication. For this reason, smoking is sometimes referred to as 'self-medicating' (Dalack, Healy & Meador-Woodruff, 1998; Goff, Henderson & Amico, 1992). The ability to attend, and to process information selectively – skills often impaired in people with schizophrenia – are known to be improved when smoking (Alder et al., 1998). These effects complicate efforts to reduce or give up smoking.

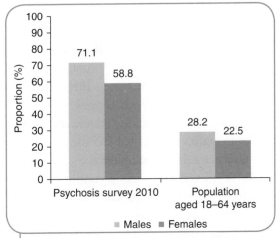

Figure 8.4 Tobacco consumption and population comparison

It is important that the advice given by health professionals to assist smoking cessation is consistent. Such advice is known to motivate individuals to seek further treatment and advice (Kreuter, Chheda & Bull, 2000; Sutherland, 2003). There is some evidence that people with SMI are less likely to receive smoking-cessation advice than other clients in primary health consultations (NHS Smokesfree, 2001).

Urinary incontinence

People with SMI have heightened risk for urinary incontinence. A number of psychotropic medications appear to be implicated, specifically anti-psychotics, benzodiazepines and antidepressants (Tsakiris, Oelke & Michel, 2008). Over-sedation and confusion are associated with the increased risks of anti-psychotics, sedatives and hypnotic agents. Clozapine, a second-generation anti-psychotic medication, is recognised as increasing urinary incontinence, especially nocturnal incontinence (Warner, Harvey & Barnes, 1994). Anti-cholinergic and antidepressant medications are associated with urinary retention and overflow.

Other factors that increase risk for urinary incontinence among those with SMI are mobility limitations, poor manual dexterity, impaired eyesight and unsuitable footwear and clothing (Chester, 1996). There is incomplete evidence of an association between urinary incontinence and depression. Melville and colleagues (2002) found major depression and panic disorder highly prevalent in women with urinary incontinence.

Carers' expectations have been recognised as an independent contributing factor. They may develop an expectation of the inevitability of incontinence. Such a belief can perpetuate a cycle of incontinence (Melville et al., 2002).

The effects of urinary incontinence are multifactorial. Individuals may be less able to advocate for active investigation and treatment of this physical health issue, and so do not have access to expert services. This may cause additional damage to self-esteem, already affected by the incontinence. Incontinence can be experienced at an early age due to the introduction of medications. This can cause additional alienation from peer groups. Additionally, staff may be challenged by urinary incontinence among in-patients and may be rejecting in their attitudes. Stigma and stereotypes can be reinforced by incontinence. When living on a restricted income or in poverty, the cost of seeking treatment and incontinence aids can be prohibitive.

It is important that incontinence screening and treatment be routinely incorporated into the physical health care of people with mental illness. Active approaches when clozapine is prescribed should be taken to manage or minimise the development or problems of incontinence. Standard assessment tools, such as 24-hour urine collections and bladder diaries, can prove difficult for some people with mental illness. Tools may need to be adapted or developed to better serve people with these problems.

Dental health

A review of published literature addressing oral health advice for people with SMI (Khokhar et al., 2011) reported that people with mental illness had worse oral health than the general population (Griffiths et al., 2000; Khokhar et al., 2011). It has been noted that people with SMI experience greater prevalence of oral disease and find accessing care for this difficult (Cormac & Jenkins, 1999; Khokhar et al., 2011.

Until 2012, dental care in Australia was not covered by universal health cover, meaning that except for a very limited range of services provided under stringent criteria, individuals had to finance their own interventions. However, over the five-year period until 2017, a planned introduction of a universal dental scheme will be integrated into public health cover. Private health insurance schemes offer dental care as an additional level of insurance after paying for basic hospital cover, for an additional fee. For many people with mental illness, this arrangement acts as a barrier to accessing routine dental care.

In addition to this financial impediment for good dental care, mental illness can result in difficulties with organisation required for preventative dental activities, such as routine cleaning and dental visits. The side-effects from medications (for example, **xerostomia**) can create a poor oral environment, and poor dietary and nutritional habits may also contribute.

> **xerostomia**
> dry mouth that may be a result of a number of different causes, such as adverse affects of medications and salivary gland dysfunction from a variety of causes, including radiotherapy and fluid balance

The effects of poor oral health are multiple. Poor oral health can affect a person's everyday functioning, as pain or discomfort from poor dentition can affect the ability to eat. People's diet may be restricted in response to this, and when coupled with low economic resources, may even result in nutritional deficits. Appearance may also be affected by poor oral health. Missing or discoloured teeth and halitosis can reduce social acceptability. In turn, self-esteem may be reduced.

Poor oral health has been associated with coronary heart disease (Montebugnoli et al., 2004). Good oral health is part of overall good health.

Xerostomia (dry mouth) is a side-effect of many psychotropic medications, including anti-psychotics, antidepressants and mood stabilisers. Reduction in salivation is an uncomfortable experience. It increases the risk of periodontal diseases, such as gingivitis, that can lead to tooth loss (Friedlander & Marder, 2002). Xerostomia may also affect the capacity to swallow food. The mechanical ability to chew food and create a bolus for swallowing becomes impaired. Saliva is essential in this process. The bolus produced may be large and dry. This increases the risk of choking – a cause of death among people with SMI that occurs with greater frequency than in the general population.

Limor and Anne are mental health nurses who actively developed programs to address physical health. They have both taken preventative approaches to help reduce prevalence of comorbidities.

Consumer narrative Limor's story: Developing an oral care program

As a nurse working with older residents in long-term mental health facilities, one has to be exceptionally innovative to overcome challenges faced from day to day. This population group is unique because people bring with them not only mental illnesses, but also secondary physical morbidities. In a rehabilitation ward of psycho-geriatric residents it is common for the people residing there to have psychotic disorders, major affective disorders, behavioural disturbances and history of drug and alcohol problems, and at times they might present with an intellectual disability. In addition, physical illnesses like obesity, malnutrition, cardiovascular diseases, pre-diabetes and diabetes, constipation, eating disorders, dysphasia, osteoporosis and psychogenic polydipsia are experienced.

I work in such a ward. It is a large, 30-bed facility for people who have all the above issues. This is a major challenge for staff, as each resident is unique with different needs, abilities and cognitive functioning.

Two issues that staff on the ward have been aware of as major, interrelated problems, were oral care and meal-time enjoyment. How do you make sure that all 30 residents have the oral care they need and have a nutritional, balanced meal they can enjoy?

Among the 30, mostly self-sufficient residents, some people still have most of their teeth, some only have a few or no teeth left and others have dentures. Some of the residents need assistance or special utensils to provide oral care and to help them eat their meals, and many have special diets because they may be overweight or malnourished, diabetic or be at risk of choking.

To overcome these problems, we came up with two simple, innovative ideas: for oral health we created an individualised oral care plan and an oral health trolley.

continued ›

Consumer narrative continued >

Each resident now has a box with his or her name on it, with all the appropriate tools the person needs for her or his own specific, beneficial oral hygiene. This innovation has ensured that appropriately tailored oral care is provided twice a day to all residents. It allows able residents to keep their independence, while at the same time providing the not-so-able residents with assistance with oral care.

A success story: one woman with few teeth and an upper denture used to carry her toothbrush in her handbag (with who knows what else in the bag). She might have brushed her teeth from time to time, but she did not seem to do a very good job with that, especially with her denture, which never left her mouth to be cleaned properly. Since the introduction of the oral health trolley she has gained independence in cleaning her few teeth twice a day and now takes her denture out of her mouth to be cleaned with the appropriate tools.

For meal enjoyment we created a special clipboard, which hangs above each resident's table, showing the person's name, any risk he or she may have (such as choking), whether any special utensils are needed and the type of diet required; for example, diabetic, soft, minced, thickened fluids, or any other diet recommended by the dietitian and/or speech pathologist. This simple innovation has helped to calm the chaos experienced in the dining room, as the correct setting and diet are now routinely and consistently available for residents, even when the person on duty is a casual staff member.

Consumer narrative   Reducing dysphagia part one: Joe's nurse

My first meeting with Joe was when I was a student psychiatric nurse in the late 1980s. I was working on a long-stay rehabilitation ward, working a 12-hour shift. In those days we did not have personal duress alarms and communication was by telephone. I was called to Joe's ward to help with a medical emergency. A patient was choking while eating meatballs and pasta. Unfortunately, the patient could not be revived.

Fifteen years on and in a different hospital I caught up with Joe. I was escorting Joe to a specialist orthopaedic appointment at a large teaching hospital. We had the first appointment for the day but the surgeon had been called away to an emergency. Joe and I spoke of the days at the other hospital and he recalled other patients and nurses I had completely forgotten about. The conversation then flowed onto the choking incident, and Joe mentioned that he thought he would die a similar death. When questioned, he said that

continued >

Consumer narrative continued ›

he had always had a fear of choking. I asked him whether he had problems with his eating and he said no, although he felt it was always a rush to eat his food. I advised him to sit up straight and not eat his food quickly. Joe then dismissed my concerns and asked if he could have a cigarette (you were still allowed to smoke outside hospitals back then!).

I spoke with staff about Joe's concerns, and various staff members stated they had also had a similar conversation with him, although no one could recall Joe exhibiting any signs of coughing or choking while eating. I then thought about my 30 years of nursing in various areas, including on a medical ward that admitted stroke patients, and thought I had never witnessed a severe choking episode in any other area of nursing other than mental health.

A few years on, and a medical emergency was called one evening. Joe was found with a head laceration, unresponsive and not breathing. The coroner's report showed death from asphyxiation with a food bolus lodged in his larynx. Whether Joe had suffered a seizure that caused him to asphyxiate or whether he asphyxiated and then fell will never be determined. What we do know is that Joe left the dining room with food in his mouth.

by Anne

Reflective questions

- Consider Limor's and Anne's stories. What were critical elements of their projects?
- Consider the possible role of health professionals' attitudes and beliefs as they relate to changing practice. How will these affect the outcome of such projects?

Dysphagia

Dysphagia is a problem that has been recognised as occurring more commonly among people with mental illness than among the general population. It is estimated that 32 per cent of people with a mental illness experience dysphagia, compared with 6 per cent of the general population (Regan, Sowman & Walsh, 2006). This seems to be related to behavioural factors and adverse reactions to anti-psychotic medications (Bazemore, Tonkonogy & Ananth, 1991). Fast-eating syndrome is the most common behavioural cause of choking among people with mental illness (Applebaum et al., 1992). It is compounded by people taking large mouthfuls of food, gorging and pocketing (saving) food in the cheek (McMannus, 2001). An Australian study of choking deaths reported that people who had died from choking were 20 times more likely to have a medical diagnosis of schizophrenia than others who had died from choking (Ruschena, Mullen & Burgess, 1998). Indeed, the risk of non-aspiration choking was 30 times greater in people with schizophrenia than the general population (Warner, 2004).

Consumer narrative   Reducing dysphagia part two

Twenty years later, after having worked in various other areas of nursing, including medical/surgical, I was once again called to a medical emergency with a very similar scenario of choking (see part one), although on this occasion with a positive outcome.

During my 30-year nursing career, the only time I have witnessed choking has been within mental health nursing. Why is this so? Could the cause be the medications, the environment or something else? While working within a large public health mental health facility over a period of 12 months there had been quite a few serious incidents of choking, and therefore a clinical practice improvement (CPI) project was commenced to ascertain what could be done about this problem. The project initially commenced with a literature search, which revealed that the problem was common across the world within the mental health field. The literature revealed various reasons this has been occurring and emphasised the role of medications and environmental factors. Researching the role of anti-psychotic medications, I discovered that there were serious choking risk factors associated with many anti-psychotic medications, both typical and atypical.

As the clients we were caring for were often people who had illnesses that did not respond to current treatments and many were stable after years of constant changes in medication, the CPI concentrated on changing the environmental factors. This involved quite a few changes and required staff to be educated and willing to change. Food service staff also needed to understand the seriousness of this problem and be accepting of the change. The environment was changed to one of a homely atmosphere, with the menu for the meal displayed outside the dining room. Music was played in the dining room in an attempt to create a relaxed environment. Tablecloths were placed on tables. The occupational therapist assessed the correct height of chairs and tables with correct utensils for each client. Clients were served one course at a time and encouraged to drink between courses, and some clients who were assessed as being at high risk of choking were encouraged to eat small mouthfuls. Clients were also involved in the change, with pre and post-evaluations undertaken. Tea and coffee were served at the end of the meal, in an attempt to stop clients leaving the dining room with a mouth full of food. The time for meals was extended to at least 20 minutes, instead of the quick 5–10 minutes it had been. Staff members were encouraged to sit with clients and engage in conversation, in an effort to slow down eating. Drinking of water was also encouraged to aid mastication of food. Incidents of choking were reduced from eight per year prior to the implementation of the CPI to nil incidents in the 12 months following.

Interventions

Physical health care for people with mental illness has been recognised as a neglected field. Mental health leaders, both in Australia and New Zealand (Muir-Cochrane & Wand, 2005) and overseas (Gournay, 2005) have recognised the need and the responsibility of those working in this field to address these issues. By the end of the first decade of the 21st century, government policies were in place to ensure that this need was no longer overlooked (Mental Health and Drug and Alcohol Office, 2009).

Initiatives to address the physical health care needs of people with mental illness must encompass approaches that will be adequately flexible. People may have cognitive deficits or poor levels of motivation (Gournay, 2005), or may be subject to limitations to access due to a range of socio-economic factors, including stigmatisation and poverty.

Nurses and other staff working with people who have mental illness recognise that extending care to include physical health interventions is an important part of holistic care (Happell et al., 2012). However, a range of other factors also act as barriers to ready adoption of this as part of day-to-day practice, including the manner in which work is organised (that is, models of care). Happell and colleagues (2012), in a study of the adoption of exercise in mental health care, suggested that such barriers may operate at both the individual and systemic levels, and may include factors such as geography, financial and social circumstances, current state of health and stigma. They acknowledged that these factors were significant barriers to most people in changing behaviours to adopt healthier levels of exercise, but pointed out that the situation of those with SMI, in particular, is difficult.

Increasingly, mental health services are developing so-called 'wellness' or 'lifestyle' clinics to address these challenges. Such clinics take many forms, responsive to the needs and desires of their recipients. They may be found in in-patient, forensic and community settings, and increasingly in primary health settings, and may take a particular focus on a part of the lifespan, such the elderly or adolescents (Wynaden et al., 2012). Studies are beginning to demonstrate the efficacy of this approach to overcome the barriers to participation previously described (Happell, Davies & Scott, 2012; Hodgson, McCulloch & Fox, 2011). Interventions for young people experiencing their first episode of psychosis are recognised as critical, as comorbid physical conditions rapidly become evident (McCloughen et al., 2012).

A range of screening tools is being introduced in different practice settings, in an attempt to deliver screening interventions where and when people with mental illness are encountered in health or mental health services. These tools include prompts to help clinicians recall the most important physical health tests to administer and questions to ask. Examples include the United Kingdom Physical Health Checklist (Phelan et al., 2004) and the Health Improvement Profile (White, Gray & Jones, 2009). In Australia, a standardised tool is being developed for introduction to public mental health services (MHDAO, 2012). All of these tools share certain characteristics: an annual list of recommended health screening checks, prompt questions about general lifestyle factors and a symptom checklist.

The nurse is well placed to be the agent for these interventions (Hardy & Thomas, 2012). Nurses are prepared educationally with the knowledge, skills and attitudes to perform these screening interventions and arrange follow-up if required. In addition, nurses work in many of the contexts in which people with mental illness are to be found. Ensuring that physical screening is a routine component of any intervention should be part of every nurse's practice. Any services redesigned or developed to address the physical health needs of those with mental illness must incorporate the opinions, desires and insights of those for whom the services are being developed (Chadwick et al., 2012).

Figure 8.5 summarises the data collected by Morgan and colleagues (2011) and described earlier in the chapter. In the course of one year prior to data being collected in 2010, almost all participants (97.4 per cent) had undergone one or more of eight different types of assessments to monitor the status of their health. For most people (85.6 per cent) this was a blood pressure check, and approximately 75 per cent had waist or weight measures taken. However, approximately two-thirds (67.3 per cent) had had a physical examination in the previous year and 63.3 per cent had had a blood test.

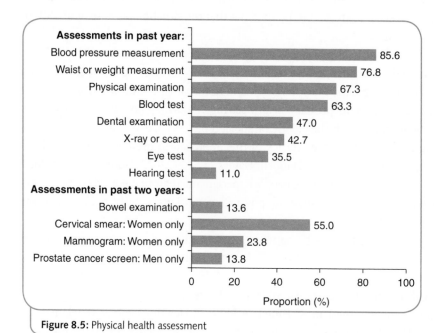

Figure 8.5: Physical health assessment

Interprofessional connections

A friend of mine, a credentialled mental health nurse, has recently commenced working with a non-government service that supports people seeking asylum in Australia. Many of these people have experienced traumatic events and, as a consequence, may have developed mental illnesses. The uncertainty of their wait to determine the outcome of their applications for refugee status and the precarious conditions under which they live are other sources of stress.

The position my friend is developing with her employer is new, but recognises the special capacity a mental health nurse has to contribute to care of asylum seekers through the facilitation of interprofessional collaboration. Her work involves comprehensive assessment of the client and then assessment of suitable services to meet her or his needs.

Recently, a new client was seen at the centre who was 34 weeks pregnant and had type 2 diabetes (but had received no treatment for this during her pregnancy). As the woman did not speak English, the interpreter service was engaged, and this added to the stress she was experiencing, along with a very different health system and culture than she has previously been accustomed to. She had only recently arrived in Australia and had had blood tests in her homeland, but no antenatal care in Australia. A range of services needed to be organised and was coordinated primarily by the mental health nurse. These services included legal services, antenatal care at the local hospital, a diabetes educator, endocrinologist, doula, dietitian, social worker at the local antenatal clinic and a social worker within the centre to find appropriate housing and financial support for her. As the woman was separated from her husband and family due to a recent upheaval in her homeland, coupled with recent traumatising events she had witnessed, the mental health nurse organised a pro bono psychologist to assist her during this difficult time.

The woman did not have access to Medicare but was applying for a protection visa, and this entitled her to access to antenatal care within a public hospital. Initially, the nurse had to clarify where the client would be living for the following six weeks, as she could not be booked into a public hospital if she was not living within its local health district .The nurse booked the woman into the hospital, then consulted with the social worker from the antenatal clinic. As the woman had minimal emotional support, the nurse contacted the local doula society, which organised a doula to support her (free of charge). The social worker at the centre organised financial support for the interim, with assistance from various non-government organisations. Although all disciplines played a major role within the care for this woman, the mental health nurse took the role of overseeing care.

The antenatal clinic organised for the woman to see a diabetes educator and endocrinologist, as her blood glucose levels were high. She was given a glucometer and explained how to use it and the importance or taking her blood levels four times a day. Afterwards the woman presented back to the centre and told the mental health nurse she did not know what she had to do with the glucometer. With the assistance

continued ›

Interprofessional connections continued ›

of the telephone interpreter service, the nurse discovered that the client was indeed experiencing a high level of stress and anxiety, which made it very difficult for her to retain new information. The nurse demonstrated how to take a blood glucose level and reinforced the importance of recording the results of each test. The nurse then asked the interpreter to go through the details again and the woman wrote them in her language to avoid confusion later.

Chapter summary

- People with mental illness experience higher rates of metabolic syndrome than the general population, resulting in higher prevalence of cardiovascular diseases and type 2 diabetes.
- Other physical illnesses and conditions are also over-represented among people with mental illnesses; these include some cancers, poor dental health, sexual dysfunctions and dysphagia.
- Routine integration of screening, assessment and referral of physical health issues for people with mental illness is critical in addressing premature morbidity.
- Services should be flexible to meet the needs and desires of individuals and should be developed in collaboration with them and their carers.

Critical thinking/learning activities

1 Evidence of effective preventative factors for the metabolic syndrome are not clear and people who are being treated with some common anti-psychotic medications develop the precursors (weight gain, insulin resistance). What approach could be given to promote physical health?

2 Sexuality is an aspect of health that is affected by the experience of mental illness. Nominate some of the reasons sexuality may be negatively affected, and some possible remedies.

3 Many psychotropic medications affect the swallowing reflex, raising orthodox treatment recommendations of dietary modification. People with enduring mental illnesses may face an indefinite future with texture-modified diets. Discuss the consequences for consumers and possible responses to support attaining the best possible quality of life.

Learning extension

Design a series of posters addressing the physical health needs of people experiencing a mental illness. Discuss which services should be targeted and which disciplines this could involve. For example, primary health posters might be designed that have GPs as their target audience. Posters may be designed for emergency department staff, to encourage comprehensive health assessment for people presenting with mental illness that also incorporates physical health. Brochures could be produced for consumers of mental health services and their carers about the risks of metabolic syndrome.

Further reading

Australian Dietary Guidelines: www.nhmrc.gov.au/guidelines/publications/n55

These were developed by the National Health and Medical Research Council from current best evidence. It is the most authoritative source in this highly contested field and should be the basis of understanding, advice and evaluations made of dietary habits.

Australian Resource Centre for Healthcare Innovations: www.archi.net.au/resources/safety/clinical/hamilton-dysphagia

Further details are available on the dysphagia CPI project described by Anne. Listening to the different professionals of different disciplines (nursing, dietetics, and speech pathology) shows how effective work is best done in a collaborative and inclusive manner.

Recovery Devon: www.recoverydevon.co.uk/index.php/recovery-in-action/as-practitioners/80-recovery-orientated-prescribing-and-medicines-management

Steph's writing addresses the human rights framework and need for collaborative approaches to all aspects of care. This includes the use of medication. The link provided is to an advisory paper addressing considerations relevant to establishing a recovery orientated approach to medications in mental health care.

Rethink Mental Illness: www.rethink.org/resources/m

This is an opportunity to familiarise yourself with a comprehensive health screening tool developed for use with people experiencing SMI.

Physical Health Care of Mental Health Consumers: www0.health.nsw.gov.au/policies/gl/2009/GL2009_007.html

Guidelines for physical health care of people with mental illness.

References

Addington, J., el-Guelbaly, N., Campbell, W., Hodgins, D. C. & Addington, D. (1998). Smoking cessation treatment for patients with schizophrenia. *The American Journal of Psychiatry*, *155*(7): 974–6.

Alder, L. E., Olincy, A., Waldo, M., Harris, J., Griffith, J., Stevens, K. & Freedman, R. (1998). Schizophrenia, sensory gating and nicotinic receptors. *Schizophrenia bulletin*, *24*(2): 189–202.

Allebeck, P. (1989). Schizophrenia: A life-shortening disease. *Schizophrenia Bulletin*, *15*: 81–9.

Applebaum, K. L., Bazemore, P., Tonkonogy, J., Ananth, R. & Shull, S. (1992). Privilege & discharge decisions for psychiatric inpatients with dysphagia. *Hospital and Community Psychiatry*, *43*: 1023–5.

Arrufo, J. F., Coverdale, J. H., Chako, R. C., Dworkin, R. J., & Rosalind, J., (1990). Knowledge about AIDS among women psychiatric outpatients. *Hospital and Community Psychiatry*, *41*: 326–8.

Australian Bureau of Statistics (ABS) (2008). *National Survey of Mental Health and Wellbeing. Summary of results 2007*. Canberra: Author.

(ABS) (2012). *Causes of Death, Australia, 2010*. Canberra: Author.

Australian Institute of Health and Welfare (2009). *Analysis of the 2007–2008 National Health Survey*. Retrieved from www.aihw.gov.au/overweight-and-obesity/prevalence.

Basson, B. R., Kinon, B. J., Taylor, C. C., Szymanski, K. A., Gilmore, J. A. & Tollefson, G. D. (2001). Factors influencing acute weight change in patients with schizophrenia treated with olanzapine, haloperidol, or risperidone. *The Journal of Clinical Psychiatry*, *62*(4): 231–8.

Bazemore, P. H., Tonkonogy, J. & Ananth, R. (1991). Dysphagia in psychiatric patients: Clinical and videofluroscopic study. *Dysphagia*, *6*(1): 2–5.

Berner, M. M., Hagen, M. & Kriston, M. (2007). Management of sexual dysfunction due to antipsychotic drug therapy. *Cochrane Database of Systematic Reviews*, *1*(Art. no.: CD003546). DOI: 10.1002/14651858. CD003546.pub2.

Blank, M. B., Mandell, D. S., Aiken, L. & Hadley, T. R. (2002). Co-occurrence of HIV and serious mental illness among Medicaid recipients. *Psychiatric Services*, *53*(7); 868–73.

Blythe, J. & White, J. (2012). Role of the mental health nurse towards physical health care in serious mental illness: An integrative review of 10 years of UK Literature. *International Journal of Mental Health Nursing*, *21*(3): 193–201.

Busche, B. & Holt, R. (2004). Prevalence of diabetes and impaired glucose tolerance in patients with schizophrenia. *British Journal of Psychiatry*, 184 (Suppl): s67–71.

Chadwick, A., Street, C., McAndrew, S. & Deacon, M. (2012). Minding our own bodies: Reviewing the literature regarding the perceptions of service users diagnosed with serious mental illness on barriers to accessing physical health care. *International Journal of Mental Health Nursing*, 21(3): 211–19.

Chester, R. (1996). Towards continence: Approaches to continence in homes for older people. *Nursing Times*, 96(31): 15–17.

Cormac, I. & Jenkins, P. (1999). Understanding the importance of oral health in psychiatric patients. *Advances in Psychiatric Treatment*, 5: 53–60.

Cournos, F., McKinnon, M. A. & Sullivan, G. (2005). Schizophrenia and comorbid human immunodeficiency virus or hepatitis C virus. *Journal of Clinical Psychiatry*, 66(S6): 27–33.

Craig, C., Marshall, A., Sjöström, M., Bauman, A., Booth, M., Ainsworth B. … & Oja, P. (2003). International physical activity questionnaire: 12-country reliability and validity. *Medicine and Science in Sports and Exercise*, 35: 1381–95.

Dalack, G. W., Healy, D. J. & Meador-Woodruff, J. H. (1998). Nicotine dependence in schizophrenia: clinical phenomena and laboratory findings. *American Journal of Psychiatry*, 155: 1490–501.

Davison, J. & Huntington, A. (2010). 'Out of sight': Sexuality and women with enduring mental illness. *International Journal of Mental Health Nursing*, 19: 240–9.

de Leon, J., Becona, E., Gurpegui, M., Gonzalez-Pinto, A. & Diaz, F. J. (2002). The association between high nicotine dependence and severe mental illness may be consistent across countries. *Journal of Clinical Psychiatry*, 63(9): 812–16.

Deegan, P. E. (2001). Human sexuality and mental illness: Consumer viewpoints and recovery principles. In P. Buckley (ed.), *Sexuality and Serious Mental Illness* (pp. 21–33). Amsterdam: Harwood Academic Publishers.

Deng, C., Weston-Green, K. & Huang, X.-F. (2010). The role of histaminergic H1 and H3 receptors in food intake: A mechanism for atypical antipsychotic-induced weight gain? *Progress in neuro-psychopharmacology & biological psychiatry*, 34(1): 1–4.

Department of Health (2001). *Diabetes National Service Framework*. London: Author.

Department of Health. (2011). *No Health Without Mental Health*. London: Author.

Dyer, J. & McGuiness, T. (2008). Reducing HIV risk among people with serious mental illness. *Journal of Psychosocial Nursing*, 46(4): 26–34.

Elliott, D. M., Mok, D. S., & Briere, J. (2004). Adult sexual assault: Prevalence, symptomatology, and sex differences in the general population. *Journal of Traumatic Stress*, 17(3), 203–211.

Foley, D. & Morley, K. I. (2011). Systematic review of early cardio-metabolic outcomes of the first treated episode of psychosis. *Archives of General Psychiatry*, 68(6): 609–16.

Fortier, P., Mottard, J. P., Trudel, Q. & Even, S. (2003). Study of sexuality-related characteristics in young adults with schizophrenia treated with novel neuroleptics and in a comparison group of young adults. *Schizophrenia bulletin*, 29(3): 559–72.

Friedlander, A. & Marder, S. (2002). The psychopathology, medical management and dental implications of schizophrenia. *Journal of the American Dental Association*, 113: 603–10.

Glozier, N. (2012). *Physical health in mental illness: Improving health, reducing risk factors, managing medication. A Contributing Life: The 2012 National Report Card on Mental Health and Suicide Prevention*. Retrieved from www.mentalhealthcommission.gov.au/media/42027/Lit%20review%20-%20Physical%20Health.pdf.

Goff, D. C., Henderson, D. C. & Amico, E. (1992). Cigarette smoking in schizophrenia: relationship to psychopathology and medication side effects. *American Journal of Psychiatry*, 149(9): 1189–94.

Goodwin, V. & Happell, B. (2007). Consumer and carer participation in mental health care: The carer's perspective: Part 2 – barriers to effective and genuine participation. *Issues in Mental Health Nursing*, 28(6): 625–38.

Gough, S. & Peveler, R. C. (2004). Diabetes and its prevention: Pragmatic solutions for people with schizophrenia. *British Journal of Psychiatry*, 184(Suppl. 47): s106–11.

Gournay, K. (2005). The changing face of psychiatric nursing: Revisiting… Mental health nursing. *Advances in Psychiatric Treatment*, 11(1): 6–11.

Gregorian, R.S., Golden, K.A., Bahce, A., Goodman, C., Kwong, W.J. & Khan, Z.M. (2002). Antidepressant-induced sexual dysfunction. *The Annals of pharmacotherapy, 36*(10): 1577–89.

Griffiths, J., Jones, V., Leeman, I., Lewis, D., Patel, K., Wilson, K. & Blankenstein, R. (2000). Oral health care for people with mental health problems: Guidelines and recommendations. *British Society for Disability and Oral Health, 1*(1): 1–20.

Hall, W. (2012). *Harm Reduction Guide to Coming Off Psychiatric Drugs,* 2nd edn. Northampton, MA: The Icarus Project and Freedom Center. Retrieved from www.theicarusproject.net/downloads/ComingOffPsych DrugsHarmReductGuide2Edonline.pdf.

Happell, B., Davies, C. & Scott, D. (2012). Health behaviour interventions to improve physical health in individuals diagnosed with a mental illness: A systematic review. *International Journal of Mental Health Nursing, 21*(3): 236–47.

Happell, B., Scott, D., Platania-Phung, C. & Nankivell, J. (2012). Nurses' views on physical activity for people with serious mental illness. *Mental Health and Physical Activity, 5*(1): 4–12.

Hardy, S. & Thomas, B. (2012). Mental and physical health comordibity: Political imperatives and practice implications. *International Journal of Mental Health Nursing, 21*(3): 289–98.

Hodgson, M.H., McCulloch, H.P. & Fox, K.R. (2011). The experiences of people with severe and enduring mental illness engaged in a physical activity programme integrated into the mental health service. *Mental Health and Physical Activity, 4*(1): 23–29.

Holt, R.I.G. & Peveler, R.C. (2005). Association between antipsychotic drugs and diabetes. *Diabetes, Obesity and Metabolism, 8*: 125–35.

Hughes, J.R., Hatsukami, D.K., Mitchell, J.E. & Dahlgren, L.A. (1986). Prevalence of smoking among psychiatric outpatients. *American Journal of Psychiatry, 143*: 993–7.

Jablensky, A., McGrath, J., Herrman, H., Castle, D., Gureje, O., Morgan, V. & Korten, A. (1999). *People Living with Psychotic Illness: An Australian study 1997–98. National survey of mental health and wellbeing: Report 4. National Mental Health Strategy.* Canberra: Australian Government.

John, A.P., Koloth, R., Dragovic, M. & Lim, S.C. (2009). Prevalence of metabolic syndrome among Australians with severe mental illness. *The Medical Journal of Australia, 190*(4): 176–9.

Jones, S., Howard, L. & Thornicroft, G. (2008). 'Diagnostic overshadowing': Worse physical health care for people with mental illness. *Acta Psychiatrica Scandinavica, 118*(3): 169–71.

Jopp, D. & Keys, C. (2001). Diagnostic overshadowing reviewed and reconsidered. *American Journal of Mental Retardation, 106*: 416–33.

Jorm, A.F., Bourchier, S.J., Cvetkovski, S. & Stewart, G. (2012). Systematic review: Mental health of Indigenous Australians: A review of findings from community surveys. *Medical Journal of Australia, 196*(2): 118–23.

Kalichman, S.C., Kelly, J.A., Johnson, J.R. & Bulto, M. (1994). Factors associated with risk for HIV infection among chronic mentally ill adults. *American Journal of Psychiatry, 151*(2): 221–7.

Kelly, C. & McCreadie, R. (2000). Cigarette smoking and schizophrenia. *Advances in Psychiatric Treatment, 6*: 327–32.

Khawaja, M.Y. (2005). Sexual dysfunction in male patients taking antipsychotics. *Journal of Ayub Medical College, Abbottabad, 17*(3): 73–5.

Khokhar, W., Clifton, A., Jones, H. & Tosh, G. (2011). Oral health advice for people with serious mental illness. *Cochrane Database of Systematic Reviews 2011,* 11. Retrieved from http://onlinelibrary.wiley.com/doi/10.1002/14651858.CD008802.pub2/pdf/standard.

Koran, D. (2004). Diabetes mellitus and schizophrenia: Historical perspective. *British Journal of Psychiatry, 184*(Suppl 47): s64–6.

Kreuter, M., Chheda, S. & Bull, F. (2000). How does physician advice influence patient behavior? Evidence for a priming effect. *Archives of Family Medicine, 9*(5): 426–33.

Lambert, T.J.R. (2011). Managing the metabolic adverse effects of antipsychotic drugs in patients with psychosis. *Australian Prescriber, 34*: 97–9.

Lambert, T.J.R. & Newcomer, J.W. (2009). Are the cardiometabolic complications of schizophrenia still neglected? Barriers to care. *Medical Journal of Australia, 190* Supplement(4): S39–42.

Maddock, S. & Hallam, S. (2010). *Recovery Begins With Hope.* London: National School of Government.

McCandless, F. & Sladen, C. (2003). Sexual health and women with bipolar disorder. *Journal of Advanced Nursing, 44*(1): 42–8.

McCloughen, A., Foster, K., Huws-Thomas, M. & Delgado, C. (2012). Physical health and wellbeing of emerging and young adults with mental illness: An integrative review of international literature. *International Journal of Mental Health Nursing, 21*(3): 274–88.

McEvoy, J.P., Lieberman, J.A., Perkins, D., Hamer, R., Gu, H., Lazarus, A., Sweitzer, D., Olexy, C., Weiden, P. & Strakowski, S. (2007). Efficacy and tolerability of olanzapine, quetiapine, and risperidone in the treatment of early psychosis: A randomized, double-blind 52-week comparison. *The American Journal of Psychiatry, 164*: 1050–60.

McMannus, M. (2001). Dysphagia in psychiatric patients. *Journal of Psychosocial Nursing, 39*(2): 24–30.

McNeill, A. (2001). *Smoking and Mental Health: A Review of the Literature*. London: ASH.

Melville, J.L., Walker, E., Katon, W., Lentz, G., Miller, J. & Fenner, D. (2002). Prevalence of comorbid psychiatric illness & its impact on symptom perception, quality of life, & functional status in women with urinary incontinence. *American Journal of Obstetrics & Gynecology, 187*(1): 80–7.

Mental Health and Drug and Alcohol Office (MHDAO) (2009). *Physical Health Care of Mental Health Consumers: Guidelines*. North Sydney: NSW Department of Health.

MHDAO (2012). *Metabolic Monitoring: A new mental health clinical documentation module*. (IB2012_024). North Sydney: NSW Department of Health: Retrieved from www0.health.nsw.gov.au/policies/ib/2012/pdf/IB2012_024.pdf.

Montebugnoli, L., Servidio, D., Miaton, R., Prati, C., Tricoci, P. & Melloni, C. (2004). Poor oral health is associated with coronary heart disease and elevated systemic inflammatory and haemostatic factors. *Journal of Clinical Periodontology, 31*(1): 25–9.

Moodie, R., Stuckler, D., Monteiro, C., Sheron, N., Neal, B., Thamarangsi, T. & Casswell, S. (2013). Profits and pandemics: Prevention of harmful effects of tobacco, alcohol, and ultra-processed food and drink industries. *The Lancet*. Online first, doi: http://dx.doi.org/10.1016/S0140–6736(12)62089–3.

Morgan, V.A., Waterreus, A., Jablensky, A., Mackinnon, A., McGrath, J.J., Carr, V. & Saw, S. (2011). *People living with psychotic illness 2010. Report on the second Australian national survey* National Mental Health Strategy. Canberra: Australian Government.

Muir-Cochrane, E. & Wand, T. (2005). *Contemporary Issues in Risk Assessment and Management in Mental Health*. South Australia: Australian and New Zealand College of Mental Health Nurses, Inc.

Narasimhan, M. & Raynor, J. (2010). Evidence-based perspective on metabolic syndrome and use of antipsychotics. *Drug Benefit Trends, 22*: 77–88.

National Health and Medical Research Council (NHMRC) (2013). *Australian Dietary Guidelines (2013)*. (Reference Number: N55). Canberra: Author. Retrieved from www.nhmrc.gov.au/guidelines/publications.

Newcomer, J.W. (2007). Metabolic syndrome and mental illness. *American Journal of Managed Care, 13*: S170–7.

NHS Smokesfree (2001). *NHS Stop Smoking Services: Service and monitoring guidance 2010/11*. London: Department of Health.

Oakley Browne, M.A., Wells, J.E. & Scott, K.M. (2006). *Te Rau Hinengaro: The New Zealand Mental Health Survey*. Wellington: Ministry of Health.

Office of the Commissioner for Human Rights (2007). *Convention on the Rights of Persons with Disabilities*. Retrieved from www.ohchr.org/EN/HRBodies/CRPD/Pages/ConventionRightsPersonsWithDisabilities.aspx.

Olfson, M., Uttaro, T., Carson, W.H. & Tafesse, E. (2005). Male sexual dysfunction and quality of life in schizophrenia. *The Journal of Clinical Psychiatry, 66*(3): 331–8.

Parker, R. (2010). Australia's Aboriginal population and mental health. *The Journal of Nervous and Mental Disease, 198*(1): 3–7.

Phelan, M., Sradins, L., Amin, D., Isadore, R., Hitrov, C., Doyle, A. & Inglis, R. (2004). The physical health check: A tool for mental health workers. *Journal of Mental Health, 13*(3): 277–84.

Quinn, C., Happell, B. & Welch, A. (2012). Talking about sex as part of our role: Making and sustaining practice change. *International Journal of Mental Health Nursing, 22*(3): 231–40.

Raedler, T.J. (2010). Cardiovascular aspects of antipsychotics. *Current Opinion in Psychiatry, 23*(6): 574–81.

Regan, J., Sowman, R, & Walsh, I. (2006). Prevalence of dysphagia in acute and community mental health settings. *Dysphagia, 2006*: 95–101.

Reiss, S., Levitan, G. & Szyszko, J. (1982). Emotional disturbance and mental retardation: Diagnostic overshadowing. *American Journal of Mental Deficiency*, *86*: 567–74.

Robson, D. & Gray, R. (2007). Serious mental illness and physical health problems: A discussion paper. *International Journal of Nursing Studies*, *44*(3): 457–66.

Roe, D. & Swarbrick, M. (2007). A recovery oriented approach to psychiatric medication: Guidelines for the practitioner. *Journal of Psychosocial Nursing and Mental Health Service*, *45*(2): 35–40.

Rosenberg, S., Goodman, L. A. & Osher, F. C. (2001). Prevalence of HIV, hepatitis B and hepatitis C in people with severe mental illness. *American Journal of Public Health*, *91*: 31–7.

Rosenberg, S. D., Drake, R. E., Brunette, M. F., Wolford, G. L. & Marsh, B. J. (2005). Hepatitis C virus and HIV co-infection in people with severe mental illness and substance use disorders. *AIDS*, *19* (S3): S26–33.

Royal Australian and New Zealand College of Psychiatrists (2005). Clinical practice guidelines for the treatment of schizophrenia and related disorders. *Australian and New Zealand Journal of Psychiatry*, *39*(1–2): 1–30.

Ruschena, D., Mullen, P. E. & Burgess, P. (1998). Sudden death in psychiatric patients. *British Journal of Psychiatric*, *172*: 331–6.

Sassi, F., Devaux, M., Cecchini, M. & Rusticelli, E., (2009). *The Obesity Epidemic: Analysis of past and projected future trends in selected OECD countries*. Paris: Organization for Economic Co-operation and Development.

Schoos, R. & Cohen, C. I. (2003). Medical health in aging persons with schizophrenia. In J. M. Meyer & H. A. Nasrallah (eds), *Medical Illness and Schizophrenia*. Vancouver: American Psychiatric Publishing.

Sewell, D. D. (1996). Schizophrenia and HIV. *Schizophrenia bulletin*, *22*: 465–73.

Simonelli-Muñoz, A. J., Fortea, M. I., Salorio, P., Gallego-Gomez, J. I., Sánchez-Bautista, S. & Balanza, S. (2012). Dietary habits of patients with schizophrenia: A self-reported questionnaire survey. *International Journal of Mental Health Nursing*, *21*(3): 220–8.

Sutherland, G. (2003). Smoking: can we really make a difference? *Heart*, *89*(Suppl 2: ii25–27), Discussion ii35–37.

Tiihonen, J., Lönnqvist, J., Wahlbeck, K., Klaukka, T., Niskanen, L., Tanskanen, A. & Haukka, J. (2009). 11-year follow-up of mortality in patients with schizophrenia: A population-based cohort study (FIN11 study). *The Lancet*, *374*(9690): 620–7.

Tsakiris, P., Oelke, M. & Michel, M. (2008). Drug induced urinary incontinence. *Drugs and Aging*, *25*(7): 541–9.

van Winkel, R., De Hert, M. & Wampers, M. (2008). Major changes in glucose metabolism including new-onset diabetes within 3 months after initiation or switch of atypical antipsychotic medication in patients with schizophrenia and schizoaffective disorder. *Journal of Clinical Psychiatry*, *69*: 472–9.

Volman, L. & Landeen, J. (2007). Uncovering the sexual self in people with schizophrenia. *Journal of Psychiatric and Mental Health Nursing*, *14*(4): 411–17.

Vos, T., Barker, B., Begg, S., Stanley, L. & Lopez, A. D. (2009). Burden of disease and injury in Aboriginal and Torres Strait Islander peoples: The Indigenous health gap. *International Journal of Epidemiology*, *38*(2): 470–7.

Warner, J. P. (2004). Risk of choking in mental illness. *Lancet*, *363*(9410): 674.

Warner, J. P., Harvey, C. A. & Barnes, T. R. E. (1994). Clozapine & urinary incontinence. *International Clinical Psychopharmacology*, *9*(3): 207–9.

White, J., Gray, R. & Jones, M. (2009). The development of the serious mental illness physical health improvement profile. *Journal of Psychiatric and Mental Health Nursing*, *16*: 493–8.

World Federation for Mental Health (2010). *Mental Health and Chronic Physical Illnesses. The need for continued and integrated care*. Retrieved from www.wfmh.org/2010DOCS/WMHDAY2010.pdf.

Wynaden, D., Barr, L., Omari, O. & Fulton, A. (2012). Evaluation of service users' experiences of participating in an exercise programme at the Western Australian State Forensic Mental Health Services. *International Journal of Mental Health Nursing*, *21*(3): 229–35.

9

Mental health of people of immigrant and refugee backgrounds

Nicholas Procter, Asma Babakarkhil, Amy Baker and Monika Ferguson

Introduction 198

What is meant by the terms refugee, immigrant and asylum seeker? 200

Temporary Protection Visas 201

Mental health of people of immigrant and refugee background 202

Culture and explanatory models in mental health 204

Isolation 207

Engagement with mainstream mental health services 208

Traumatic stress 209

Access and engagement when in distress 211

Trust and human connectedness in mental health 211

Older people of immigrant background 212

Chapter summary 213

Critical thinking/learning activities 213

Learning extension 214

Further reading 215

References 215

Learning objectives

At the completion of this chapter, you should be able to:

- Describe the mental health problems and needs of people from immigrant and refugee backgrounds.
- Identify risk and protective factors for mental health for people of immigrant and refugee backgrounds.
- Identify and discuss the implications of mental illness for people of refugee and asylum seeker backgrounds as they interact with mainstream health and mental health services.
- Identify and discuss the implications of cultural explanatory models in mental health.
- Demonstrate awareness of engagement with consumers and carers from immigrant, asylum seeker and refugee backgrounds, including enablers and barriers to meaningful engagement in mental health.

Introduction

cultural competence and responsiveness
the ability to see beyond the boundaries of one's own cultural interpretations, to be able to remain objective when faced with individuals from different cultures and to be able to interpret and understand behaviours and intentions of people from other cultures, in the context in which they occur and without bias or judgement; the term also refers to organisations and systems that function effectively and appropriately in interactions with people from diverse cultural and linguistic backgrounds

refugee
someone who leaves her or his country of origin or usual residence due to fear of persecution for reasons of race, religion, nationality, or membership of a particular group or political opinion and is unable or unwilling to return to it

asylum seeker
someone who has left his or her country of origin in search of refuge

While the health systems in Australia, New Zealand and other developed countries are regarded as some of the finest in the world, there is an ever-present need to ensure flexibility regarding **cultural competence** and cultural inclusivity across a range of practice settings. Australia, for example, has one of the most diverse populations in the world, with more than 25 per cent of its current population being born overseas (Commonwealth of Australia, 2012). If current rates of immigration to Australia continue to grow, it is estimated that by 2050 approximately one-third of Australia's population will be overseas-born (Cully and Pejozki, 2012).

This chapter examines the mental health needs of people from **refugee** and immigrant backgrounds, with particular emphasis given to **asylum seekers**. The chapter explores mental illnesses that may affect these populations and focuses on engagement between people of refugee and asylum seeker backgrounds and mainstream mental health services. The chapter seeks to deepen and broaden readers' understandings of the effects of trauma among asylum seekers, and links this to strategies that might be used by mainstream mental health clinicians and services in response.

Consumer narrative   Hanan's story: part one

My name is Hanan. I am a 51-year-old housewife and mother of two from Iraq, where I worked as a teacher for 10 years. My journey began in 1996, when I left Iraq with my family and spent time living in Jordan, Syria, Iran, Malaysia and Indonesia, then Nauru before eventually, in 2004, being granted refugee protection and permanent residence in Australia.

Traumas to my mental health started during the journey to Australia in a leaky fishing boat, upon which 270 people were squashed, including my young sons. During the boat journey I felt uncertain of my survival from one hour to the next and was in a constant state of high stress for several days. This constant fear was compounded by my children becoming ill, the lack of a bathroom (with only one toilet on board) and the smugglers constantly demanding that all passengers move around to balance the boat and stop it

continued ›

from taking on too much water and sinking. When the boat was no longer safe, I was told to wait for another ship to pick us up. We waited for seven days on the boat while it took on water. I suffered a constant fear of death.

My family spent three-and-a-half years on Nauru, where we lived in tents and, later, in rooms with tin roofs. It was very hot, dirty, and we were constantly harassed by mosquitoes. We had limited access to water, which was particularly difficult as all island inhabitants had a 30-minute window of time to use water each day, with only five bathrooms for over 1000 people. There were regularly quarrels about the use of showers. For the first two years it was very distressing as there were no schools for the children, no activities and no access to health care. It was only after the initial two years that a mental health clinic was provided and two hours of schooling per day for children. This followed repeated hunger strikes, which my husband was a part of, and some asylum seekers sewed their lips or attempted to hang themselves in their tents. It was 10 years ago that this happened, but I still feel the effects today.

During our time on Nauru, I developed anxiety over the status of my family's application for a protection visa. I was anxious and worried about my children's mental health, which was being affected by the suicides and self-mutilation of other asylum seekers. I was also anxious about my vision impairment problems, which I attribute to my constant state of distress. A specialist declared me legally blind and in need of surgery to restore my vision. This advice was ignored for over three years – the time I was held on Nauru. It was only after I arrived in Australia that I managed to get surgery to restore my vision.

Consumer narrative   Ali's story

My name is Ali. I am 19 years old, from Afghanistan and work in a metal scrap yard in Sydney. My parents were from different ethnicities. My father was killed when I was 12 years old, and I escaped Afghanistan with my mother and two younger siblings to live as refugees in Quetta, Pakistan. At age 16, I left Pakistan to come to Australia to support my family. My uncle in Russia sent $10 000 to pay people smugglers so that I could take the journey from Pakistan to Australia.

I spent six months in the detention centre on Christmas Island, after arriving by boat. Since that dangerous, frightening journey I have been scared of the ocean, and still can't go to the beach with my friends without fear and feeling tense. I refuse to go.

Most of the asylum seekers in the detention centre were Afghan and, because of my young age, the older men took care of me, keeping me company and providing me with reassurance. A few months after being released from detention, I found out that a bomb

continued ›

Consumer narrative continued ›

had exploded near my mother's house in Pakistan. I wasn't able to contact her for several days and was extremely worried and anxious because I didn't know what was going on. Three days after the bomb-blast report, I found out that my mother had been in the vicinity of the bomb, had seen the blast, was uninjured, but badly shaken from seeing other people die. She was at risk of losing her life and extremely frightened.

I felt helpless and agitated. This caused me to start thinking about life, and my sense of hopelessness grew because my intellectual disability hindered my learning of English. My mother called regularly, telling me to forget about school and to start working to fix my life and get the family to Australia. All this pressure has made me hate my mental incapacity for not being able to learn and study fast enough to save my family.

I felt that no matter what I did I kept hitting barriers. I felt hopeless and helpless to solve my problems. As the eldest son, I had pressure from family responsibility to help my family, who were in danger.

I was having more and more mental issues but refused psychological treatment, which seemed worthless to solve my problems. The pressure to make money became very important so I moved out from the foster carer into a house with other single refugee men who had come to work to support their families. Now, after much difficulty, I feel like I am doing something worthwhile and successful rather than wasting time at school, where I know I won't learn English.

What is meant by the terms refugee, immigrant and asylum seeker?

The stories of Hanan and Ali are first-person accounts of extremely difficult life circumstances, similar to those faced by many other refugees and asylum seekers. According to the United Nations Convention on the Status of Refugees, a refugee is a person who:

> … owing to a well-founded fear of being persecuted for reasons of race, religion, nationality, membership of a particular social group or political opinion, is outside the country of his nationality and is unable or, owing to such fear, is unwilling to avail himself of the protection of that country; or who, not having a nationality and being outside the country of his former habitual residence as a result of such events, is unable or, owing to such fear, is unwilling to return to it.

> United Nations High Commission for Refugees (UNHCR) 2012

At some point in time, every person who is a refugee has been an asylum seeker. In countries such as Australia and New Zealand, a person is officially designated a refugee when her or his claim for asylum has been accepted through the process of refugee status determination.

An asylum seeker is a person seeking protection under the 1951 Refugee Convention (UNHCR, 2012). Typically, an asylum seeker has left his or her country of origin and formally applied for asylum in another country, but the application has not yet been assessed. By contrast, an economic migrant is someone who has moved to another country to work. Refugees are not economic migrants.

Each year, the UNHCR publishes reports on the number and location of refugees, asylum seekers and displaced persons around the world. The 2012 report stated that there were more than 479 000 asylum applications received by 44 industrialised countries in the preceding year (UNHCR, 2013). Most applications were made by asylum seekers originating from Afghanistan, and the United States was the largest recipient of new asylum claims, for the seventh year in a row. Of the total number of applications made in 2012, a combined total of 16 110 were lodged in Australia and New Zealand. The majority of these claims (15 800) were received by Australia, and this figure represents a 37 per cent increase when compared to the number of claims made in 2011. Of the applications made in 2012, one-third of asylum seekers in Australia originated from either Afghanistan or Sri Lanka. Some other prominent countries of origin include the Islamic Republic of Iran, Pakistan and China. By comparison, there were approximately 300 applications received by New Zealand in 2012, a figure that has remained relatively stable for the past seven years. The five most popular countries of origin of these asylum seekers were the Islamic Republic of Iran, China, Sri Lanka, Pakistan and Fiji.

Temporary Protection Visas

In some jurisdictions such as Australia, asylum seekers who are found to be refugees may be granted a Temporary Protection Visa (TPV). A TPV was a document issued to people who applied for refugee status following unauthorised entry into Australia in the period 1999 to 2008. This visa entitled the person to live in Australia for three years, at which point she or he could re-apply for another TPV. For a TPV to be renewed, the applicant's circumstances would be re-assessed to determine whether it was safe enough for the person to return to her or his home country. The impermanent nature of TPVs and the processes associated with their renewal – such as the lack of certainty about when interviews to re-assess claims would occur and how safety of one's homeland would be assessed – meant that TPV holders faced considerable anxiety (Procter, 2011), mental distress and uncertainty about their continuing personal circumstances (Procter, 2005). This uncertainty, coupled with strongly held beliefs that it is unsafe to return to their country of origin resulted in substantial psychological and physical effects in some TPV holders (Procter, 2005).

Studies have suggested that temporary refugee protection contributes substantially to the risk of depression, post-traumatic stress and problems related to mental illness in refugees (Steel et al., 2006), including intrusive, anxiety based symptoms in the form of constant worrying about the possibility of being deported (Coffey et al., 2010). In the study by Coffey and colleagues (2010), asylum seekers' marginalised status arising from TPVs reinforced the sense of insecurity, powerlessness and helplessness that had characterised the experience of detention. In a study investigating the effects of temporary protection on the mental health of Mandaean refugees, temporary protection status was strongly associated with daily stresses related to financial and work difficulties and problems in accessing health care, language classes and other opportunities (Steel et al., 2006). Since TPV holders were denied the right to family reunion visas and to re-enter Australia if they travelled overseas, they were unable to assist family members to flee dangerous situations, thereby reinforcing feelings of guilt and powerlessness (Coffey et al., 2010).

Mental health of people of immigrant and refugee background

Many studies have been conducted into the mental health experiences of refugees and asylum seekers, detailing the prevalence of serious mental illnesses, particularly in refugees who have relocated to developed countries. Some of the key issues associated with refugee mental health relate to previous experiences from flight to settlement – sometimes temporary and unstable in harsh and difficult circumstances. The sense of hopelessness, loss of future aspirations and uncertainty about family and friends left behind that accompany such traumatic experiences are risk factors for self-harm, which affect mental health and the recovery process (Commonwealth and Immigration Ombudsman, 2013). A major review of mental health in displaced and refugee children and adolescents settled in low-income and middle-income countries who are forcibly displaced confirmed that exposure to violence is a well-established risk factor for mental illness (Reed et al., 2012). A recent review of studies investigating the mental health effects of immigration detention identified high levels of distress and mental illness (Robjant, Hassam & Katona, 2009). The most common conditions reported included depression, post-traumatic stress and anxiety. Behavioural responses to distress and inner turmoil expressed as self-harm and suicidal behaviour have also been reported (Commonwealth and Immigration Ombudsman, 2013).

Risk and protective factors

People of refugee and asylum seeker backgrounds are at greater risk of developing mental illness and suicidal behaviours than the general Australian population (Procter et al., 2011). Prolonged periods of being held in immigration detention are associated with poorer mental health in refugees and asylum seekers, particularly among children and young people, and those with pre-existing vulnerabilities. Typically, there is an initial improvement in mental health upon release from detention, but this is generally short-lived. In most instances there is a re-emergence of mental health problems and symptoms of mental illness within six months of release (Procter et al., 2011).

The factors contributing to increased risk of mental health problems and mental illness among people of refugee and immigrant backgrounds include:
- low English-language proficiency;
- having a clear cultural, religious and spiritual identity;
- loss of close family bonds and confidants;
- racism, discrimination and feeling marginalised and disenfranchised;
- limited knowledge of how the health system works; and
- previous exposure to trauma prior to settlement.

The most significant protective factors for mental health among people of refugee and asylum seeker backgrounds include:
- positive family relationships;
- positive peer relationships;
- verbalisation ability (self-expression);
- problem-solving and cognitive abilities;
- assertiveness;
- having confidantes;
- clear cultural and linguistic identity; and
- satisfaction with family success and acculturation.

An overall absence of previous traumatic events, a recognised professional occupation and employment in that occupation are also considered protective of mental health (Procter et al., 2011). Although employment is a *protective factor*, the conditions of employment appear to be most critical. There may also be differences between ethnic groups within on employment setting as much as across employment settings. This means that occupational setting is key to the success of employment as a protective factor (Bhui, 2008).

Reflective questions

Imagine you are working with a refugee family. They are seeking information and guidance. Consider the following questions.
- What community contacts or collaborative relationships might they want to establish with health and community services as a means of helping to manage the transition from refugee to citizen?
- Why might it be important to focus on protective factors? Outline the specific risks and protective factors associated with being of refugee and asylum seeker backgrounds.

Physical illness

People of refugee and asylum seeker backgrounds are not only at increased risk of experiencing mental illness, but also physical health conditions. A recent study was undertaken of child and adolescent refugees of Karen ethnicity who arrived from refugee camps in Thailand, situated along the Thai-Burma border, and were settled in outer metropolitan Melbourne. The study revealed high rates of nutritional deficiencies and infectious diseases (Paxton et al., 2012). The data supported the need for post-arrival health screening and accessible, funded, catch-up immunisation. A community based refugee service in Darwin undertook a retrospective clinical audit of newly arrived refugees attending for general and mental health needs (Johnston, Smith & Roydhouse, 2011). The most common diagnoses confirmed by testing were vitamin D deficiency, hepatitis B carrier status, tuberculosis infection, schistosomiasis and anaemia.

Culture and explanatory models in mental health

culture
shared and learned meanings and behaviours that are transmitted within the context of a social activity for the purpose of interpreting the world, promoting individual or societal adjustment, growth and development; cultures are subject to continuous adaptation in response to changing internal and external circumstances

explanatory model of mental health and mental illness
an approach used to explore the way an individual explains, understands or interprets her or his own or someone else's mental health problems or illness and mental well-being; a person's explanatory model will influence the way in which feelings and symptoms are presented, the nature and scope of distress, behaviour, pattern of help seeking, perception of a good outcome as well as adherence or non-adherence to treatment

The combined elements of social, **cultural** and interpersonal factors in mental health lead practitioners to consider the deeper meaning structures held by people of immigrant and refugee backgrounds. Based on the work of Kleinman and Seeman (2000), this means that clinicians must be open to the **explanatory model** used by the person in distress. This will involve looking beyond taken-for-granted assumptions associated with the way in which symptoms and experiences of health and illness are understood and presented, the way help is sought and the way care is evaluated by those who receive it. The clinical work of any health professional – no matter how willing or keen to help – will be compromised if it does not consider the person's understanding of health difficulties and what practitioners themselves consider to be differently perceived causes of illness, optimal care and culturally appropriate support and treatment. This is particularly so in the mental health arena.

All consumers make their interpretations of their health and well-being, the way in which their health is shaped by events and circumstances and the practical help they need to enable change or improve their situation. Cultural explanatory models attempt to answer these and related questions, such as what something is called, why it started when it did, as well as the severity and likely treatment outcome. The cultural awareness questions listed below are adapted from Procter (2007) and are designed to help practitioners respond to people in the context of their mental health issues and/or mental illness:

- Can you tell me about what brought you here? What do you call _____ (use the person's words for their problem)?
- When do you think it started, and why did it start then?
- What are the main problems it is causing you?

- What have you done to try and stop/manage _____ to make it go away or make it better?
- How would you usually manage _____ in your own culture to make it go away or make it better?
- How have you been coping so far with _____?
- In your culture, is your _____ considered 'severe'? What is the worst problem _____ could cause you?
- What type of help would you be expecting from me/our service?
- Are there people in your community who are aware that you have this condition?
- What do they think or believe caused _____? Are they doing anything to help you?

In thinking about cultural explanatory models, it is important to be aware that a person's cultural and linguistic background can greatly influence how concepts such as illness and well-being are understood, and therefore how health conditions should be treated. For example, in some cultures or religions, mental illness may be understood to result from reasons as diverse as karma, spiritual possession or mind–body imbalance (Nguyen, Yamanda & Dinh, 2012). The 'mind' may be considered as not separate from the body, as it tends to be within the biomedical model, and this can lead to differences in understanding and explaining a mental illness. Furthermore, in some languages there may not be a word or expression for a particular mental illness, such as depression. It is important for health professionals to be aware of such differences and to be prepared to discuss mental health and illness in alternative ways, where necessary. However, in line with the recovery approach in mental health, it is also important to acknowledge that individuals are unique and there can be distinct differences in beliefs both across and within cultures.

Consumer narrative   Hanan's story: part two

All of this experience has made me feel hopeless for myself and my family's future … helpless to escape the prison I was put in without a crime, and worthless. I cannot say strongly enough that we feel like the world has forgotten us and doesn't know we are here. We are humans, not animals. As I tell this story again, I worry about the people coming today and being put into detention centres. My husband and I regret coming to Australia and would not have come if we knew there would be such a high cost to my family's life and health. My husband and I share a great deal of ongoing guilt and self-blame for putting our two sons through this traumatic experience, which has had irreversible and lifelong consequences. I know we chose to come; they were too young to have a say.

In my life now I often go to my room and sit alone with the lights off for hours to cry. Sometimes, I feel agitated and upset with sounds of the TV and conversation, and sometimes I yell at my children or fight with my husband for no reason. My sons often try to calm me down. I respond by telling them to leave me alone and I cope

continued ›

with the situation by removing myself from the room. Afterwards, I feel bad for how I treated my family and sad that I have become like this.

I feel that I have not benefited from my treatment at the community based torture and trauma recovery service. They can't solve my problems; they just listen but don't do anything. Talking makes me feel worse. I feel sad for reliving the experiences and exhausted from crying in front of the doctor. It is always so slow. I can't read, speak or write English very well, so I need an interpreter. I also often find that this sadness manifests itself physically by making me lethargic, and causes pain in my stomach and diarrhoea. I now have limited mobility due to back problems and arthritis, but I don't like to go out anyway, as I feel reluctant and lacking energy to leave the house. My emotions fluctuate from anger to sadness and from fear and worry to hopelessness.

Reflective questions

Imagine you are working with Hanan, who tells you that getting help for her problems is useless, that her life is never going to improve and there is no point talking about the situation as no one really understand her point of view.

- What type of response would be important in this situation?
- What skills or interventions would you use to build a collaborative relationship with Hanan?

Consumer narrative   A nurse's approach

As a registered nurse working in an acute care setting and seeing someone like Hanan, my first challenge would be to try and understand her perspective. For this to happen, I would be aware of the need to have an accredited interpreter available for the initial assessment interview. From there, the key would be to try and understand the way in which Hanan's symptoms and experiences are presented, when, how and why help is being sought, and what we both might see as a good outcome. At the same time, I would consciously try to work towards helping to develop and build trust. To my mind, it is critical to look beyond taken-for-granted assumptions when working with people of immigrant and refugee backgrounds, by ensuring that such a human connection is not tokenistic and adds genuine value to the lives of people seeking assistance. Clear communication is the real key. Wherever possible, Hanan should be able to use her preferred language, especially in stressful situations. If Hanan requests an interpreter or expresses a hesitation about her language skills, a professional interpreter should always be used, but this may

continued ›

Consumer narrative continued ›

not be possible in emergency situations. In general terms, the only exception to this would be in emergency situations. Below are some additional practise tips to consider when working collaboratively in determining how well and to what extent a person speaks and understands English.

1   Ask questions the person has to answer in a sentence. Avoid questions that can be answered with a 'maybe', 'yes' or 'no'. It is preferable to use 'what' or 'why? how? when? questions, as these help to facilitate an expression of views and ideas, as well as allow for an 'opening-up'. Through this process there may be fewer obstacles for dialogue to occur.

2   Ask the person to repeat in her or his own words some information you have just given.

3   If the person cannot answer the questions easily, or is unable to repeat the information accurately, use a professional interpreter.

When working with people in this situation, it is important to remember:

1   Asking a person for his or her name, address, date of birth and other predictable information is not an adequate test of English-language skills.

2   Having social conversation skills in English does not always mean a person understands complex information in spoken or written English.

3   Active engagement with people to achieve cultural competence will depend upon the practitioner's openness and flexibility regarding cultural awareness.

Isolation

People of immigrant or refugee background may experience isolation due to a range of factors. The process of emigration often means leaving behind an established social network of some sort, and may involve other losses, such as of language and self-identity. More broadly, emigration may lead to a sense of losing one's cultural identity. Other factors may also create or contribute to a sense of isolation for people of immigrant or refugee background. Stigma and shame surrounding mental illness can be significant among some cultural groups. A high level of stigma can have a severe effect on a person's family's desire or ability to seek help, and may further isolate the person or his or her family from the community. Isolation is particularly relevant to immigrant elders. Despite living in the host country for many years, immigrant elders who live in a cultural enclave are more likely to have problems understanding the language of the host country. Immigrant elderly also appear to be at risk of social isolation, as traditional, intergenerational relationships are rapidly disappearing in Australian cultural life. The increasing urban sprawl characterising Australian cities can results in social dislocation of young and old, without adequate social support measures and extended family in place. If the immigrant elder is a refugee or displaced person, he or she is likely to arrive with only a few members of the extended family for support. As time goes on, the elder may also find that younger generations are reluctant to provide the kinds of support the elder expects (Chiriboga, Yee & Jang, 2005). Immigrant elders have described the lack of availability of members in their community of origin with whom to socialise as a profound loss (Giuntoli & Cattan, 2012).

Reflective question

Discuss the considerations that should be taken into account when collaborating with older people of immigrant and refugee backgrounds who are reluctant to seek support from others.

- What skills do mental health clinicians have that enable them to advance collaborative care?

Engagement with mainstream mental health services

Health professionals providing treatment to people from culturally and linguistically diverse (CALD) backgrounds should have and display respect for the person's cultural heritage, provide services in her or his preferred language if the person's English proficiency is limited, and needs to understand how the cultural background of the person might affect symptom manifestation, significance and treatment.

Clinical assessment, health and helping strategies for people of immigrant and refugee background must incorporate personal reflection, therapeutic sensitivity, compassion, patience and understanding. Effective communication, an important basis for building trust, means that health professionals should ascertain the person's preferred language and whether an interpreter is necessary. Lack of English proficiency should not be assumed to be the result of poor language attainment; it could be associated with dysphasia due to a current or previous stroke or other neuro-muscular disease, or due to the loss of an acquired language due to cognitive decline such as dementia. Care should be individualised to a patient's customs and beliefs, as well as practices regarding health, illness and death, and patients should be asked what *they believe* is the cause of their problem. The clinician should encourage people to talk about any concerns, needs or problems they may be experiencing in the hospital or community setting. Health care professionals should allow each patient to decide the level of family involvement and which additional networks may be available for informal support, such as religious groups or friends.

carer
a person who provides personal care, support and assistance to an individual with a mental health problem or mental illness; carers include family members, friends, relatives, siblings, neighbours, grandparents or foster carers, and in transcultural and other contexts it is important to acknowledge this through use of humanistic language in line with a recovery approach: for example, the terms 'support person or people' and 'support networks' may be preferable to the term 'carer'

This is a particularly important concern when working with people from collectivist cultures, in which the family and/or wider community are seen as key to achieving well-being and recovery.

With people from refugee and asylum seeker backgrounds presenting distinctive mental illnesses, there is a need for considered and culturally safe ways to engage consumers, **carers** and other key people who may be involved. A monocultural 'business as usual approach' should not be taken, whereby services and individuals adopt a 'one size fits all' approach to service delivery and care planning. The key issue pertaining to mental health service delivery to people of immigrant and refugee backgrounds is ensuring culturally competent and appropriate care. There is a tendency for services to put an assessment and care plan together that suits the needs of the service provider, rather than the CALD consumer.

Traumatic stress

Personal loss as well as the loss of loved ones, especially people who have had to leave their homelands involuntarily (as a result of social and political unrest), may create a context for trauma. The stories of Hanan and Ali highlight how a past experience of trauma is a notable risk factor for the development of mental illness among individuals of immigrant and refugee backgrounds. Certain traumatic experiences (for example, torture and violence) are very strongly related to mental illnesses, such as post-traumatic stress and depression, among these individuals (Steel et al., 2009). Recognising the presence of trauma symptoms and acknowledging the role that this trauma has played in a person's life is central to the recovery process. When a clinician (and the wider service system) takes this approach, it is referred to as trauma-informed care.

Trauma-informed care

Trauma-informed care has been applied to address various mental health concerns associated with varying degrees or forms of trauma. It is a relatively recent development, with its aims of accurately identifying trauma and associated symptoms; training clinicians to have an awareness of how trauma affects the person; minimising re-traumatisation; and an overarching 'do no harm' approach (Miller & Najavits, 2012). Central to trauma-informed care is the goal of ameliorating, rather than exacerbating, the negative effects of trauma (Brown, Baker & Wilcox, 2012). Providing appropriate care requires clinician education on issues related to trauma and the lived experiences and effects of trauma on the individual (Jennings, 2007). It is essential that systems are informed by, and adapted according to available knowledge of the role that trauma plays in the consumer experience of mental illness (Jennings, 2007). Such a system must recognise that trauma can contribute towards a person's vulnerability and has effects on different aspects of a person's life, throughout the lifespan. This understanding is central to designing services that are appropriate to the individual consumer.

Practising trauma-informed care allows clinicians to make decisions about necessary treatments and approaches to an individual's situation. In particular, Blanch (2008) has warned that it cannot be assumed that all refugees have been traumatised and require trauma treatment, even though they have all faced a challenging journey. Having a heightened understanding of the effects of trauma as well as symptoms of trauma allows approaches to be best suited to the individual consumer.

Elliot and colleagues (2005) described 10 principles of trauma-informed services, which are deemed necessary if services are to be both accessible and effective for those who have experienced trauma:

1   Recognise the effects of trauma on the development and coping strategies of the consumer.
2   Set recovery from trauma as a key goal.
3   Employ an empowerment model, to facilitate the person taking control of his or her life.
4   Work towards maximising the person's choice and control over the recovery process.
5   Strive for therapeutic relationships that develop safety and trust (that is, relationships that are the opposite of traumatising).
6   Create an atmosphere respectful of the person's need for safety, respect and acceptance.
7   Emphasise the person's strengths (focusing on adaptations rather than symptoms, and resilience rather than pathology).
8   Aim to minimise the possibilities of re-traumatisation.
9   Be culturally competent, understanding the person in the context of her or his life and background.
10 Encourage consumer input, in designing and evaluating services.

Barriers to talking about trauma with clinicians

The process of telling one's story is central to understanding the trauma experienced by individuals of immigrant and refugee backgrounds and working towards recovery (de Haene et al., 2012). However, there are various barriers that may prevent these individuals from discussing and disclosing their trauma experiences. In the primary care setting, for example, such barriers have been found to include feeling that it is only appropriate to discuss trauma if the clinician asks about it first; not considering the effects of trauma upon health; and a desire to not raise upsetting memories (Shannon, O'Dougherty & Mehta, 2012). These, and other such barriers, need to be addressed in order to facilitate discussion with consumers and maximise the potential for trauma-informed care.

Reflective questions

Self-assessment of beliefs and attitudes is an important aspect of working across cultures. Assessment of these issues should be interlinked and used to improve clinical-care situations. Cultural sensitivity should frame how engagement unfolds. Simply asking a question can be an opportunity for the development of a trusting and effective therapeutic relationship. To achieve these aims and ideals, clinicians working in mental health must also identify their own prejudices and biases, and what these suggested regarding their clinical practice. The following questions can guide this reflective process. Working in small groups, answer the following questions:

- What are my own views and feelings about immigrants and refugees?
- Am I comfortable working with people who are distressed and non-communicative?
- Do I fear or dislike them? Do they unsettle me? Am I ambivalent towards them and, if so, why?
- How are my ideas, thoughts and feelings about working with refugees and immigrants manifested during clinical practice?
- How do media and popular opinions regarding certain immigrant and religious groups shape my views?
- To what extent do I encourage and facilitate consumers of immigrant and refugee backgrounds and their families, where appropriate, to make key decisions about their care?

Access and engagement when in distress

Perhaps the most challenging aspect of mental health care practice is in the emergency context, with people seeking access to the health care system at the very point of their distress. From all service access points, clinicians working in mental health are able to assist refugees to make sense of an increasingly globalised and, at times, hostile world, to better understand and respond to individual need, develop culturally competent problem-solving abilities and appreciate the factors that can promote health and comfort. With an informed knowledge base of background issues in the wider world – including the sociopolitical – clinicians, people of immigrant and refugee backgrounds, their families and significant networks can work together to target strategies and support programs that seek to maximise capacity to cope on an ongoing basis and positive mental health.

Trust and human connectedness in mental health

Building trust and rapport with consumers from immigrant or refugee backgrounds, their families and/or the wider ethnic community is fundamental. Factors such as uncertainty associated with obtaining or maintaining a visa, trauma or war, and being held in detention may compromise or threaten a person's ability to trust and reach out for help when needed. Such experiences, which may have been endured by consumers over a long period of time, are quite often the contributing factors to the person's mental illness. As such, it is critical that if and when consumers are ready to share their stories, fears and hopes, that health professionals are ready to listen, be compassionate, sensitive and flexible in their approach and, most of all, have patience and a commitment to their work. These and other qualities are key to building trust and connecting with consumers from immigrant and refugee backgrounds, their families and wider supports.

Older people of immigrant background

Procter and Baker (in press) described how the existing cultural and linguistic diversity of older people necessitate the development of an appropriate policy and service response. *The World Health Report 2010* highlights that particular attention must be paid to the difficulties ethnic and migrant groups face in accessing health services (World Health Organization (WHO), 2010). In 2000, there were 600 million people worldwide aged 60 and older, and the WHO has estimated that there will be 1.2 billion by 2025 and 2 billion by 2050 (WHO, 2006). In addition:

- About 66 per cent of all older people are living in the developing world; by 2025, it will be 75 per cent.
- In the developed world, the very old (age 80 years and older) is the fastest-growing population group.
- Women outlive men in virtually all societies; consequently, in very old age, the ratio of women to men is 2:1.

Future projections of ageing populations in the United States, Canada, Australia and across Europe reveal increasing heterogeneity of immigrant elders, and it is anticipated that numbers will increase even more extensively than that of non-immigrant elders. In Australia, for example, the population is ageing at a fast rate, and it is estimated that by 2056, 23–5 per cent of the population will be older than 65 years (Australian Bureau of Statistics, 2008). These statistics are similar to other developed nations.

Older people of immigrant and refugee backgrounds are exposed to unique risk factors for mental health. The *Framework for Mental Health in Multicultural Australia* (Mental Health in Multicultural Australia, 2013) highlights the following key concerns. That older people of refugee and immigrant backgrounds:

- have reduced access to mental health services when compared with other Australians;
- are over-represented in involuntary admissions and acute in-patient units; and
- are exposed to more quality and safety risks due to cultural and linguistic barriers.

Mental health clinicians working in health and human services face two intertwined challenges: how to assist immigrant elders with their mental health needs and how to develop the cultural competence skills to be able to meaningfully engage, assess and treat patients, accepting both the challenges and opportunities posed by diversity (Procter & Baker, in press).

Chapter summary

- People from immigrant and refugee backgrounds are at greater risk of developing mental illness and suicidal behaviours. Some of the factors that may contribute to the manifestation of mental illness among people of immigrant and refugee backgrounds include isolation, pre-migration experiences such as trauma and displacement, and stigma of mental illness in some cultures.
- Risk factors for mental illness among people of immigrant and refugee backgrounds include low English-language proficiency, loss of support networks and prior trauma. Protective factors for mental health include positive relationships, strong cultural and linguistic identity, and ability to express concerns.
- Mainstream health and mental health service providers need to consider and enact culturally safe and appropriate ways to engage with consumers from immigrant and refugee backgrounds and their supports. Such care needs to be consumer and recovery-focused and committed to addressing barriers, such as language barriers, which prevent or hinder access to good quality care.
- Cultural explanatory models provide pathways for discovering a range of issues related to a person's mental health, such as consumers' interpretation of their well-being, their beliefs as to why the problem started and what would help to improve the situation.
- Engaging with consumers and carers from immigrant, asylum seeker and refugee backgrounds involves avoiding a monocultural, 'one size fits all' approach to service provision. To enable engagement, it is important that health professionals take time to listen to consumers and understand their stories, are flexible and consider the potential involvement of others, such as family and community supports, who may be important to the person's recovery.

Critical thinking/learning activities

1   On your own, think about a time when you or someone you are close to experienced a mental illness or distress. Brainstorm some reasons you think this occurred. Then, in small groups, share and compare your suggested reasons for the occurrence of mental illness. Discuss any differences and how you developed your individual views about mental illness.

2   In pairs, role-play how you might discuss mental health issues or concerns in a culturally aware manner. To do this, first discuss what you understand by the term 'culturally aware'. Second, imagine that one of you is a clinician and the other is a person of refugee or immigrant background.

3   In pairs, role-play how you might go about determining the extent to which a consumer speaks and understands English, and whether or not the person requires assistance from an interpreter. To do this, imagine that one of you is a clinician and the other is a person of refugee or immigrant background.

4   After reading the stories of Hanan and Ali, brainstorm a list of key challenges faced by individuals of immigrant and refugee backgrounds. In small groups, discuss (a) What might be mental health protective factors to help favourably shift risk associated with mental distress and/ or illness, and (b) How protective factors might contribute to an increased ability to cope with adversity and reduce risk of mental illness.

5   In pairs, take turns to describe an experience that you have had at some point in your life that was particularly traumatic or distressing for you. After you have done this, write down how you felt when discussing this experience. Can you identify some factors that were barriers to discussing this experience? Can you identify some factors that made talking about this experience easier?

Learning extension

Consider the following story.

I am a nurse working with Thanh, a 27-year-old single man who arrived from Vietnam to Australia about 10 years ago. He has no family in Australia, and moves from one Housing Trust home to another. Thanh was diagnosed with schizophrenia about three years ago. He is currently on oral anti-psychotic medication. Thanh has been seeing me in my capacity as a community nurse for the past 12 months. Last week, he had a dental problem and was required to have follow-up treatment. He requested practical support from the Vietnamese community. In response, a community elder provided transport to attend the appointment that day. However, due to the complexity of the dental work required, the support Thanh needed had to be extended for another two days.

Thanh asked the community elder for two more days of practical support. The elder has discussed this with me and together we decided that I would pick up Thanh on the second day only. For the return trip of the second day and on the third day, Thanh and I agreed that he needed to make his own arrangements and take care of himself. The community elder informed Thanh about this decision. However, Thanh did not seem to hear the elder. Thanh was unhappy about this decision and kept ringing the elder several times during the day and night, demanding support. Thanh sounded very worried and confused. He told the elder that he felt he could not make it to treatment on his own on the second day. Thanh also became verbally aggressive and threatened both me and the elder for not helping him.

The following morning, I turned up at Thanh's home. Thanh was disoriented, restless, shaky, confused (for example, about the time and date) and talking very loudly. He was in a rush, leaving his home without knowing where the keys were. He was concerned that he had lost his keys. He also said things that did not make sense (for example, words were spoken in a confused and non-logical progression), worried that he was going to be locked up and suspicious others were 'out to get him'. He also mentioned that he had not taken his medication that morning.

I tried to reassure Thanh and attempted to do some practical problem-solving for the situation (I reassured him that it was okay to close the door, see the dentist first then look for the keys later on). I then drove Thanh to the dentist for treatment. Afterwards, Thanh got home by himself. Since this day the elders and I have found it very difficult to work with Thanh. We are reluctant to visit his home and do not want to see him on our own – especially at his home. Thanh continues to be suspicious, accusing and hostile. I am now left feeling unsure about what to do next. I am also unsure about how to engage with him. I am concerned for my safety.

Consider the following questions:

- What questions would you like to ask Thanh and the community elder to be able to understand what everyday life is really like for them?
- List what you consider to be the cultural considerations that have shaped the interaction between Thanh, the nurse and the community elder?
- What are 'culturally safe practices'? What skills should the clinician use to enhance access and utilisation of health care services for immigrant groups?

Further reading

Australasian Society for Traumatic Stress Studies: www.astss.org.au/news/podcast/podcasts-and-vodcasts-downloads
Mental Health in Multicultural Australia Project: www.mhima.org.au
National Mental Health Commission: www.mentalhealthcommission.gov.au/news-events/our-news/shining-a-light-on-culturally-and-linguistically-diverse-%28cald%29-communities.aspx
Victorian Transcultural Psychiatry Unit: www.vtpu.org.au.
Working with Interpreters – Guidelines: www.health.qld.gov.au/multicultural/interpreters/guidelines_int.pdf

References

Australian Bureau of Statistics (2008). *Population Projections, Australia (2006–2011) (No. 3222.0)*. Canberra: Author.

Bhui, K. (2008). Migration and mental health. In H. Freeman & S Stansfeld (eds), *The Impact of the Environment on Psychiatric Disorder* (pp. 184–209). New York: Routledge.

Blanch, A. (2008). *Transcending Violence: Emerging models for trauma healing in refugee communities.* Alexandria, VA: National Center for Trauma Informed Care.

Brown, S. M., Baker, C. N. & **Wilcox, P.** (2012). Risking connection trauma training: A pathway toward trauma-informed care in child congregate care settings. *Psychological Trauma: Theory, Research, Practice, and Policy, 4*: 507–15.

Chiriboga, D. A., Yee., B. W. K. & **Jang, Y.** (2005). Minority and cultural issues in late-life depression. *Clinical Psychology: Science and Practice, 12*: 358–63.

Coffey, G. J., Kaplan, I., Sampson, R. C. & **Tucci, M. M.** (2010). The meaning and mental health consequences of long-term immigration detention for people seeking asylum. *Social Science & Medicine, 70(12)*: 2070–9.

Commonwealth of Australia (2012). *Cultural Diversity in Australia*. Canberra: Australian Bureau of Statistics.

Commonwealth and Immigration Ombudsman (2013). *Suicide and Self-harm in the Immigration Detention Network*. Canberra: Commonwealth of Australia.

Cully, M. & **Pejozki, L.** (2012). Australia unbound? Migration, openness and population futures. In J. Pincus & G. Hugo,(eds) *A Greater Australia: Population, policies and governance* (pp. 60–71). Melbourne: Committee for Economic Development in Australia.

de Haene, L., Rober, P., Adriaenssens, P. & Verschueren, K. (2012). Voices of dialogue and directivity in family therapy with refugees: Evolving ideas about dialogical refugee care. *Family Process, 51*: 391–404.

Elliot, D. E., Bjelajac, P., Fallot, R. D., Markoff, L. S. & Glover Reed, B. (2005). Trauma-informed or trauma-denied: Principles and implementation of trauma-informed services for women. *Journal of Community Psychology, 33*: 461–477.

Giuntoli, G. & Cattan, M. (2012). The experiences and expectations of care and support among older migrants in the UK. *European Journal of Social Work, 15*: 131–47.

Jennings, A. (2007). Blueprint for Action: Building Trauma-informed Mental Health Service Systems (Draft). Retrieved from www.theannainstitute.org/2007%202008%20Blueprint%20By%20Criteria%202%2015% 2008.pdf.

Johnston, V., Smith, L. & Roydhouse, H. (2011). The health of newly arrived refugees to the Top End of Australia: Results of a clinical audit at the Darwin Refugee Health Service. *Australian Journal of Primary Health, 18*: 242–7.

Kleinman, A. & Seeman, D. (2000). Personal experience of illness. In G. L. Albrecht, R. Fitzpatrick & S. C. Scrimshaw (eds), *Handbook of Social Studies in Health and Medicine* (pp. 230–43). London: Sage Publications.

Mental Health in Multicultural Australia (2013). *Framework for Mental Health in Multicultural Australia*. Retrieved from www.mhima.org.au/framework.

Miller, N. A. & Najavits, L. M. (2012). Creating trauma-informed correctional care: A balance of goals and environment. *European Journal of Psychotraumatology. 3*: 17246.

Nguyen, H. T., Yamanda, A. M. & Dinh, T. Q. (2012). Religious leaders' assessment and attribution of the causes of mental illness: An in-depth exploration of Vietnamese American Buddhist leaders. *Mental Health Religion & Culture, 15*: 511–27.

Paxton, G. A., Sangster, K. J., Maxwell, E. L., McBride, C. R. J. & Drewe, R. H. (2012). Post-arrival screening in Karen refugees in Australia. *PLoS ONE, 7*: e28194.

Procter, N. G. (2005). Providing emergency mental health care to asylum seekers at a time when claims for permanent protection have been rejected. *International Journal of Mental Health Nursing, 14(1)*: 2–6.

Procter, N. G. (2007). Mental health emergencies. In K. Curtis, C. Ramsden & J. Friendship (eds). *Emergency and Trauma Nursing*. New York: Elsevier Press.

Procter, N. G. (2011). Providing mental health support for protection visa applicants in Australian immigration detention: Partnering mental health support and migration law consultation. *Psychiatry, Psychology and Law, 18(3)*: 460–5.

Procter, N. G. & Baker, A. (in press) Immigrant elders. In M. Mezey, M. Bottrell, B. Berkman, C. Callahan, T. Fulmer, E. Mitty, G. Paveza, E. Siegler and N. Strumph (eds), *The Encyclopaedia of Elder Care*, 3rd edn. New York: Springer.

Procter, N. G., Williamson, P., Gordon, A. & McDonough, D. (2011). Refugee and asylum seeker self-harm with implications for transition to employment participation: A review. *Suicidologi, 16*: 30–8.

Reed, R. V., Fazel, M., Jones, L., Panter-Brick, C. & Stein, A. (2012). Mental health of displaced and refugee children resettled in low-income and middle-income countries: Risk and protective factors. *Lancet, 379*: 250–65.

Robjant, K., Hassam, R. & Katona, C. (2009). Mental health implications of detaining asylum seekers: Systematic review. *British Journal of Psychiatry, 194*: 306–12.

Shannon, P., O'Dougherty, M. & Mehta, E. (2012). Refugees' perspectives on barriers to communication about trauma histories in primary care. *Mental Health in Family Medicine, 9*: 47–55.

Steel, Z., Chey, T., Silove, D., Marnane, C., Bryant, R. A. & van Ommeren, M. (2009). Association of torture and other potentially traumatic events with mental health outcomes among populations exposed to mass conflict and displacement. *Journal of the American Medical Association, 302*: 537–49.

Steel, Z., Silove, D., Brooks, R., Momartin, S., Alzuhairi, B. & Susljik, I. (2006). Impact of immigration detention and temporary protection on the mental health of refugees. *British Journal of Psychiatry, 188(1)*: 58–64.

World Health Organization (WHO) (2010). *The World Health Report: Health systems financing. The path to universal coverage*. Geneva, Switzerland: Author. Retrieved from www.who.int/whr/2010/en/index.html.

WHO (2011). *Global Health and Ageing*. Geneva, Switzerland: Author. Retrieved from www.who.int/ageing/ publications/global_health/en/index.html.

United Nations High Commission for Refugees (UNHCR) (2012). *Convention Relating to the Status of Refugees*. Retrieved from www.unhcr.org/pages/49da0e466.html.

UNHCR (2013). *Asylum Trends 2012: Levels and trends in industrialised countries*. Retrieved from www.unhcr.org/5149b81e9.html.

10

Gender, sexuality and mental health

Helen P. Hamer, Joe MacDonald, Jane Barrington and Debra Lampshire

Introduction 218
Gender and health 223
Culturally competent human
connectedness 224
Interpersonal abuse and psychological
trauma 229
Interpersonal trauma and mental health 231

Trauma-informed care 233
Chapter summary 239
Critical thinking/learning activities 239
Learning extension 240
Further reading 240
References 240

Learning objectives

At the completion of this chapter, you should be able to:

- Understand the continua of sexual orientation and gender identity.
- Define the difference between sexual orientation and gender identity.
- Reflect on the notion of culturally competent care for gender and sexually diverse populations.
- Understand the effects of hetero-normativity, cis-normativity, homophobia, trans-phobia, and violence and abuse on peoples' mental health.
- Reflect on the complexities of privilege and oppression in relation to gender and sexuality as well as ethnicity, class and ability.
- Develop skills and confidence in providing trauma-informed nursing care.

Introduction

In this chapter we focus on the cultural diversity of genders and sexualities, and the effects of marginalisation and interpersonal abuse on people's mental health. We describe the ways in which mental health nurses are able to practise empathically and effectively in gender and trauma-informed mental health nursing. Throughout the first part of the chapter we will be reading Riley's story to help us understand how mental health services can be more supportive and accepting of gender and sexual diversity.

Continua of sexuality and gender

sexual orientation
denotes a person's sexuality relative to her or his own sex (homosexual, heterosexual or bisexual)

gender identity
an aspect of identity that can be understood as one's psychological sex and may not correspond to one's physical sex

The Australian (2011) and New Zealand Human Rights Commissions (2008) refer to a broad and diverse range of **sexual orientations** and **gender identities**. Many people are familiar with the idea that there exists a range of sexual orientations. One way to conceptualise gender as more than a binary of male and female is to imagine a continuum of gender identity (United Nations High Commissioner for Human Rights, 2012), with heterosexual or straight at one end and lesbian or gay at the other. Many people position themselves at either end, while others place themselves at a myriad places in between. Some people move along the continuum over the course of their lifetime. It is less commonly acknowledged that there is also a wide range of gender identities. Some terms that people might use include transgender, transsexual, intersex, gender-queer, woman or man.

'Transgender' is a term that encompasses a range of identities for people who do not identify with the sex they were assigned at birth. Some of these people identify as transmen (assigned female at birth, identify as male) or as transwomen (assigned male at birth, identify as female). Some people do not identify with the binary concept of male or female, and may use terms like gender-queer. Gender-queer people identify as both male and female, or as neither. This is different to intersex, which is a general term used for a variety of conditions in which a person is born with a reproductive or sexual anatomy that does not fit the typical biological definitions of female or male. Some people identify as transsexual, which often refers to a person whose gender identity is opposite to the physical sex he or she was assigned at birth, and who has changed or is in the process of changing her or his physical sex to conform to this gender identity. Some gender-diverse people identify as gender conforming, as within the binary of male and female, woman and man. Other gender-diverse people identify as gender non-conforming, as outside or beyond the binary of male and female, woman and man. People who are transgender, transsexual,

sexuality
whom you love and whom you desire romantically or sexually

intersex, gender-queer and gender diverse also have sexual orientations, which can be straight, gay, bisexual, lesbian, queer and so on.

It is important to note the distinction between sexual orientation and gender identity. Sexual orientation is about **sexuality**. Gender identity is about your own gender: who you are and how you identify your gender. There are socially determined norms about both sexuality and gender. With regard to sexuality, people are generally expected to be heterosexual; to be attracted to people of the opposite sex. For example, a woman is expected to be attracted exclusively to men. With regard to gender, people are generally expected to identify with the sex they are assigned at birth; for example, an infant who is assigned female at birth is expected to grow up to identify as a woman. However, many people do not follow the patterns of these social expectations.

The social pressure exerted through these expectations about sexuality is called **hetero-normativity** and the equivalent for gender is **cis-normativity**. Cis-normativity also assumes that being cis-gender is superior and more desirable than being transgender, transsexual or intersex.

Examples of cis-normativity in a nursing context
You are working in an acute mental health unit:
1   A person who is female assigned at birth walks in wearing masculine clothes. You could assume that this person is a 'butch' lesbian. However, the person may identify as a transman, and not as a woman or as a lesbian. If you have assumed that the person is 'female' and a 'lesbian', then you will probably use female pronouns such as 'she' and 'her'.
2   This is problematic because if the person identifies as a transman the person will probably prefer male pronouns such as 'he' and 'him'.
3   A person who is male assigned at birth, whom you have assumed to be a man, starts wearing women's clothes in the acute unit. You could assume that this person is a 'cross-dresser' and encourage the person to only wear men's clothes. This person may identify as a woman, or as a transwoman. Inclusive nursing practice would involve asking the person whether she or he would prefer to be in a women-only room or dormitory. Also check if the person would prefer to be known as 'she', and check if the person uses a different name on a day-to-day basis (regardless of whether this is his or her legal name).

Most people, regardless of how they identify, experience the pressure of social norms in relation to gender and sexuality. Different cultures frame gender and sexuality in different ways. In the Māori context there is less distinction between gender identity and sexual orientation, and the Māori term *takatāpui* is used collectively to refer to both men and women. *Takatāpui* can include anyone who has a diverse sexuality and/or gender. This flexibility is not found in paradigms of gender and sexuality that dominate in the non-indigenous populations of Australia and New Zealand.

There are too many labels for both gender identity and sexual orientation for a comprehensive list to be provided here, and relying on labels, categories or acronyms such as LGBTTIQ (lesbian, gay, bisexual, transgender, *takatāpui*, intersex and queer) risks alienating or excluding people whose terms are not included, or who do not identify with any of the terms offered. In this chapter we prefer to use a more inclusive term, gender and sexual diversity (GSD), which includes the widest possible range of genders and sexualities.

hetero-normativity
a concept that represents punitive rules (social, familial, and legal) that compel individuals to conform to dominant heterosexual standards of identity

cis-normativity
the expectation that all people are cis-gender, that people assigned male at birth always grow up to be men and those assigned female at birth always grow up to be women

Self-identification

It is crucial to respect the self-identification of any person. With regard to sexual orientation, this means acknowledging how a person experiences and describes her or his sexuality. Respect the words the person uses to identify himself or herself, regardless of assumptions you may have made about the person's sexual orientation. Similarly, respecting self-identification in relation to gender means acknowledging how a person experiences and describes her or his gender. For some people, gender correlates to the sex they were assigned at birth. The term currently used for this is 'cis-gender', which is a companion and contrasting term to transgender, so that people do not talk about 'transgender' and 'normal gender', because this further entrenches cis-normativity.

For some people, the sex they were assigned at birth does not match how they feel, or how they would identify their gender. Sometimes this leads to a gender transition, which is a process of changing one's gender from male to female or from female to male. This process may involve any combination of social, legal and medical elements. It may be purely social; changing one's name and gendered pronouns such as 'he' and 'she', and may include legal changes of name or sex, or may involve medical support such as hormone therapy or surgery. Some gender-diverse people do not transition, or do not identify as part of a binary system of male and female. Gender-diverse people often face barriers when accessing medical services because of the potential disjunction between how they experience and identify their gender and how it is recorded on public documents or medical records.

Intersex

When an infant is born, the medical team assigns a sex that is recorded on the birth certificate. Usually, female or male is recorded on the birth certificate; however, 'indeterminate' or 'intersex' (an umbrella term that is used to include a range of bodily expressions, identities and conditions) are terms used to describe a person whose reproductive and sexual anatomy do not fit the typical definitions of male or female (Human Rights Commission of New Zealand, 2008). When a clinical term is necessary, the most common is Disorders of Sex Development (DSD). There is a continuing negotiation between intersex communities and medical institutions about the medicalisation of intersex identities and embodiments. The most controversial issue is the continued use of invasive genital surgery on intersex infants to enable a clear determination of male or female (for information and resources see the Intersex Trust of Aotearoa New Zealand: www.ianz.org.nz). In recent years some countries have been considering amending their laws regarding the recording of births, deaths and marriages to extend the options under gender and include intersex or indeterminate (ACT Law Reform Advisory Council, 2012).

Consumer narrative   Riley's story

I was assigned female at birth, but I identify as male. I was a really happy kid, and even a happy girl, until I was about 20 years old. I had come out as a dyke when

continued >

Consumer narrative continued ›

I was 15 years old and felt really comfortable in my sexuality. But I had some discomfort about the assumptions people made about my gender. When thinking about my body, I could honestly say that I felt comfortable in it for the most part, but that socially other people didn't seem to understand what my body meant. I didn't think that having breasts should mean I was female, but when other people saw my chest they assumed I was a girl. The problem was not me; it was the assumptions of the people around me who knew nothing more than the binary of male and female.

Fluidity of gender

The idea that gender can be fluid, can change over time or move beyond the binary of male and female is increasingly evident in younger populations. Recent collections of creative work about non-binary gender (Bornstein & Bergman, 2010) demonstrate the challenge that gender non-conforming people, who may or may not identify as transgender, present to the dominant paradigm.

Consumer narrative   Riley's story

I explored different ways of 'doing' my gender from when I was about 20 years old, until I was about 25 years old. I found some excellent support from the queer communities I was already part of, where there were lots of different people, some who identified as transgender, some as gender-queer, some as man or woman – it was clear to me that there was a wide range of options.

When I turned 25 years old I decided it was time to investigate what my options were if I wanted medical support with my transition. I wanted to go on testosterone medication because I wanted to look more masculine; however, I had to see a psychiatrist before the endocrinologist would proceed with treatment.

The psychiatrist at Student Health was someone I knew. I had worked with her doing diversity training workshops for staff and students, so I felt comfortable being honest with her. We talked for almost an hour, about my desire to transition and what that might involve for me. She asked about my childhood, about my relationship with my body, about my sexuality and how I currently identified my gender. We talked about the continuum of gender, and I said that I had started life at the female end of the continuum, and now identified as being more towards the male end. I felt distressed that my boyhood wasn't seen by other people very often, apart from my close friends and in some queer circles.

I mentioned that I liked using words like 'gender-queer', because for me that was about moving beyond a binary understanding of being either male or female. I understand that the binary system works for some people, but it doesn't work for me. And I know there are other cultures that have more expansive understandings of gender, because gender is culturally specific and socially constructed.

Pathologising gender and sexual diversity

Theoretical positions on human sexuality have been historically understood through the dominance of the male/female, masculine/feminine and heterosexual/homosexual binaries. For many years the diagnosis of gender identity disorder (GID) (American Psychiatric Association (APA), 2000) required the person to identify as heterosexual. GID will be renamed 'gender dysphoria' in the DSM-5 (APA, 2013). Along with these changes will be the creation of a separate gender dysphoria in children, adolescents and adults. The grouping will be given its own category.

The perpetuation of social stigma towards same-sex attracted people resulted in the category of homosexuality being moved from the realm of religious and moral understandings to the realm of pathology (Monro, 2000; Monro & Warren, 2004) or immaturity (Rudman & Glick, 2012). Homosexuality was thus perceived as a behaviour rather than an identity, and therefore classified as a mental illness in the first edition of the *Diagnostic and Statistical Manual of Mental Disorders* (APA, 1952), DSM-1. However, social changes precipitated by equal rights movements led to gay rights activists pressuring the medical establishment to remove homosexuality from the DSM-3 in 1973. Gay and lesbian activism in New Zealand also led to the decriminalisation of homosexuality in 1986, through the *Homosexual Law Reform Act, 1986* (NZ). Nonetheless, gender diversity continues to be pathologised, particularly non-binary genders. In order to access health care, especially health care relevant to gender transition, most gender-diverse people have to submit to the pathologising medical paradigm, which treats diversity as something to be treated and fixed. It is proposed that further legislative changes will have a positive effect on the well-being of GSD. The passing of the recent Marriage Amendment Bill in New Zealand (2013) has afforded same-sex couples the same rights as heterosexuals; for example, queer partners are now able to make health care decisions for their partners as their next of kin.

Intersex people face a different challenge because medical interventions on intersex bodies often occur when the infant or child is too young to understand the situation. The medicalisation and subsequent surgical interventions upon intersex infants and children remains an ongoing human rights issue (United Nations High Commissioner for Human Rights, 2012).

Hetero-sexism and hetero-normativity

Hetero-sexism is described as the predisposition to considering heterosexuality as normal, and is biased against people from other sexual orientations (Ministry of Health, 2002). In his story, Riley uses the word 'queer'; a term that has been regarded as derogatory in the past but has been reclaimed by queer theorists (Sedgwick, 1990; Seidman, 2002; Spargo, 1999) to explain that the understandings of normal sexuality lie within a frame of hetero-normativity. Hetero-normativity also shapes how perceptions of otherness are constructed, and who deserves to be accepted in society. Queer analysis therefore highlights that hetero-normative understandings of gender diversity are embedded within the context of power and that such dominant heterosexual and gender roles exist in order to regulate social life (Vitulli, 2010).

Genders, sexualities and power

Foucault (1979) argued that as sexual subjects humans are the object of power. Communities interpret biological differences between men and women to create a set of social norms and behaviours that are considered appropriate for these genders. These norms determine men's and women's access to their rights, resources, influence and power within society, such as health care. Although the specific nature and degree of these differences vary from one society or ethnicity to the next, they typically favour men, creating an imbalance in power and gender inequality that perpetuate; for example, family violence (New Zealand Family Violence Clearinghouse, 2009) and the wage gap (Oostendorp, 2009). The notion of intimacy within a relationship assumes that there is equal power between partners (Timmerman, 1991), yet the influence of social norms and gender roles can affect the sharing of equal power. P.J. Adams (2012) argued that traditionally men have maintained dominance in many aspects of society, such as work and the home, by sharing a collective masculine identity and central belief that men should be 'in charge' (p. 14). Such hostile and benevolent sexism and misogyny (Anderson, 2008) within society affects all people, perpetuates negative stereotypes against men and women, and creates an environment that supports and perpetuates gender violence (WHO, 2005). As nurses it is important that we are aware of these structural inequalities that inform the experiences of consumers, such as how women are socialised, the effects of pathologising difference, stigma, labelling and hetero-normativity (Davison & Huntington, 2010).

Gender and health

Gender roles, norms and responsibilities are some of the social determinants of mental health in men and women. For example, the feeling that one lacks autonomy over one's life increases the risk of developing a depressive disorder, particularly in women. Similarly, the socialisation of men not to show certain emotions also puts them at risk of developing mental and physical health problems when faced with the loss of a partner (WHO, 2002). Women experience considerably more psychological distress and mental illness associated with reproductive health than men (WHO, 2002). Pregnancy and child birth also place women at greater risk of mental illness; for example, one in three to one in five women in developing countries and one in 10 in developed countries experience depression and anxiety during and after childbirth (WHO, 2008).

Mental health nurses have an important role to play in the well-being of mothers and babies, and have developed specialist practice within the area of maternal mental health. Nurses in this specialty offer a broad range of interventions, such as the assessment and support of women who have serious and enduring mental illness, and guidance and advice on medication during the pregnancy trimesters and when breastfeeding. Nurses are also instrumental in preparing women and their partners in caring for the new baby. Other treatments provided by these specialist nurses are evidence-based talking therapies, such as cognitive behavioural therapy for the individual mother or couple, group work and family therapy. Support for both the partner and the wider family is also essential at this stage of human development. The nurse must also avoid making hetero-normative assumptions about who is the mother's partner and who is the father of the baby. The number of lesbian and gay-led families within New Zealand is increasing (Gunn & Surtees, 2009), and therefore nurses need to work within a culturally inclusive way in order not to further marginalise GSD groups (O'Neill (Roache), Hamer & Dixon, 2012).

Reducing the risk of mental distress during the perinatal period is achieved when the maternal mental health nurse works collaboratively with the midwife to provide comprehensive care and support to mothers and their significant others. One in three women who have a history of sexual violence are likely to experience a post-traumatic stress disorder; therefore, careful consideration must be given to developing a suitable birth plan for the mother that is trauma-informed. In so doing, the risk factors are decreased for the mother and promote maternal bonding and overall welfare of the new baby (Madrid, Skolek & Shapiro, 2006).

Culturally competent human connectedness

Cultural competence within nursing practice ensures that nurses have the appropriate cultural knowledge and skills to deal with all cultural encounters (Campinha-Bacote, 2002). Increasing one's awareness of the historical, social and political influences on health will foster the development of relationships that engender trust and respect (Gibbs, 2005).

It is equally important for nurses to reflect on their own gender and sexual orientation and to consider the inherent assumptions and values derived from their socialisation within a predominantly hetero-normative environment. Essentially, if the nurse does not use inclusive language then she or he cannot be regarded as providing safe care (Flemmer et al., 2012). Within a culturally competent human connectedness (CCHC) framework, the nurse is able to demonstrate an understanding of the specific needs of the cultural group in question. However, the mental health system is not immune to the power structures that perpetuate hetero-sexist and homophobic attitudes. Reflections on the nurse's own cultural safety are paramount, and support from senior nurses who are also challenging and changing such discriminatory practices will reduce the moral distress that is present in the everyday practice of nurses.

Exploring the relationship of gender identity and sexual orientation with mental distress is important to the person's recovery journey. However, GDS users of mental health services have reported that the majority of health professionals they encountered did not include questions about their sexual orientation within the standard mental health assessment (Ministry of Health, 2002). When health professionals do ask and respond positively to disclosures of sexual orientation, it increases the person's sense of safety and acceptance, rather than feelings of invisibility, fear and alienation.

How to talk to people about sexual orientation and gender diversity

Human connectedness is fostered when the nurse puts the person at ease at the beginning of the assessment process. Some of the following suggestions will help nurses learn how to ask these important questions:

- An open and safe approach is to tell people that it is 'standard policy' to ask questions about gender and sexuality because they are important topics for many people. You could say: 'Some people want to talk about gender identity or sexual orientation. Is there anything about those topics you would like to discuss?' Or: 'When we are discussing your personal history, this is a safe place to talk about gender or sexuality, if you want to.'
- Check the person's gender identity by asking: 'We have you recorded on the referral form as female/male (as relevant). Is this how you would like me to record your gender?'
- When collecting information about sexual orientation or gender identity, it is always important to respect privacy and check with the person whether he or she is comfortable with you recording details of the conversation, or disclosing this information to other staff members. Use the person's preferred name and pronouns ('he' or 'she' or 'they'), as requested, in conversation and note-taking.

Reflective question

- Many people who are attracted to people of the same sex do not want to attach a label to their sexual orientation. Why might this be so?

- If the person asks why you are asking the above questions, one response could be: 'We ask about sexuality and gender as they can be an important yet difficult issues to discuss in our society and it is important people know they can discuss these issues here without being judged.' What are some other responses you can think of?
- If the person says: 'I look like a woman, but I feel like a man', how would you respond?
- When you ask about relationships, ask: 'Do you have a partner?' and if so, 'What do they do?', rather than 'Are you married?'
- The former response demonstrates openness and acceptance. What other, similar, inclusive assessment questions might you ask?
- In sum, hetero-nomativity and cis-normativity are often perpetuated through language, unintentionally, and perpetuate the person's experience of being treated as 'not normal' or 'lesser' in some way. Therefore, it is good practice to use gender-

neutral language as much as possible, especially with regard to relationships, such as use of the term 'partner' rather than 'husband' or 'wife', which some people find exclusive.

Questions sourced from Birkenhead and Rands (2012), and Semp (2006).

Consumer narrative   Riley's story

I talked about the continuum of gender with my psychiatrist because I wanted her to understand the variety of options that I had seen out in the queer worlds. I wanted to bring that expansiveness into this medical encounter. None of my answers matched the criteria in the DSM.

I told the psychiatrist that I knew that there was a clash between the white, Western medical paradigm, which only acknowledges the existence of binary male and female genders, and my lived experience. My experience, and my own identity, had taught me that gender is a complicated dance of self and body within a wider context of social recognition. There is a vast array of genders, but often people experience violence because they do not fit into either male or female, or are considered not 'masculine enough' or 'feminine enough'.

I said that I knew that sexuality was more complex than we generally admit, and I knew many people who did not identify as simply gay or straight. When she asked me about my sexuality, I said, 'I am attracted to people'. I specified that gender-diverse or queer people were usually the ones I was more attracted to, but there isn't a label for that, except maybe 'queer'.

In the end, the psychiatrist looked at me, sighed, and said with some resignation: 'I cannot diagnose you with gender identity disorder, or gender dysphoria'.

I agreed, enthusiastically! She asked what we should do. I suggested that she write a letter to the endocrinologist, stating that I was mentally healthy and capable of making this decision. She did so, right there in front of me. I was so impressed by that.

We basically used an 'informed consent' model, instead of a diagnostic model. She still needed to know that I understood all the risks, and had realistic expectations about what testosterone injections would do to my body. She needed to know that I also had support from family and friends.

In this encounter with the psychiatrist, Riley knew that there was a tension between the continuing influences of the biomedical view of homosexuality and psychiatric treatment that may still exist for some medical practitioners, particularly that the person can be viewed as a passive recipient of care. In contrast, the informed consent model accepts that Riley has full capacity to make an informed choice and therefore represents a rights-based approach to practice. The power of Riley's narrative in the encounter with the psychiatrist helped to change the outcome because the psychiatrist heard and validated

Riley's informed opinions. Riley's explanation was accepted as his truth and not translated into a biomedical paradigm. Such an example of CCHC between the psychiatrist and Riley sustained his autonomy and ability to take the lead in directing future medical interventions that were appropriate to him.

Consumer narrative   Riley's story

Although the psychiatrist and I composed the letter to send to the endocrinologist, I noticed she was using female pronouns in reference to me in the letter. I asked if she could change them to male pronouns, which was what most of my friends were using for me. She said no, because 'it would only confuse the doctor'. I didn't want to push my luck, so I said okay. Later I reflected on how frustrating it was that I was asking to be recognised as the person that I already knew I was (even if that is somewhat ambiguous, because we're all in the process of 'becoming' all the time). I was being asked to identify as male, in order to access testosterone therapy, but in the same hour I was told I couldn't have male pronouns in a referral letter because other medical professionals would get 'confused'.

I felt powerless in that moment, as if I had offered to show a very vulnerable part of myself, and someone had said, 'No, you do not get to decide who you are'. I got the impression that I could only be 'he' when I looked 'typically male'. It felt to me as though I was 'not allowed' to be 'he' while I still looked, to them, like an androgynous, queer girl. It was sad and frustrating because I had talked about identifying as a boy, and how I felt more comfortable with 'he' rather than 'she', but it was assumed (by a lot of people, my psychiatrist included) that until I had completed some kind of medical transition, I could not legitimately be a boy.

I could only expect to be recognised as myself, and be treated as a boy, when I was no longer 'confusing'. Instead of expanding the understanding of my medical support people (psychiatrist, GP, nurses, endocrinologist), I felt like I had to shrink myself down to fit into the narrow criteria of acceptable masculinity. I had to wait for them to respect how I identified, wait until I looked male enough that they wouldn't feel too troubled calling me 'he'.

Reflective question

In pairs, discuss the psychiatrist's decision to use the 'she' pronoun and the possible link to cis-normativity (and to a lesser extent hetero-normativity) within the medical profession.
- If the psychiatrist had used the 'he' pronoun, do you think it would have confused the endocrinologist?

Effects of homophobia and trans-phobia

Although the Yogyakarta Principles (International Commission of Jurists, 2007) embody the rights of GSD to attain similar standards of physical and mental health as heterosexuals, the effects of **homophobia** (de Graaf, Sandfort & ten Have, 2006) and **trans-phobia** continue to have a profound effect on the mental health of GSD (Cochran & Mays, 2009). For example, lesbians and gays have higher rates of mental illness, self-harm and suicide attempts than heterosexuals (King et al., 2003; King et al., 2008). Further, lesbians and gays who experience higher levels of homophobia are significantly more likely to use drugs and alcohol (Weber, 2008) and four times more likely to develop a substance abuse disorder (Cochran et al., 2004; McCabe et al., 2010). Given that GSD groups experience higher levels of mental distress (Adams, Dickinson & Asiasiga, 2012) than their heterosexual counterparts, it should be of concern to all nurses that this vulnerable population continues to avoid seeking health care due to hetero-normative and homophobic attitudes within health settings (Cox, Holden & Sagovsky, 1987; Daley, 2006; Markowitz, 1999; O'Neill (Roache) et al., 2012).

homophobia
the fear of or aversion to homosexuals

trans-phobia
a feeling of disgust towards individuals who do not conform to society's gender expectations

Consumer narrative   Riley's story

Throughout this process with my psychiatrist I also reflected on how my privilege, as a well-educated *pākeha* (a non-Māori New Zealander) with white skin, had greatly improved my chances of being understood and being recognised as an expert on my own experience. I got what I needed from this medical encounter, and my endocrinologist accepted the informed consent letter that my psychiatrist had written. I knew that if I hadn't been as confident and articulate, if I hadn't known all the right academic and community terms to use, I would've had a much harder time. I felt grateful that I had successfully negotiated a way to access the treatment I needed, without relying on the DSM. But I was also left with a feeling of frustration about how the medical system failed to recognise my complex, or 'confusing', gender. It was my privilege that enabled me to get the support I needed. I feel worried about a medical system that relies on us having this level of privilege, since many of us are not white or middle-class and do not go to university. What happens then?

Reflective question

In pairs, discuss the role of the nurse in influencing a safe passage through the health system for people who are perceived as not fitting the norm.
- How will you establish trusting relationships with people who have not had positive experiences with clinical staff in the past?

Interpersonal abuse and psychological trauma

The final section of this chapter looks at the nature of abusive interpersonal experiences many people have endured and survived, and the ways in which such experiences can manifest as psychological distress and mental illness. Suggestions are made about how nurses might create safe interpersonal spaces in which to engage with peoples' narratives of interpersonal abuse, helping to avoid re-traumatisation and promoting recovery.

Developing a therapeutic relationship is a fundamental skill or technology in nursing. It creates a safe space within which the person can talk about his or her life, worries, current challenges and hopes and dreams for the future. The therapeutic relationship creates the place in which the unspeakable may be spoken, and in which the unspoken can be expressed in symbolic language or behaviour and can be recognised and accepted. In listening to accounts of interpersonal abuse the nurse helps the person to find understanding, meaning, acceptance and compassion for herself or himself. It is the profound human connection between the person and the nurse that enables a sharing and co-construction of a personal narrative that constitutes the work of recovery. For many people we work with, psychological distress often arises from terrible experiences of abuse caused by a known and often loved and trusted person. Our witnessing of these accounts is part of the work of the mental health nurse.

As nurses we bring our own experiences to our work, and few of us have not experienced the distress of bereavement, broken relationships or betrayal of trust. We also bring to our work our own human vulnerabilities, so before reading the following section on trauma and trauma-informed care (TIC), take a moment to think about self-care. Remember, it takes courage for people to tell us their stories and courage for us to listen to them.

Self-care

Being with people whose reality is imploding or fragmenting and who are overwhelmed with terror is honourable but also very challenging work. In order to sustain this work we need to care for ourselves. Observe your own limits; be aware of your own emotional and psychological well-being, to minimise the potential for vicarious traumatisation (Trippany, White Kress & Wilcoxon, 2004) or compassion fatigue (Jenkins & Baird, 2002), which describes the erosion of our capacity to care associated with our exposure to accounts of another person's traumatic experiences. If you begin to feel vulnerable and out of balance, talk to a trusted colleague or a professional supervisor about the support services that are available in your workplace or university.

Interpersonal abuse

Interpersonal abuse occurs in the context of an interpersonal relationship or situation that is distressing and harmful. Interpersonal abuse occurs among people who know each other; for example, partners, family members, friends, colleagues, teachers and religious leaders. Most interpersonal abuse is said to be perpetrated by men upon women and children, although women have also been shown to be abusers (McNulty, 2012). Despite the progress of human rights legislation, a male sense of entitlement to power, control and the privilege of access to female bodies for sexual and domestic services remains pervasive. The

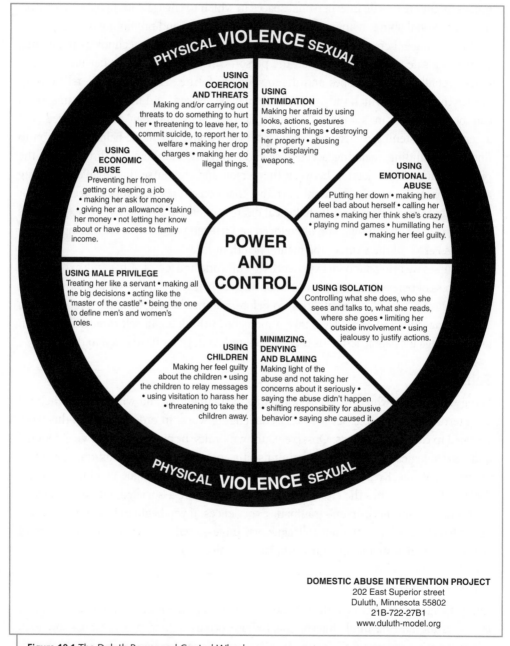

Figure 10.1 The Duluth Power and Control Wheel

Source: Reproduced with permission from the Duluth Domestic Abuse Intervention Projects, 2011.

Duluth model of power and control (Duluth Domestic Abuse Intervention Projects, 2011) (Fig. 10.1) summarises the strategies used to achieve compliance and acquiescence within interpersonal relationships, which Sheffield (1989, p. 483) described as 'sexual terrorism'.

Family and partner violence

Female victims are often held responsible for violent acts of sexual terrorism against them and because these assaults often are not taken seriously by authorities; it as been estimated that 90 per cent of victims do not report these crimes to police (Ministry of Justice, 2009). In New Zealand, in has been reported that one in three women has experienced family or partner violence (Fenrich & Contesse, 2009). In recognition of this high rate of family and partner violence, screening has been made the responsibility of all health professionals (Feldhaus et al., 1997; Koziol-McLain et al., 2008). It is of note that family and partner violence are evident in GSD populations, and though this is an area that requires more research, Edwards and Sylaska (2012) have reported that minority-group stress, such as victimisation, stigma and internal homo-negativity, may play a part in family and partner violence.

Currently, in New Zealand, all women aged 16 to 65 years who present to any health service are screened for family or partner physical violence in the first instance. Three standard questions that are perceived as non-threatening and safe are recommended and should be asked in the context of an overall assessment. These are:

1 Have you been hit, kicked, punched or otherwise hurt by someone within the past year? If so, by whom?
2 Do you feel safe in your current relationship?
3 Is there a partner from a previous relationship who is making you feel unsafe now?

The screening focuses on current *physical* abuse and safety rather than historical abuse and its effects. Screening for histories of abuse and trauma in all GSD people who present to mental health services is discussed in the following section.

Interpersonal trauma and mental health

Many people across the range of genders and sexualities present with histories of physical, psychological, emotional and sexual abuse. The seminal work by Finkelhor and Browne (1985) conceptualised four core traumagenic dynamics as a result of the sexual abuse of children. These are traumatic sexualisation, betrayal, stigmatisation and powerlessness.

Nurses encounter a range of expressions of these dynamics; for example, persistent anxiety, fearfulness, difficulties with trust and feeling safe in the world, passivity, loss of autonomy and loss of hope. The person may engage in unsafe behaviours such as unsafe sex, substance misuse/abuse or addiction, anti-social behaviour, and difficulty with intimacy, interpersonal and sexual relationships. The person may also re-experience her or his trauma in flashbacks, nightmares or psychotic episodes. The person may have a self-concept of being flawed or damaged, and may have difficulty establishing an identity acceptable to herself or himself. The person may be filled with shame and self-stigma, may isolate himself or herself, and may fail to reach potential in many areas of life, such as education and employment. Traumatised people are more likely to have longer and more frequent admissions to an acute mental health facility, spend more time in seclusion, relapse more frequently, be given psychotropic medications and attempt suicide and engage in self-harm than the general population (Read, 1998).

The effects of abuse may be reduced by the presence of consistent, loving relationships; for example with grandparents or pets, and by early disclosure of the abuse where the child is believed, supported and protected. However, interpersonal abuse most often remains a secret as children often feel responsible for the abuse or fear the negative consequences of disclosure (Goodman-Brown et al., 2003).

The longer-term, adverse effects of abuse are increased the younger the age of the person at the time at which it begins. These effects are closely associated with the severity and frequency of the abuse and the person's relationship to the abuser. If the abuser is a parent then this leads to a betrayal of trust. Berliner and Conte (1990) found that many abusers employ a technology of abuse involving deliberate strategies for grooming the child into the abuse, in order to decrease the child's resistance and increase compliance. The abuse may start out with pleasant events such as fun games, and gradually the games become sexualised. The abuser may use threats to ensure that the child keeps the secret, such as threatening to kill the child's pet. Herman (2001) suggested that because abuse often remains secret, traumatic events surface not as a verbal narrative, but as a cluster of symptoms that become transformed into diagnoses; for example, borderline personality disorder and schizophrenia.

Understanding of the traumatic effects of interpersonal abuse has emerged only in recent decades in response to social movements such as gay rights and civil rights, and more recently the service user movement (Lakeman, McGowan & Walsh, 2007), and has created a space for the voices of survivors of abuse to be heard. Understandings of trauma within the biomedical paradigm have largely been focused on external traumatic events that occur to otherwise healthy adult individuals; for example, witnessing a murder or the effects of warfare. Although the diagnostic category of post-traumatic stress disorder (PTSD) was included in the DSM-III (1980), it reflected trauma knowledge drawn from the survivors of military combat. The DSM-5 (APA, 2013) description of diagnosis of PTSD describes four major effects of trauma, summarised here as:

- hyper-arousal and anxiety;
- intrusive phenomena such as flashbacks and nightmares;
- Avoidance of triggers (places, people, smells, sights, sounds) that precipitate memories of the trauma and numbing; and
- negative thoughts and mood or feelings.

However, there has been criticism that this conceptualisation of the effects of trauma is of limited use when attempting to understand the effects of interpersonal abuse. Herman (1992) suggested a diagnostic category that captures the dynamics of interpersonal abuse, which she calls Complex-PTSD, and has utility in describing the presentation of a person who is experiencing the traumatic effects of interpersonal abuse.

Complex-PTSD requires a history of subjection to totalitarian systems of control, such as within sexual and domestic life, and includes domestic battering, childhood abuse and organised sexual exploitation over a prolonged period of time. Herman (1992) identified and elaborated several categories of alterations in the victim/survivor's way of being and experiencing life. These alterations are found in the person's affect or mood regulation, consciousness, self-perception, perception of the perpetrator, relationships with others and systems of meaning and faith.

Trauma-informed care

What makes mental health nursing practice trauma-informed is recognition of the high prevalence of neurological, biological, psychological and social effects of abuse and trauma on a person's development and life. In the biomedical paradigm, emphasis is usually placed on mapping a person's pathology, making a diagnosis and prescribing the relevant psycho-pharmacological treatment. The DSM has been criticised for fitting individuals into standard, predefined categories (Bloom & Farragher, 2011; Holmes & Warelow, 1999) and focusing on the individual's flaws or deficits. In trauma-informed care (TIC), the focus and question moves from 'What is wrong with you?' to 'What happened to you?' (Bloom, 1997; Bloom & Farragher, 2011; Bloom & Reichart, 1998). TIC assumes that understanding and meaning can be made of the person's trauma and subsequent distress, and that it is within the person's capability to recover (Chandler, 2008; Elliott et al., 2005). TIC aims to protect the traumatised person from further harm, such as labelling and shaming, powerlessness, invalidation, restraint, seclusion and other coercive practices. It aims to provide safe spaces in which people can begin to construct a narrative account of the events in their lives and make meaning of their distress or illness.

trauma-informed care when a human service program takes the step to become trauma-informed, every part of its organisation, management and service-delivery system is assessed and potentially modified to include a basic understanding of how trauma affects the life of an individual seeking services and how traditional service-delivery approaches and programs can be more supportive and avoid re-traumatisation.

The nurse's role

According to Jennings (2004), 80 per cent of adults and 82 per cent of young people in psychiatric hospitals have experienced physical or sexual abuse. Therefore, nurses are likely to encounter people with histories of abuse and trauma. However, in our clinical experience, many practitioners report feeling anxious about 'opening a can of worms' or 'stirring things up' for the person by talking about abuse and with no apparent benefit to the person in them doing so. Although some mental health nurses work as specialists in interpersonal trauma recovery, most nurses are not specialised in trauma work and have only brief periods of time working with a person; for example, during a period of hospitalisation when acutely ill. The following are some suggestions for implementing TIC and facilitating the person's recovery within any context in which that care occurs.

The fundamental role of the nurse is to listen compassionately and to respond to the needs of the distressed person at that moment. Be aware that every experience of human connectedness is powerful and contributes to recovery. You do not need to 'fix' the person. The person will do the work of healing over time as she or he progresses through recovery. Recovery from interpersonal abuse and trauma is considered as taking place in three sequential but overlapping stages (Herman, 2001):

1 safety and stabilisation;
2 trauma resolution: remembrance and mourning; and
3 social reconnection.

The ways in which mental health nurses can support the person's work at each of these stages are discussed in the following part of this chapter.

Stage 1: Safety and stabilisation

Safety and stabilisation of the person's mental state and environment is the first therapeutic task. The provision of safe places and safe people to be with is paramount, as most highly distressed people are likely to be at this first stage of recovery. TIC requires the practice of 'universal precautions' (National Executive Training Institute, 2005, p. 27). Just as we carry a high awareness of pathogens in physical health care in order not to spread them, likewise nurses are required to treat every person *as though the person carries* a history of interpersonal abuse and its effects. This assists us to avoid re-traumatising the person and to be open to what is helpful or unhelpful. We only know that there is no history of abuse once the person has a safe-enough relationship with us to tell us so.

The person must be asked about his or her experiences of abuse and trauma, but this should be done in the context of a wider assessment in which other information is being gathered, in order to position it as something that is important but not shameful (Read, Hammersley & Rudegeair, 2007). People often wait to be asked about their abuse history on the basis that when we are ready to ask the question we are ready to hear the answer. To tell staff members who may disbelieve them, judge them or pathologise them is a huge risk for any person; therefore, it is important to note that even if a person says 'no' in the first instance, she or he may disclose later with someone trusted.

Once the person has been asked about his or her experiences of abuse and trauma, and replies recorded in the person's notes, the question should only be asked again as needed, as it can be re-traumatising to be asked many times by people one has only just met. Use the skills of the therapeutic relationship, particularly respect, empathy and being non-judgemental. If someone decides to tell you about a painful experience it is appropriate to reply 'I'm sorry that happened to you'.

Supporting the stabilisation and safety of the person is fundamental; it is only when a person feels safe enough in the present, has learned skills in managing stress and distress, and has been educated about trauma and the trauma recovery process, that she or he is resourced and ready to venture back into the terrors of the past. If the person chooses to talk to you about painful experiences, let her or him take the lead on what and how much to disclose. This respects the person's autonomy, the pace of talking about his or her experiences and self-protection mechanisms.

It is this re-experiencing – known as exposure – that is central to healing from trauma for all people. Talking to you about her or his experiences is one of the ways that the person may use the therapeutic relationship with you. Proceeding cautiously in these conversations is a way of preventing the person from being overwhelmed. This pacing can be difficult to manage; sometimes the story and the feelings that are associated with the story simply tumble out, so just do your best. Going too far, too fast, is the greatest pitfall in trauma work. The tortoise, not the hare, is the role model for trauma work!

Inform yourself about what is known about the person's trauma history from his or her clinical notes and by talking to your colleagues. Use this information sensitively to care for the person and to prepare yourself to talk to the person about the abuse and its traumatic effects when, and if, the person opens up the conversation. Let her or him tell their story rather than you telling it. Your role is to listen compassionately. The person's role is to be the expert on herself or himself, and to do the work of recovery.

Let the person know that you are interested in helping him or her to achieve a sense of safety. You can ask general questions like 'Do you feel safe in your room or in this unit?' or 'Is there anything we can do to help you feel safe and comfortable here?' Be aware of the person's safety strategies to manage her or his fear of being harmed again in an interpersonal situation; for example, needing to be near a door for a fast escape from a situation. By being aware of these needs you can assist the person to manage the environment within what is possible in that clinical setting and reduce his or her levels of distress.

Use the least coercive practices possible. Draw on nursing skills in de-escalation, sensory modulation (Champagne & Sayer, n.d.) and interventions that are set out in the person's advance directives, in order to avoid restraint and seclusion. Being held down or locked up can be overwhelmingly re-traumatising for people who experienced these events in their past. Anxiety and distress are very common among traumatised people and manifest in many ways, including self-harm. It is important to understand the effectiveness of self-harm in its many forms – such as cutting, overdosing and drug or alcohol abuse. Self-harm is helpful to people in different ways, such as promoting dissociation from painful memories and feelings, or locating the pain in the physical body rather than in the heart or mind. Support the person to reduce distress through self-soothing skills or medications he or she finds helpful until the person's skill levels increase. Referral to structured therapies such as dialectical behaviour therapy (Linehan, 1993) can provide effective skills for relief of symptoms of anxiety.

Be authentic and trustworthy; do what you say you are going to do. Trust feels like a dangerous risk if your life experience is one of betrayal by those who are supposed to nurture and love you. Take care not to judge the abusive people or their life experiences; it is for the person to do that if she or he chooses. The work of making sense of loving someone, and hating what he or she did to you, takes time. Validate the person authentically. This means giving genuine feedback and care. Interpersonal abuse is a strong form of invalidation, so any form of validation is healing. Genuine, constructive feedback is usually very helpful to someone who is struggling with constructing an identity beyond shameful victim or mad person and creating a narrative account of his or her life in which the person's strengths, character and talents can emerge and shine.

Use collaborative investigation and discovery, not of the details of the abuse, but of abuse-related issues that may be present, such as grief, loss, anger, hopelessness or low self-esteem. Making sense and meaning of the person's experience is part of the process of recovery, as are gaining understanding and processing anger, and grieving for the many losses associated with interpersonal abuse.

Suspend judgement about the truth of accounts of interpersonal abuse you may hear. Many health professionals find they are unable to believe that people can treat each other so cruelly, and question whether what they hear or read in clinical notes is indeed true. It is not our role to investigate the truth of these experiences; that would be the role of the legal system. In Australia, the Royal Commission into Institutional Responses to Child Sexual Abuse (2013) has been commissioned to hear accounts of abuse of children in institutions such as churches. As these large numbers of accounts emerge, they will provide a broader context for understanding the many ways in which abusers harm their fellow humans.

We need to record the person's accounts of abuse in her or his notes as accurately as we can, in the person's own words and without judgement. Some people may want to report the abuse to legal authorities. This is often because the person wants to stop the offending and protect other children from the abuser. There are complex judgements to be made about how to proceed, so consult with your team and your supervisor if a person raises this with you. What most people want in order to resolve their traumatic experiences is acknowledgement that it happened, not denial and secrecy, and that it was the responsibility of the abuser, that it was harmful to him or her and that some repair is made such as acknowledgement and apologies from those who abused and those who failed to protect the person from abuse (NSW Health Education Centre Against Violence, 2013).

Safety is a paramount value in mental health nursing. Be prepared to let the person know that if she or he tells you that she or he, or another person, is unsafe in some way, you will need to share that information with others. Never try to deal with complex problems alone. You need to consult with the team about how to proceed if you learn of someone at risk. We must always act in situations of risk; the skilful part is to respond effectively to get the best outcome for the person and/or other person at risk, and this is where the wisdom of the team is needed. Check what current policies there are in your clinical area about the detection and reporting of abuse of children, adults and older adults.

Consider ways in which you can increase your knowledge and skills in caring for abused and traumatised people. Reflect on accounts of interpersonal abuse in the news; understand the ways in which power plays out in interpersonal relationships and the attitudes and values that have led to them occurring. This provides a larger context of understanding the experiences of people and, indeed, ourselves.

Stage 2: Trauma resolution

Over time, once a person has achieved safety and stability she or he is able to move to the next stage: trauma resolution. In this stage, the person works with a trusted therapist to process his or her traumatic memories through graded exposure by telling and retelling his or her story within a safe, therapeutic space. The person is supported to make sense of her or his experiences and of herself or himself; something the person may have thought impossible because the person considers himself or herself to be 'mad'. The person may have been told that she or he was mad by others as a way of keeping the abuse secret; constructing the teller of the story as 'crazy' also constructs the person as an unreliable historian who is not to be believed. At this stage of recovery, the person is able to focus on constructing a narrative account that makes connections between past experiences, symptoms of mental illness and behavioural patterns.

The role of the mental health nurse at this stage is to support the work of therapy by following the plans of the therapist, which guide the nursing care and skill development of the person. You can make a great contribution to the person's recovery by being active and skilful in liaison and communication with his or her therapist or the crisis team to help the health system to work smoothly and effectively for him or her.

Stage 3: Social reconnection

In this stage the person reviews his or her social context and makes choices about who to have in his or her life; reconnects with education and employment and seeks the ordinary joy and happiness of life. At this point many people will experience freedom from their symptoms of psychological distress or mental illness because the source of these problems, past abuse and the trauma that ensued have been resolved. Many people make wonderful recoveries and contribute their knowledge of the experience of both abuse and recovery to the support of others on the recovery journey. This is known as the 'survivor mission'.

While TIC provides a pathway of recovery for many people, there are also people who do not wish to revisit their past or who do not attribute their current distress or problems to interpersonal life events. Each person will have her or his own narrative account of her or his experiences of mental ill health, which we must respect. Trauma-informed mental health nursing practice is helpful for all people, regardless of how and where they experience their distress or illness. It respects their right to least-coercive care, is focused on therapeutic relationship and empathic care, supports the development of skills for managing distress, and works for the creation of a narrative that makes meaning of the past in the present.

Consumer narrative   Jane's story

I recall the anxiety I felt as a new mental health nurse when I read a consumer's 'history' before working with her or him for the first time in the in-patient unit. Accounts of intense psychological distress and references to past abuse and chaotic life circumstances would often feel overwhelming to me. As a new nurse, what did I have to offer this person? Would I say the right things or make things worse? How would I meet my professional responsibilities as a mental health nurse? Over time I discovered for myself the wisdom of mental health nursing's focus on therapeutic relationships. The key to my anxiety as a new nurse was learning how to create a safe therapeutic space. While 'history' can provide a helpful context for meeting the person, it is usually not written by that person. I needed to build a therapeutic relationship in which the person could speak of his or her hopes and needs.

The moment would come when I would need to introduce myself and explain my role. I would remind myself of the values of being authentic, respectful, non-judgemental, trustworthy and compassionate. I would take some deep breaths, greet the person, and listen to him or her with all my mind and heart. What had begun as a daunting professional challenge would become a conversation between two people grappling with the challenges of life, health and recovery. As time went by I brought more knowledge and skills to my conversations with consumers; however, the foundation of therapeutic relationship always remained essential and powerful. Experience helps us to build confidence, but a little anxiety will always remain because we meet each consumer anew and are challenged to understand and engage with his or her uniqueness as a human being and with his or her unique recovery experience.

Chapter summary

This chapter has presented stories and information, supplemented by activities designed to deepen understanding of:

- the diversity of sexual orientation and gender identities;
- the skills in practising culturally safe and inclusive care;
- how the power of language, behaviour and the structures within society and the health system can have an effect on peoples' mental health;
- the required knowledge, skill and confidence to provide a safe and compassionate environment by adopting trauma-informed nursing care; and
- the importance of the narrative within the text so that we can hear the 'real-world' voice of the users of the services we provide.

Critical thinking/learning activities

1. Re-read the definition of hetero-normativity and then make a list of what you perceive to be the traditional gender roles within couple relationships that are perpetuated; for example, by the cinema and print media. Compare these roles to the changes, if any, that you are witnessing in society or within your social circle.

2. In the first section of Riley's narrative he told us that the 'problem was not me; it was the assumptions of the people around me who knew nothing more than the binary of male and female'. What may be some of the similar assumptions and actions that nurses may engage in that could be disrespectful of Riley and his gender identity?

3. Riley also said: 'I feel worried about a medical system that relies on us having this level of privilege, since many of us are not white or middle-class and do not go to university. What happens then?' If you were able to continue this conversation with Riley and respond to his question, what may be some of the key points that you would like to discuss and debate with him in response to his concerns?

4. The Duluth model of power and control (Figure 10.1) summarised the strategies used to achieve compliance and acquiescence within interpersonal relationships. Either individually or with one of your peers, reflect on these strategies and note any that may apply to people you know, or even to yourself.

5. In the TIC section we talked about the importance of our own human vulnerabilities and the need to consider our self-care. Having reflected and discussed the above activities, now pay attention to the helpful strategies that you are currently using, or can use in the future, that promote your own mental and physical well-being.

Learning extension

Riley explained that even though there is a vast array of genders, people continue to experience violence because they do not fit into either male or female gender roles, or are not 'masculine enough' or 'feminine enough'. Make a list of the negative words commonly used to describe people who do not fit the above stereotypes. Write a paragraph answering the following reflective questions:

- How would you feel if these terms were applied to you, your friends or your family?
- How might nurses assist in challenging and changing this hurtful language in our personal and work lives?

Further reading

Barbara, A. M., Doctor, F. & Chaim, G. (2007). *Asking the Right Questions 2: Talking with clients about sexual orientation and gender identity in mental health, counselling and addiction settings.* Toronto, Canada: Centre for Addiction and Mental Health. Retrieved from http://knowledgex.camh.net/amhspecialists/Screening_Assessment/assessment/ARQ2/Documents/arq2.pdf.
This manual is very practical and applicable in both the mental health and substance abuse services and relevant to the Australasian setting.

Read, J., Hammersley, P. & Rudegeair, T. (2007). Why, when and how to ask about childhood abuse. *Advances in Psychiatric Treatment, 13*(2): 101–10.
This paper gives an excellent account of how to ask questions safely about trauma and how to respond to disclosure.

References

ACT Law Reform Advisory Council (2012). *Beyond the Binary: Legal recognition of sex and gender diversity in the ACT.* Retrieved from www.justice.act.gov.au/publication/view/1897/title.

Adams, J., Dickinson, P. & Asiasiga, L. (2012). *Mental Health Promotion and Prevention Services to Gay, Lesbian, Bisexual, Transgender and Intersex Populations in New Zealand: Needs assessment report.* Retrieved from www.mentalhealth.org.nz/file/downloads/pdf/file_459.pdf.

Adams, P.J. (2012). *Masculine Empire: How men use violence to keep women in line.* Auckland: Dunmore Publishing Ltd.

American Psychiatric Association (APA) (1952). *Diagnostic and Statistical Manual of Mental Disorders.* Washington, DC: Author.

APA (2000). *Diagnostic and Statistical Manual of Mental Disorders: DSM-IV-TR,* 4th edn. Washington, DC: Author.

APA (2013). *Diagnostic and Statistical Manual of Mental Disorders: DSM-V* (5th edn). Washington, DC: Author.

Anderson, E. (2008). 'I used to think women were weak': Orthodox masculinity, gender segregation, and sport. *Sociological Forum, 23*(2), 257–80.

Australian Human Rights Commission (2011). *Addressing Sexual Orientation and Sex and/or Gender Identity Discrimination: Consultation report.* Retrieved from http://humanrights.gov.au/human_rights/lgbti/lgbticonsult/report/index.html

Berliner, L. & Conte, J. (1990). The process of victimisation: The victim's perspective. *Child Abuse and Neglect*, *14*(11): 29–40.

Birkenhead, A. & Rands, D. (2012). *Let's Talk about Sex (Sexuality and Gender): Improving mental health and addiction services for rainbow communities*. Auckland: District Health Board.

Bloom, S. L. (1997). *Creating Sanctuary: Toward the evolution of sane societies*. New York: Routledge.

Bloom, S. L. & Farragher, B. (2011). *Destroying Sanctuary :The crisis in human service delivery systems*. New York: Oxford University Press.

Bloom, S. L. & Reichart, M. (1998). *Bearing Witness: Violence and collective responsibility*. New York: Haworth Maltreatment and Trauma Press.

Bornstein, K. & Bergman, S. B. (eds). (2010). *Gender Outlaws: The next generation*. Berkeley, CA: Seal Press.

Campinha-Bacote, J. (2002). The process of cultural competence in the delivery of healthcare services: A model of care. *Journal of Transcultural Nursing*, *13*(3): 181–4.

Champagne, T. & Sayer, E. (n.d.). *The Effects of the Use of the Sensory Room in Psychiatry*. Retrieved from www.ot-innovations.com/pdf_files/QI_STUDY_Sensory_Room.pdf.

Chandler, G. (2008). From traditional inpatient to trauma-informed treatment: Transferring control from staff to patient. *Journal of the American Psychiatric Nurses Association*, *14*(5): 363–71.

Cochran, S. D., Ackerman, D., Mays, V. M. & Ross, M. W. (2004). Prevalence of non-medical drug use and dependence among homosexually active men and women in the US population. *Addiction*, *99*(8): 989–98.

Cochran, S. D. & Mays, V. M. (2009). Burden of psychiatric morbidity among lesbian, gay, and bisexual individuals in the California Quality of Life Survey. *Journal of Abnormal Psychology*, *118*(3): 647–58.

Cox, J. L., Holden, J. M., & Sagovsky, R. (1987). Detection of postnatal depression. Development of the 10-item Edinburgh Postnatal Depression Scale. *British Journal of Psychiatry*, *150*: 782–6.

Daley, A. (2006). Lesbian and gay health issues: OUTside of Canada's health policy. *Critical Social Policy*, *26*(4): 794–816.

Davison, J. & Huntington, A. (2010). 'Out of sight': Sexuality and women with enduring mental illness. *International Journal of Mental Health Nursing*, *19*(4): 240–9.

de Graaf, R., Sandfort, T. G. M. & ten Have, M. (2006). Suicidality and sexual orientation: Differences between men and women in a general population-based sample from the Netherlands. *Archives of Sexual Behavior*, *35*(3): 253–62.

Duluth Domestic Abuse Intervention Projects (2011). *Domestic Abuse Intervention Programs*. Retrieved from www.theduluthmodel.org.

Edwards, K. M. & Sylaska, K. M. (2012). The perpetration of intimate partner violence among lgbtq college youth: The role of minority stress. *Journal of Youth and Adolescence*, *1*(11). Online first.

Elliott, D. E., Bjelajac, P., Fallot, R. D., Markoff, L. S. & Reed, B. G. (2005). Trauma-informed or trauma-denied: Principles and implementation of trauma-informed services for women. *Journal of Community Psychology*, *33*(4): 461–77.

Feldhaus, K. M., Koziol-McLain, J., Amsbury, H. L., Norton, I. M., Lowenstein, S. R. & Abbott, J. T. (1997). Accuracy of 3 brief screening questions for detecting partner violence in the emergency department. *Journal of the American Medical Association*, *277*(17): 1357–61.

Fenrich, J. & Contesse, J. (2009). *'It's not ok': New Zealand's efforts to eliminate violence against women*. New York: Leitner Centre for International Law and Justice.

Finkelhor, D. & Browne, A. (1985). The traumatic impact of child sexual abuse: A conceptualization. *American Journal of Orthopsychiatry*, *55*(4): 530–41.

Flemmer, N., Doutrich, D., Dekker, L. & Rondeau, D. (2012). Creating a safe and caring health care context for women who have sex with women. *Journal for Nurse Practitioners*, *8*(6): 421–96.

Foucault, M. (1979). *The History of Sexuality, Volume 1: An introduction*. New York: Vintage.

Gibbs, K. A. (2005). Teaching student nurses to be culturally safe: Can it be done? *Journal of Transcultural Nursing*, *16*(4): 356–60.

Goodman-Brown, T. B., Edelstein, R. S., Goodman, G. S., Jones, D. P. H. & Gordon, D. S. (2003). Why children tell: A model of children's disclosure of sexual abuse. *Child Abuse & Neglect*, *27*(5): 525–40.

Gunn, A. & Surtees, N. (2009). *We're a Family: A study of how lesbians and gay men are creating and maintaining family in New Zealand*. Retrieved from www.familiescommission.org.nz/publications/research-reports/we%E2%80%99re-a-family.

Herman, J. L. (1992). Complex PTSD: A syndrome in survivors of prolonged and repeated trauma. *Journal of Traumatic Stress*, *5*(3): 377–91.

Herman, J. L. (2001). *Trauma and Recovery*. New York: Pandora.

Holmes, C. A. & Warelow, P. (1999). Implementing psychiatry as risk management: DSM-IV as a postmodern taxonomy. *Health, Risk & Society, 1*(2): 167–78.

Human Rights Commission of New Zealand (2008). *Sexual Orientation and Gender Identity*. Retrieved from www.hrc.co.nz/human-rights-environment/sexual-orientation-and-gender-identity.

International Commission of Jurists (2007). *Yogyakarta Principles: Principles on the application of international human rights law in relation to sexual orientation and gender identity*. Retrieved from www.unhcr.org/refworld/docid/48244e602.html.

Jenkins, S. R. & Baird, S. (2002). Secondary traumatic stress and vicarious trauma: A validational study. *Journal of Traumatic Stress, 15*(5): 423–32.

Jennings, A. (2004). *The Damaging Consequences of Violence and Trauma: Facts, discussion points, and recommendations for the behavioral health system*. Retrieved from www.nasmhpd.org/docs/publications/archiveDocs/2004/Trauma%20Services%20doc%20FINAL-04.pdf.

King, M., McKeown, E., Warner, J., Ramsay, A., Johnson, K., Cort, C. & Davidson, O. (2003). Mental health and quality of life of gay men and lesbians in England and Wales: A controlled, cross-sectional study. *British Journal of Psychiatry, 183*: 552–8.

King, M., Semlyen, J., Tai, S., Killaspy, H., Osborn, D., Popelyuk, D. & Nazareth, I. (2008). A systematic review of mental disorder, suicide, and deliberate self harm in lesbian, gay and bisexual people. *BMC Psychiatry, 8*(1). Online only, doi: doi:10.1186/1471–244X-8–70.

Koziol-McLain, J., Giddings, L. S., Rameka, M. & Fyfe, E. (2008). Intimate partner violence screening and brief intervention: Experiences of women in two New Zealand health care settings. *Journal of Midwifery & Women's Health, 53*(6): 504–10.

Lakeman, R., McGowan, P. & Walsh, J. (2007). Service users, authority, power and protest: A call for renewed activism. *Mental Health Practice, 11*(4): 12–16.

Linehan, M. M. (1993). *Skills Training Manual for Treating Borderline Personality Disorder*. New York: Guilford Press.

Madrid, A., Skolek, S. & Shapiro, F. (2006). Repairing failures in bonding through EMDR. *Clinical Case Studies, 4*(4): 271–86.

Markowitz, J. C. (1999). Developments in interpersonal psychotherapy. *Canadian Journal of Psychiatry, 44*(6): 556–61.

McCabe S., Bostwick, W., Hughes, T., West, B. & Boyd, D. (2010). The relationship between discrimination and substance use disorders among lesbian, gay, and bisexual adults in the United States. *American Journal of Public Health, 100*(10): 1946–52.

McNulty, E. A. (2012). Transcription and analysis of qualitative data in a study of women who sexually offended against children. *Qualitative Report, 17*(47): 1–18.

Ministry of Health (2002). *Family Violence Intervention Guidelines: Child and partner abuse*. Wellington: Author. Retrieved from www.health.govt.nz/publication/family-violence-intervention-guidelines-child-and-partner-abuse.

Ministry of Justice (2009). *Te toiora mata tauherenga: Report of the task force for action on sexual violence incorporating the views of Te Ohaakii a Hine* – National network ending sexual violence together – task force for action on sexual violence. Retrieved from www.justice.govt.nz/policy/supporting-victims/taskforce-for-action-on-sexual-violence/policy-and-consultation/taskforce-for-action-on-sexual-violence/documents/tasv-report-full.

Monro, S. (2000). Theorizing transgender diversity: Towards a social model of health. *Sexual and Relationship Therapy, 15*(1): 33–45.

Monro, S. & Warren, L. (2004). Transgendering citizenship. *Sexualities, 7*(3): 345–62.

National Executive Training Institute (2005). *Training Curriculum for Reduction of Seclusion and Restraint. Draft curriculum manual*. Alexandria, VA: National Association of State Mental Health Program Directors & National Technical Assistance Center for State Mental Health Planning.

New Zealand Family Violence Clearinghouse (2009). *Family Violence Statistics Fact Sheet*. Retrieved from www.nzfvc.org.nz/sites/nzfvc.org.nz/files/factsheet-statistics-2009–1.pdf.

NSW Health Education Centre Against Violence (2013). *Recovering From Adult Sexual Assault: Navigating the Journey*, 3rd edn. Parramatta, NSW: Author. Retrieved from www.ecav.health.nsw.gov.au/pdf/NavigatingJourney2013.pdf?pg=0&s=R.

O'Neill (Roache), K. R., Hamer, H. P. & Dixon, R. (2012). 'A lesbian family in a straight world': The impact of the transition to parenthood on couple relationships in planned lesbian families. *Women's Studies Journal*, 26(2): 39–53. Retrieved from www.wsanz.org.nz/journal.

Oostendorp, R. H. (2009). Globalization and the gender wage gap. *The World Bank Economic Review*, 23(1): 141161.

Read, J. (1998). Child abuse and severity of disturbance among adult psychiatric inpatients. *Child Abuse & Neglect*, 22(5): 359–68.

Read, J., Hammersley, P. & Rudegeair, T. (2007). Why, when and how to ask about childhood abuse. *Advances in Psychiatric Treatment*, 13(2): 101–10.

Royal Commission into Institutional Responses to Child Sexual Abuse (2013). Viewed at www.childabuseroyalcommission.gov.au/our-work/about-the-royal-commission.

Rudman, L. A. & Glick, P. (2012). *Social Psychology of Gender: How power and intimacy shape gender relations*. New York: Guilford Press.

Sedgwick, E. K. (1990). *Epistemology of the Closet*. Berkeley, CA: University of California Press.

Seidman, S. (2002). *Beyond the Closet: The transformation of gay and lesbian life*. New York: Routledge.

Semp, D. (2006). A Public Silence: Discursive practices surrounding homosexuality in public mental health services in Aotearoa/New Zealand. Unpublished PhD thesis, University of Auckland.

Sheffield, C. J. (1989). The invisible intruder: Women's experiences of obscene phone calls. *Gender & Society*, 3(4): 483–8.

Spargo, T. (1999). *Foucault and Queer Theory*. Cambridge, UK: Icon Books.

Timmerman, G. M. (1991). A concept analysis of intimacy. *Issues in Mental Health Nursing*, 12(1): 19–30.

Trippany, R. L., White Kress, V. E. & Wilcoxon, S. A. (2004). Preventing vicarious trauma: What counselors should know when working with trauma survivors. *Journal of Counseling & Development*, 82(1): 31–7.

United Nations High Commissioner for Human Rights (2012). *Born Free and Equal: Sexual orientation and gender identity in international human rights law*. Retrieved from www.ohchr.org/Documents/Publications/BornFreeAndEqualLowRes.pdf.

Vitulli, E. (2010). A defining moment in civil rights history? The employment Non-Discrimination Act, trans-inclusion, and homonormativity. *Sexuality Research and Social Policy*, 7(7): 155–67.

Weber, G. N. (2008). Using to numb the pain: Substance use and abuse among lesbian, gay, and bisexual individuals. *Journal of Mental Health Counseling*, 30(1): 31–48.

World Health Organization (WHO) (2002). *Gender and Mental Health*. Retrieved from http://whqlibdoc.who.int/gender/2002/a85573.pdf.

WHO (2005). *WHO Multi-country Study on Women's Health and Domestic Violence Against Women: Summary report of initial results on prevalence, health outcomes and women's responses*. Retrieved from www.who.int/gender/violence/who_multicountry_study/en.

WHO (2008). *Millennium Development Goal 5: Improving maternal mental health*. Retrieved from www.who.int/mental_health/prevention/suicide/Perinatal_depression_mmh_final.pdf.

11

Mental health of children and young people

Rhonda L. Wilson and Serena Riley

Introduction 245
Respect for young people 245
Developing a rapport with young people 246
Developmental stages 248
Reducing risk and vulnerability 249
Mental health promotion, prevention and early intervention for young people 252

Common mental health conditions in young people 256
Chapter summary 258
Critical thinking/learning activities 258
Learning extension 258
Acknowledgement 259
Further reading 259
References 259

Learning objectives

At the completion of this chapter, you should be able to:

- Consider the developmental needs of young people and how this influences their mental health.
- Identify youth-friendly environments and contexts that enhance mental health care.
- Identify some enablers and barriers to developing therapeutic rapport with young people.
- Recognise the importance of hopefulness and resilience in young people and how this influences their recovery experiences.
- Identify some common mental health problems experienced by young people.

Introduction

This chapter outlines a developmental orientation to understanding the mental health of children and young people. It examines the implications for mental health in children and young people in relation to the environment, nature and nurture, and brain development in the context of vulnerability or risk, and resilience or protection. The chapter explores mental health promotion for young people, drawing from two real stories about bullying and altered eating patterns, including anorexia nervosa and bulimia, which include experiences of depression, anxiety and psychosis. Emphasis is given to prevention, promotion and early intervention for mental illness, including social media and e-mental health interventions for young people in relation to non-suicidal self-injury or suicide crisis, and popular public health initiatives to reduce suicide, such as RUOK Day, headspace and other online services.

Respect for young people

Health professionals providing mental health care to children and young people should do so in a way that conveys respect and genuine concern. For children and young people, the first occurrence of a mental illness is likely to be a very confusing and perhaps a frightening experience. An important priority is for health care professionals to develop a strong initial therapeutic rapport with the young people they are helping. Young people are unsure of what to anticipate in mental health care, especially if it is their first appointment, or their first experience of a mental illness (Watson, Rickwood & Vanags, 2013; Wilson, Cruickshank & Lea, 2012). Health professionals can do a great deal to allay the confusion, anxiety and apprehension that may accompany a first experience of gaining mental health care, simply by creating a respectful and trusting relationship from the outset (Coughlan et al., 2011; Wilson, et al., 2012).

Most mental health problems are first encountered during the ages of 12–25 years, and approximately 20 per cent of the world's young people are affected (Wei et al., 2013). It is very important to promote mental health, provide accessible, youth-focused early intervention when it is needed, and to support the recovery care of young people, because we know that the earlier mental health care is initiated, the more likely will be the success of recovery (Boyd et al., 2011; Coughlan et al., 2011; McAllister & Handley, 2008; Wilson, 2007; Wilson, et al., 2012). Early commencement of mental health care reduces periods of disruption to the important developmental stages of growth, educational and vocational attainment, and social functioning (Coughlan et al., 2013; McAllister & Handley, 2008).

A shift towards a stronger focus on the mental health and well-being of young people is gaining international momentum (Coughlan, et al., 2013). The objectives of the Youth Mental Health Declaration include:

- authentically involving young people and their families in meaningful youth mental health service development;
- improving the understanding of youth mental health within communities;

youth-friendly
services, settings and health professionals in which authentic respect, care and congruence with the young person and her or his culture are conveyed

- improving accessibility of **youth-friendly** mental health services and supports;
- the adoption of youth-focused, strength-based mental health care; and
- focusing on developing resilience, hope and recovery.

Developing a rapport with young people

Health professionals working with young people need to be aware of the dynamics of culture for young people. It is important to understand the language, social context, values and beliefs of young people so that a relevant and appropriate therapeutic relationship can be established (Wilson et al., 2012). In particular, it is important to ensure that the behaviours of the health professionals do not represent a barrier to young people engaging with mental health care providers (Wilson et al., 2012). An authentic and respectful relationship will need to develop so that mental health care is achieved (Conradson, 2003; McAllister & Handley, 2008).

Health professionals should not try to become like a young person by adopting the behaviours or popular language of young people; however, neither should they be shocked or unaware of the real-life experiences and culture of young people. Health professionals should maintain a fluid knowledge of the dynamics of young people's cultures, and should inform themselves about trends, spaces and places in which young people feel most comfortable (Conradson, 2003). In addition, clinicians should position themselves to find a point of congruence or agreement, operate with a positive regard for the person, and with warm empathy so that a helping relationship can be developed and maintained (Rogers, 1980). The following lists, while not exhaustive, represent some barriers and enablers to authentic engagement with young people, and offer some practical assistance to students in their preparations for clinical placement or in transition to registration as a practitioner.

Barriers

- Clinical uniforms can present an overly pathological environmental context (Conradson, 2003).
- Formal clothes, out-dated fashions and/or poor hygiene may repel young people (for example, the contemporary fashion faux pas in the wearing of jeans and running shoes together). Young people make subjective judgements about trustworthiness and emotional connections based on decisions that may lack logic or reason, because they are still learning the social skills of extending respect and regard to others (Conradson, 2003). Therefore, clinicians will need to take this developmental factor into consideration as part of their professional preparation for working with young people.

- Inauthentic use of the social language of young people. It is not considered 'cool' by young people for older people to use their language, or to assume intimate knowledge of their language, without having gained social permission and creditability to do so.
- Laughing at the culture of young people or suggesting that 'they will grow out' of an undesirable stage is not helpful.
- Sarcasm and lecturing about what is 'right' and 'wrong' are unhelpful and demeaning to the person. Avoid taking an authoritarian approach.
- Long and drawn-out assessment appointments with multiple health professionals in attendance can be daunting for young people, and is likely to be counter-productive to an accurate mental health assessment.
- Try to avoid demanding that young people adhere to rules.
- Alienating settings and attitudes within health services, such as treating adolescents like children rather than as emerging adults, labels like 'typical teenager issues' and admission to an adult facility can hinder recovery (Coughlan et al., 2011).
- A previous bad experience of mental health care and long waiting times or lists are detrimental to young people's engagement and recovery (Coughlan et al., 2011; McAllister & Handley, 2008; Wilson et al., 2012).

Enablers

- Always introduce yourself and do so in a way that describes your role and availability to the young person. Introduce the young person to any other person who is involved in her or his care. It is appropriate to use first names in introductions because this represents contemporary culture, but it is equally important that the young person is informed about the delegation and roles of the people who are in helping positions.
- Health professionals wearing contemporary and age-appropriate, smart casual, logo-free and modest clothing will convey respect and authenticity to young people. Young people are quick to identify 'fake' or imposter-like affiliation with their culture, and they have a low regard for it.
- Use respectful plain language that is not laden with professional jargon, or with the casual lingo of young people. Keep yourself informed about the casual vocabulary of young people, because it is the role of health professionals to be able to interpret and understand the communication of the people they are trying to help (Wilson et al., 2012). It is appropriate to ask the young person to offer a definition of any term her or she uses that you may be unfamiliar with, because this will convey respect and interest in the person.
- Convey respect by responding appropriately to young people so that they feel they have been heard and that their experiences are regarded seriously (McAllister & Handley, 2008; Wilson et al., 2012).
- Sharing humour with young people (not laughing at them) and talking with (not at) the young person is ideal. Position yourself to journey with the young person towards recovery.

- Build and maintain a general awareness of the popular music, TV, internet and social media preferences of young people. Perhaps engage in some of these activities (at least occasionally) in order to gain some first-hand experience of these important social and cultural characteristics of young people's behaviour. This is of particular importance in regard to social media, because it has become a primary communication tool for young people, and on occasion can be a source of some discomfort as well (for example, cyber-bullying) (Christenson, 2007; Christenson & Petrie, 2013a, 2013b; Department of Health and Ageing, 2012).
- Check with young people about whether their basic needs have been met (for example, when was the last time they ate, had a drink, a change of clothes and a safe place to sleep?). If the young person is hungry, then providing a simple sandwich and drink can convey care and will assist in establishing therapeutic rapport and trust.
- Provide opportunities for breaks in assessment sessions, so that engagement is optimised. Ensure that the young person has a support person present (preferably of her or his choosing) if the young person would like that.
- Negotiate an agreement of shared responsibility, behaviours and actions that are achievable and safe for both the young person and the mental health professional/s, and that are based on the rights and responsibilities of both. Make clear what the consequences might be for breaking the agreement (for example, mandatory reporting of abuse, the use of the Mental Health Act to promote and ensure safety etc). Include young people and their families in the decision-making about mental health care interventions (Coughlan et al., 2011; McAllister & Handley, 2008).
- Develop some basic skills in appropriate social activities; for example, playing electronic board games of interest to young people, sporting activities (for example, shooting basketball hoops or pool/ snooker, or ten pin bowling). There is no need to be proficient in any of these activities, but it is ideal to create an opportunity for young people to teach you how to develop skills in some of these types of activities. The reciprocal nature of learning and caring promotes horizontal rather than hierarchal relationships, which have helpful therapeutic qualities.

Developmental stages

There are a number of seminal theorists whose work explains the developmental stages of children and young people. A general knowledge of these developmental concepts assists mental health clinicians to understand the related implications for mental health, recovery and well-being (McAllister & Handley, 2008). The psychological, intellectual and moral development of children and young people has been described across the lifespan, and with stages specifically relating to the need for successful schooling and cohesive social relationships (Erikson, 1968; Kolberg, 1963; Piaget, 1952; Vogel-Scibilia et al., 2009). Neurological developmental explanations are also relevant because the physiological development of the brain continues until about 22 years of age for humans, and thus cognitive abilities and capacities in young people are still forming at an early adult life stage (Blows, 2011; Geake, 2009).

It is equally important to consider the ecological systems that influence human development, and particularly any effects that magnify risk, vulnerability, strength and resilience in regard to the mental health and well-being of young people (Bronfenbrenner, 1986, 2005). Young people need an environment in which they can be nurtured and in which their fundamental physical, social and psychological needs are met, in order to become robust individuals who are resilient and able to cope and thrive in all life domains (Candlin, 2008; Harms, 2010; Stein-Parbury, 2009).

Reducing risk and vulnerability

Mental health promotion is about reducing the risk factors and vulnerabilities that may predispose young people towards mental illness. A strengths-based focus is concerned to increase opportunities to build psychological, physical and social strengths, because in doing so they offer protection and a buffer to various risks and vulnerabilities, and thus the effects of adverse conditions are minimised. Promoting sufficient support to families who care for children and young people is especially important in this regard, because healthy family contexts represent an ideal environment for children and young people to thrive (Lourey, Holland & Green, 2012).

Drug and alcohol misuse

Alcohol abuse is highest among young people aged 16–24 years age, with 11.1 per cent of the total Australian youth population affected, which represents a significant vulnerability for the developing brains of people in this age group (Teesson et al., 2010). Cannabis use represents a further vulnerability for this age group, because it is the next most common drug used, with a first-use average age of 18 years, and it is associated with a risk for developing comorbid psychosis and/or anxiety and/or depression (Australian Institute of Health and Welfare (AIHW), 2011; Mental Health Council of Australia, 2006). More than one-third of people over 14 years of age use drugs in any given year in Australia, which is similar to other English-speaking countries (AIHW, 2011). This topic is further discussed in Chapter 7 of this book, and it is relevant for students to read that chapter in conjunction with this chapter to further explore the drug and alcohol implications for young peoples' mental health.

Trauma and abuse

We know that it is far better that trauma or abuse should never occur, but if it has occurred, the younger the age at which it has occurred, the more likely it is that the effects will be less overall than at older ages. This acknowledgement does not trivialise the experience of trauma or abuse at any life stage, but it does indicate that resilience and recovery is more strongly aligned with a younger exposure to adverse conditions (Harms, 2010). Trauma and abuse can take many forms (for example, physical, sexual, refugee, war etc.) and bullying can be one such trauma for children and young people. The following exercise and real-life story helps to explore the mental health dynamics related to bullying in a school setting.

Reflective questions

There is a school-yard saying that goes like this: 'Sticks and stones might break my bones, but words will never hurt me.'

- Have you heard that saying? Do you agree or disagree with the sentiment?
- What effects do you think unkind, unfair or disrespectful words have had on your own life?
- Have you developed some resilience to cope with unkind words when they are directed at you?
- What if hurtful words and actions occurred in your life on most days? How would you feel? What might you do? How do you think it might affect your mental health?

Bullying – what it is like to be 12 years old and bullied

The following is a real-life recount by Clare, who came to know a 12-year-old school boy during her usual volunteering as a parent-helper at her local primary school. Some of the language in this story is very strong and unpleasant, but we have retained it because it is important that health clinicians who work in both general and mental health settings are aware of the challenges that young people face in their daily lives. It is relevant that health professionals should develop an appreciation of how uncomfortable some of their clients' circumstances of daily life can be. This is one such example.

Consumer narrative   Clare's story

He didn't have any hope that anything would change, but said the pill would hopefully make him care less about it.

Jason is an extraordinary boy. I met him late last year when I was a parent-helper on a school excursion for Year 5 and 6 kids. Jason was in Year 6 in the combined Year 5/6 selective opportunity class for gifted children. He was and is an incredibly handsome kid; tall, olive skin and bright sparkly eyes. I immediately assumed he must be very popular because he was so well mannered and personable, along with being cute and clever. But it became clear that he was a loner.

continued ›

I found Jason by himself a few times during the excursion, and asked him why he wasn't off with the other boys. He told me they didn't like him and called him names, and it was easier for him to be by himself. I asked him what sort of names – he said 'Queer, retard, gay, dancing queen, cock-sucker, faggot'. That's when I discovered that he had been dancing for several years (ballet, jazz, hip-hop). He said he really enjoyed dancing and that it kept him fit and flexible, and he seemed quite proud to show me his particularly muscular legs. But, clearly, some of the other boys at the school were merciless and relentless in their teasing. They didn't dare call him things when a teacher was around, but there were plenty of times when a teacher was not around. In addition, he told me that he was often shoved, had things thrown at him, was picked last and laughed at when he simply walked past those boys. He was sensitive to all the bullying behaviour.

I asked Jason if his mum and dad knew about it. He said they didn't know how bad it was, and just told him to ignore them. I told him he really needed to tell his teacher and his parents, and that I'd go with him to tell the teacher if he wanted that support. He said didn't want to upset his mum more at that time. She was already crying a lot about his dad going overseas to work for 12 months. I urged him to tell his mum, ASAP! I also had a quiet word with his teacher.

Anyway, that was last year, and I didn't see Jason again until yesterday. He looked flat. There was no sparkle in his eye anymore. I asked him how he was finding high school and the selective gifted program there. That's when he told me about the five boys who have continued on from primary school to the same high school as him, and how the teasing had worsened, and that he had been in a fight with one of them on Friday. He said one boy had hidden behind a pole and had kicked at him 'like a total coward'.

It was clear to me that Jason had initiated the fight, that he was just so angry and he really wanted to hurt that other boy. Jason said: 'He wouldn't even come out and fight like a man! And he calls me a sissy poofter!' I just thought that this poor, tortured kid, who is just a little boy on the inside, is alone and trying to prove his manhood. Jason said he was in trouble because of the fight, and on the weekend he had tried to kill himself. He had been in hospital all weekend, and was kept home on Monday and Tuesday, and then yesterday (Wednesday) was his first day back at school. Already that same boy Jason had tried to punch (the boy who had kicked out at him from behind the pole) had teased him again. He told me the name of the antidepressant he was on, the pill that he took with breakfast, how it was supposed to make him feel happier and how he would have to keep going back to see the psychologist for a while. He didn't have any hope that anything would change, but said the pill would hopefully make him care less about it.

Mental health promotion, prevention and early intervention for young people

A focus on young people's mental health has gained some momentum in Australia in recent years, with a particular emphasis on the development of early intervention and youth-friendly services for people aged 15–24 years. The Australian government has sought to expand its *headspace* initiatives, which are considered by some to be flagship, integrated youth mental health services (Cohen et al., 2009; Hodges, O'Brien & McGorry, 2007; McGorry et al., 2007). However, the number of these centres is limited and there are many communities that lack these mental health services for young people, due to financial restraints. This significantly limits the availability and accessibility of youth-friendly services for young people, despite the aspirations and recognised need for appropriate mental health services for all young people (Boyd et al., 2011; Coughlan et al., 2011; Wilson et al., 2012).

e-Mental health

e-Mental health for young people is a concept that has the capacity to assist with some of the geographical limitations in service accessibility (Christenson & Petrie, 2013b; Griffiths, 2013; Smith, Skrbis & Western, 2012; Usher, 2010; Wilson et al., in review). Some evidence-based online services are now available, including:

- **www.reachout.com** A number of resources are available for young people, including the mobile app 'Smiling mind', which is a relaxation tool designed to promote wellness in young people using mindfulness meditation. Providing an app such as this for download to a smartphone creates a convenient resource in the pockets and bags of young people, to draw upon for self-care in relation to simple stress.
- **www.beacon.anu.edu.au** A clearinghouse of peer-reviewed, therapeutic tools such as a cognitive behavioural therapy interventions.
- **www.youthbeyondblue.com** A website that provides information and assists young people and their families to locate appropriate mental health help.
- In addition, there many are many support groups, community mental health promotion initiatives and mental health organisations that connect with young people through social media (for example, Facebook and Twitter), to promote a positive community conversation about mental health (www.facebook.com/ruokday? Or #RUOK; www.facebook.com/suicidecallbackservice or #SCBS). Access to these supports can be achieved by 'Liking' the group on Facebook or by 'following' the group on Twitter).
- SMS texts are also a useful real-time tool to consider for use in future mental health care for young people. Lublin (2012) presented an interesting perspective about using real-time communications by mobile phone to assist young people with mental health crises, suggesting that it might be a revolutionary approach to saving lives and even comparable with the effects of the discovery of penicillin in society. View the short presentation by Lublin (2012) and consider the implications for innovative use of texting in regard to young peoples' mental health promotion.

Reflective questions

Briefly explore some of the websites and social media identified above.

- Think about the young people you know among your family and friends – do you think e-mental health and mental health promotion in social media would appeal to them? Why? Or why not?
- Would you use these resources yourself?
- What do you notice that is appealing or repelling about these sites? Do you think they are useful as part of a national mental health strategy?
- Might they be helpful to someone like Jason? His parents? Or Clare?

What is it like to be a young person experiencing a mental illness?

Serena is a young woman who has been able to tell her story of experiencing a mental illness that was very disruptive in her life. She shares her experiences and, in doing so, illustrates some important aspects that helped her towards recovery.

Consumer narrative   Serena's story: A journey through darkness and a personal story of recovery

For eight years I had struggled with anorexia nervosa and bulimia, never letting anyone know the secret that was killing me. From 13 to 20 years of age I was consumed by an undiagnosed mental illness. Self-harm, eating disorders, post-traumatic stress disorder (PTSD) and depression were my life, but nobody knew. In December 2010 I realised that I needed help. I told someone close to me about my feelings and set about searching for treatment. A process that started with hope ended in disappointment and despair as I searched without success for an eating disorder treatment facility in Australia.

On a morning in April 2011, I gave up. I could see no way out of the darkness I was in and no hope for a future. I felt so consumed and defeated by my problems that I attempted to end it all. After swallowing 40 Panadol tablets, my 12-month journey through mental health hospitals began. My first encounter was the emergency department after my overdose. In a state of confusion, depression and physical shutdown, I was assessed by a very empathetic nurse. She explained what was happening as my liver began to fail and my vital signs dropped. But most importantly, she shared that she had been in my position five years earlier but was now better, and that planted a tiny flicker of hope for a future free from mental illness.

In contrast, the doctor on the ward that night treated me without respect or compassion. There was no understanding of mental illness and I felt like a disgrace and shamed, wishing I was dead more than ever. One of the hardest things about that year was the shame of surviving. I experienced some nurses, doctors, family and friends who regarded me as simply an illness, a 'crazy', unstable, suicidal young girl, instead of as a *person*. But inside I was *me*, scared, hopeless, *but still me*.

continued ›

The months that followed, in ICU, low-security and high-security mental health wards, were like a bad dream. Even now I wonder if it really happened. My body was failing and I was told that I could have a heart attack at any minute due to the eating disorders. My body was deteriorating but I was trying to hold on through it all. In the hospitals there were nurses who understood, and those who didn't. After experiencing a psychotic event and badly cutting my arm, I was helped by a compassionate nurse. She showed me care and kindness. There was an understanding of my situation. An understanding that I was still just a girl, trapped in the disorders, *just as scared of myself as others were of me*.

As I was tossed around between psychiatrists, doctors, occupational therapists, dietitians, psychologists and nurses, I witnessed a range of treatment and care. From the moment I entered the hospital I was started on a mixture of anti-psychotics, anti-convulsants and antidepressant medications. High doses of strong medications designed to treat schizophrenia, psychosis, borderline personality disorders and the like. It took months and much trial and error to find the right drugs. It was a horrible time, in which I had many adverse reactions that resulted in trips to emergency departments. For months I felt like a drugged-up zombie forced into a world of disturbed drowsiness by the medication. Although the sedation seemed to protect me from myself, it encouraged me to isolate and withdraw while reducing my appetite further.

One day in hospital, after fasting for 11 days due to the anorexia, I was made to eat. After the meal I couldn't cope. While vomiting in the bathroom a nurse pulled me out and dragged me through the ward to be tossed in the isolation room, all the while telling me how disgusting and shameful I was. While I agree that the action of self-induced vomiting is disgusting and shameful, *I as a person am not*. But at that time, in that vulnerable state, *I believed I was*. The words of that nurse instilled in me more self-hatred and encouraged my decline into further depression. The difficulty with my situation was that, although my depression and PTSD were understood, my self-harm, eating disorders and related psychosis were not. The staff lacked understanding and knowledge of my conditions, and I often felt judgement from them. The contrast between health care practitioners who treated me as a person as opposed to a misunderstood illness was enormous. The words they spoke and ways they treated me affected me greatly, by either building up hope or ripping it away. The thing is, somewhere inside the shell of that broken, sick, depressed person was me. *I was still there, not a word spoken or action taken toward me went unnoticed by my fragile inner-self*.

When I spent some time out of hospital I was confronted with the stigma in the community about mental illness. Among many people the topic of my illness was avoided. Within my church, however, a project was commenced without my knowledge to create for me a quilt. While working on the project the members were freely discussing mental illness in an attempt to educate themselves and break the stigma associated with it. This meant a lot to me as it removed some of the shame and judgement I had been feeling.

continued >

Consumer narrative continued ›

For the final three months of in-patient treatment I was moved to an eating disorder-specific mental health hospital, where I was treated for my anorexia, bulimia, self-harm, depression and PTSD. It was a rough journey to break the cycle of illness, but the staff was equipped to deal with the situations that arose. Understanding and knowledge allowed the nurses to treat me with dignity and informed care. There were still terribly hard times in which I thought I would break, but through therapy, support, faith in God and care from staff I was able to push through toward recovery.

After a year in and out of hospital I returned home, more stable than I had been for the previous eight years. I was on medication that worked and had journeyed through a tough re-feeding program. The year that followed commenced with twice-weekly psychologist appointments and regular visits to my dietitian and GP. We worked on intense trauma therapy to overcome the PTSD as well as continuing work on dealing with the roots of depression and self-harm in my life. As the year continued, with only a couple of small relapses, the appointments were spread out further with my dietitian, and then they stopped altogether. Through strong family and therapeutic support, and my belief in a God who encourages self-worth, I was able to step out and start living my life. I had found a new confidence to make friends and a drive to give everything my all. In the past month I have been assessed and declared to be in remission from the eating disorders, with assessment scores putting me above the average population and in the recovered sector. My moods are also stable and I am beginning to wean myself off some of the more aggressive medications. My self-harm has been under control for over a year now, and the PTSD is also in remission. I know there is still further to go, *but I will make it*, as I am determined never to go back to that darkness that stole my adolescence and nearly ended my life.

Instilling hope

In Serena's story, she indicated that hope for the future was an important aspect in her recovery journey. Instilling hope for the future is a very important mental health care intervention, and one that all members of the interdisciplinary team are responsible for developing (Early Psychosis Writing Group, 2010; Kylma et al., 2006; Lourey et al., 2012). Serena described how some conversations and events developed a sense of hope for the future in her, and yet others diminished a sense of hopefulness while unhelpfully reinforcing stigma and feelings of shame and hopelessness. The list below provides some practical examples of ways in which health professionals can work towards fostering hope in the lives of other children and young people:

- Adopt a respectful and unhurried approach to listening.
- Sit next to the person. Physically and mentally position yourself to demonstrate care and interest in the person.
- Use words and language that are easily understood – avoid jargon. Explain what is happening and what will happen next so that there are no uncomfortable surprises.

- Ask about what the person is looking forward to in the future (today, next week, next year).
- Validate and reaffirm achievable, positive aspirations and goals for the future.
- Make sure basic immediate needs are met: safety (physical and psychological), enough good-quality food and drink, housing with a bed, appropriate clothing and privacy.
- Avoid flippant and judgemental comments – rather, reframe problems with a positive solution focus (Wand, 2010). Help the person to find a way to see the 'glass half full, not half empty'.

Common mental health conditions in young people

Suicide

More than 20 per cent of all deaths in young men and women in Australia are by suicide, making it a leading cause of death for young people (Lourey, et al., 2012). While suicide is not an illness but a behaviour, the determinants of suicide are closely associated with mental illness. Chapter 13 in this book addresses this topic in further detail, and students should read these sections concurrently. Suicide risk is accentuated by risk factors such as unemployment, social isolation, depression, recent bereavement, financial stress, disconnection from family and friends, and drug and alcohol misuse and abuse (Lourey et al., 2012). The greater the experience and accumulation of psychological stresses in a person's life, the greater the experience of suicidal thinking in that person's life (Lourey et al., 2012). Conversely, there are also protective factors that buffer individuals against suicide; for example, being connected with family and friends, being connected with culture, school and community, having another person care about their well-being, having a positive outlook on life, being creative with problem solving, experiencing sound financial stability, keeping physically fit and well, and being able to access mental health support when it is needed (Harms, 2010; Lourey et al., 2012).

Non-suicidal self-injury

Non-suicidal self-injury can be described as the deliberate destruction of body tissue without any suicidal intentions (Martin et al., 2010). Non-suicidal self-injury is considered a risk factor for suicide (Martin et al., 2010). All self-injury should be carefully considered on each occasion, and should instigate a thorough mental health assessment. It is never appropriate to dismiss self-injury as a benign 'call for help'. Clearly, it is a sign that the person's mental health is compromised and that distress is occurring and is interfering with a healthy lifestyle, and that the person is likely to benefit from mental health assessment and related interventions. Some examples of non-suicidal self-injury behaviours may include cutting, scratching, biting, burning or hitting (Martin et al., 2010). The motivation for non-suicidal self-injury includes emotional regulation and management, or self-punishment (Martin et al., 2010). Recalling Serena's story earlier in this chapter, it is clear that health professionals can influence hope for the future in regard to non-suicidal self-injury, through their actions and words.

non-suicidal self-injury
the deliberate destruction of body tissue without any suicidal intentions

Psychosis

Psychosis is most likely to be first experienced at around 18 years of age (Amos, 2012; Early Psychosis Writing Group, 2010), and this age represents an important developmental stage in the life of young people as they transit between school and vocation or training, as young adults. This is sometimes a period of stress, important decision-making and participation in risk-taking behaviours that sometimes include drug and alcohol misuse, and these activities may constitute risk factors for some people in regard to developing one or more episodes of psychosis (Early Psychosis Writing Group, 2010). Alcohol and cannabis consumption are both commonly noted in association with an onset of psychosis, and can be considered risk factors; however, it is not clear that any causal relationship is apparent (Early Psychosis Writing Group, 2010; Gregg, Barrowclough, & Haddock, 2007; Henquet et al., 2006; Mental Health Council of Australia, 2006). Early intervention that addresses all life domains to support a young person with psychosis has been found to be highly successful and cost-effective (Amos, 2012; Killackey et al., 2006; Yung, 2013).

> **psychosis**
> a symptom of mental illness that affects a person's thinking, behaviours and emotions; in early phases it is difficult to pinpoint and can seem as though 'something is not quite right'. The experiences of psychosis are sometimes similar to a normal developmental phase of adolescence. The problems become acute when disorganised thinking and/or hallucinations, and/or a deterioration in maintaining social relationships becomes apparent and disrupts daily life adversely

Depression and anxiety

Depression and anxiety can affect young people, with the average onset of depression at about 25 years of age (that is, half of all people affected will have had their first experience of depression or anxiety as a young person) (Slade et al., 2009). Depression and anxiety problems affect the emotions, thoughts, behaviours or motivation and physical health of people. A sustained lack of pleasure in life and a lack of hope for the future are some identifiable suicide risk factors. A range of psychological therapeutic actions can be administered by mental health clinicians to improve the mental health of people who experience depression and or anxiety (Ekers & Webster, 2012). A range of self-help and e-mental health resources with a growing body of supporting evidence is also useful (Christenson & Petrie, 2013a; Griffiths & Christensen, 2007).

Reflective questions

You have read about the experiences of some young people, and some information about types of mental health difficulties that some young people may experience.

- Can you imagine what it must be like to be a young person who is experiencing a first episode of any type of mental illness?
- How do you think you would like to be helped, if this were you?
- What would be the most helpful things a mental health professional (for example, a nurse) might do to assist you in getting help, and in recovering?

Chapter summary

- Understanding the developmental changes and dynamics that occur in young people assists mental health professionals to also understand the implications for development in regard to mental health promotion, well-being and recovery for young people.
- Ensuring that youth-friendly services, environments and relationships exist between young people and health professionals enhances timely engagement in mental health care by young people, when it is needed.
- Developing a therapeutic rapport with young people is especially important so that good experiences of care enable recovery and well-being, while barriers to engaging in mental health care should be avoided and minimised wherever possible.
- The development of resilience and hope for the future underpins successful recovery for young people.
- Common mental illnesses in young people respond well to a range of mental health care interventions, and best recovery and well-being are most likely where early intervention can be achieved.

Critical thinking/learning activities

1 List some practical ways in which you could find a point of congruence or agreement with a young person. How could you find some common area of interest that allows you to demonstrate empathy and warmth towards a young person with a mental illness?
2 List some features of a youth-friendly environment in which to deliver mental heath care.
3 List some ways in which a therapeutic rapport might be developed and maintained with young people.
4 In what ways does hope for the future (or lack of it) affect the recovery journey for a young person?
5 Visit some of the websites provided in this chapter. Which one appeals to you more? Why?

Learning extension

Visit the website of Children of Parents with a Mental Illness (COPMI) at www.copmi.net.au or the COPMI Facebook page at www.facebook.com/COPMIorg. These resources are designed to support and foster resilience while buffering vulnerability in children who are sometimes the carers of their parents with mental illness. In addition, the siblings of children with disabilities often also share the burden of caring for their siblings. An expert and carer group with representatives from Australia and New Zealand has developed a beginning discussion about this newly identified dynamic and an initial report advocates for support for vulnerable siblings (The Royal Australian & New Zealand College of Psychiatrists, 2010).

Listen to this podcast from Radio National's All In the Mind program, which discusses the physical and mental health care of young people: www.abc.net.au/radionational/programs/allinthemind/newdocument/4689134.

Acknowledgement

We thank Sandy Butler for contributing some ideas to the development of this chapter.

Further reading

Children of Mentally Ill Consumers (COMIC): www.howstat/comic/Home.asp
Hope for Life Suicide prevention: www.suicideprevention.salvos.org.au
MindHealthConnect: www.mindhealthconnect.org.au
A range of online tools and online therapy for a range of mental illnesses.
The International Declaration on Youth Mental Health: www.inspireireland.ie/international-declaration-on-youth-mental-health

References

Amos, A. (2012). Assessing the cost of early intervention in psychosis: A systematic review. *Australian and New Zealand Journal of Psychiatry*, **46**(8): 719–34.

Australian Institute of Health and Welfare (AIHW) (2011). *2010 National Drug Strategy Household Survey Report*. Drug Statistics Series No.25. Cat. no. PHE 145. Canberra: Author.

Blows, W. T. (2011). *The Biological Basis for Mental Health Nursing*, 2nd edn. New York: Routledge.

Boyd, C. P., Hayes, L., Nurse, S., Aisbett, D. L., Francis, K., Newnham, K., et al. (2011). Preferences and intention of rural adolescents toward seeking help for mental health problems. *Rural and Remote Health*, 11(1582): 1–13.

Bronfenbrenner, U. (1986). Ecology of the family as a context for human development: Research perspectives. *Developmental Psychology*, 22(6): 723–42.

Bronfenbrenner, U. (2005). Ecological systems theory. In U. Bronfenbrenner (ed.), *Making human beings human: Bioecological perspectives on human development* (pp. 106–73). Thousand Oaks: Sage Publications.

Candlin, S. (2008). *Behaviour Change in Adolescence. Therapeutic communication: A lifespan approach*. Frenchs Forest, NSW: Pearson Education Australia.

Christenson, H. (2007). Internet-based Mental Health Interventions for Young Australians. Paper presented at the New South Wales Early Psychosis Forum, Westmead Hospital, Sydney.

Christenson, H. & Petrie, K. (2013a). Information technology as the key to accelerating advances in mental health care. *Australian and New Zealand Journal of Psychiatry*, 47(2), 114–16.

Christenson, H. & Petrie, K. (2013b). State of the e-mental health field in Australia: Where are we now? *Australian and New Zealand Journal of Psychiatry*, 47(2): 117–20.

Cohen, A., Medlow, S., Kelk, N. & Hickie, I. B. (2009). Young people's experiences of mental health care. Implications for the headspace national youth mental health foundation. *Youth Studies Australia*, 28(1): 13–20.

Conradson, D. (2003). Spaces of care in the city: The place of a community drop-in centre. *Social and Cultural Geography*, 4(4), 507–25.

Coughlan, H., Cannon, H., Shiers, D., Power, P., Barry, C., Bates, T. et al. (2011). *The International Declaration on Youth Mental Health*. Association of Child and Adolescent Mental Health Special Interest Group in Youth

Mental Health in Ireland, 1–5. Retrieved from www.inspireireland.ie/wp-content/uploads/2011/10/YMH-Declaration_full-version_september-2011.-11.pdf.

Coughlan, H., Cannon, H., Shiers, D., Power, P., Barry, C., Bates, T., et al. (2013). Towards a new paradigm of care: The mental health declaration on youth mental health. *Early Intervention in Psychiatry*, 7: 103–8.

Department of Health and Ageing (2012). E-Mental Health Strategy for Australia. Canberra: Australian Government. Retrieved from www.health.gov.au/internet/main/publishing.nsf/Content/D67E137E77F0CE90CA257A2F0007736A/$File/emstrat.pdf.

Early Psychosis Writing Group (2010). *Australian Clinical Guidelines for Early Psychosis*, 2nd edn. Melbourne: Orygen Youth Health.

Ekers, D. & Webster, L. (2012). An overview of the effectiveness of psychological therapy for depression and stepped care service delivery models. *Journal of Research in Nursing*, 18(2): 171–84.

Erikson, E. (1968). *Identity, Youth and Crises*. New York: WW Norton.

Geake, J. G. (2009). *The Brain at School. Educational neuroscience in the classroom*. Berkshire: Open University Press.

Gregg, L., Barrowclough, C. & Haddock, G. (2007). Reasons for increased substance use in psychosis. *Clinical Psychology Review*, 27: 494–510.

Griffiths, K. M. (2013). A virtual mental health community: A future scenario. *Australian and New Zealand Journal of Psychiatry*, 47(2): 109–10.

Griffiths, K. M. & Christensen, H. (2007). Internet-based mental health programs: A powerful tool in the rural medical kit. *Australian Journal of Rural Health*, 15: 81–7.

Harms, L. (2010). *Coping with Stress. Understanding human development: A multidimensional approach*. South Melbourne, Vic.: Oxford University Press.

Henquet, C., Krabbendam, L., Spauwen, J., Kaplan, C., Lieb, R., Wittchen, H. et al. (2006). Prospective cohort study of cannabis use, predisposition for psychosis, and psychotic symptoms in young people. *British Medical Journal*, 330(11): 1–5.

Hodges, C. A., O'Brien, M. S. & McGorry, P. D. (2007). headspace: National youth mental health foundation: Making headway with rural young people and their mental health. *Australian Journal Rural Health*, **15**, 77–80.

Killackey, E. J., Jackson, H. J., Gleeson, J., Hickie, I. B. & McGorry, P. D. (2006). Exciting career opportunity beckons! Early intervention and vocational rehabilitation in first-episode psychosis: Employing cautious optimism. *Australian and New Zealand College of Psychiatry*, 40: 951–62.

Kolberg, L. (1963). The development of children's orientations toward moral order: Sequence in the development of moral thought. *Vita Humana*, **6**(11), 33–173.

Kylma, J., Juvakka, T., Nikkonen, M., Korhonen, T. & Isohanni, M. (2006). Hope and schizophrenia: An integrative review. *Journal of Psychiatric and Mental Health Nursing*, 13: 651–64.

Lourey, C., Holland, C. & Green, R. (2012). *A Contributing Life: The 2012 national report card on mental health and suicide prevention*. Sydney: National Mental Health Commission. Retrieved from www.mentalhealthcommission.gov.au.

Lublin, N. (2012). Texting that saves lives. TED talks. Ideas worth spreading. Retrieved from www.ted.com/talks/nancy_lublin_texting_that_saves_lives.html.

Martin, G., Swannell, S., Harrison, J., Hazell, P. & Taylor, A. (2010). *The Australian National Epidemiological Study of Self-injury* (ANESSI). Brisbane: Centre for Suicide Prevention Studies.

McAllister, M. & Handley, C. (2008). Promoting mental health. In M. Barnes & J. Rowe (eds), *Child, Youth and Family Health: Strengthening communities* (pp. 166–88). Marrickville, NSW: Elsevier.

McGorry, P. D., Tanti, C., Stokes, R., Hickie, I. B., Carnell, K., Littlefield, L. K. et al. (2007). headspace: Australia's national youth mental health foundation – where young minds come first. *Medical Journal of Australia*, 187(7): S68–70.

Mental Health Council of Australia (2006). *Where There's Smoke… Cannabis and mental health*. Melbourne: ORYGEN Youth Mental Health Service.

Piaget, J. (1952). *The Origins of Intelligence in Children* (M. Cook, trans.). New York: International Universities Press.

Rogers, C. (1980). *A Way of Being*. Boston: Houghton Mifflin.

Slade, T., Johnstone, A., Teesson, M., Whiteford, H., Burgess, P., Pirkis, J., et al. (2009). *The mental health of Australians 2: Report on the 2007 national survey of mental health and wellbeing*. Canberra: Department of Health and Ageing.

Smith, J., Skrbis, Z. & Western, M. (2012). Beneath the 'Digital Native' myth. *Journal of Sociology*, 49(1): 97–118.

Stein-Parbury, J. (2009). *Challenging Interpersonal Encounters with Patients. Patient & person: Interpersonal skills in nursing*, 4th edn. Chatswood, NSW: Churchill Livingstone Elsevier.

Teesson, M., Hall, W., Slade, T., Mills, K., Grove, R., Mewton, L. et al. (2010). Prevalence and correlates of DSM-IV alcohol abuse and dependence in Australia: Findings of the 2007 National Survey of Mental Health and Wellbeing. *Addiction*, 105(12): 2085–94.

Royal Australian & New Zealand College of Psychiatrists (2010). *Addressing the Needs of Siblings of Children with Chronic Conditions*. Melbourne, Vic. Retrieved from www.ranzcp.org/Files/ranzcp-attachments/Resources/siblings_report-pdf.aspx.

Usher, W. (2010). Australian health professionals' social media (Web 2.0) adoption trends: Early 21st century health care delivery and practice promotion. *Australian Journal of Primary Health*, 18: 31–41.

Vogel-Scibilia, S. E., McNulty, K. C., Baxter, B., Miller, S. & Dine, M., Frederick, J. F. (2009). The recovery process utilizing Erikson's stages of human development. *Community Mental Health Journal*, 45: 405–14.

Wand, T. (2010). Mental health nursing from a solution focused perspective. *International Journal of Mental Health Nursing*, 19: 210–19.

Watson, C., Rickwood, D.J. & Vanags, T. (2013). Exploring young people's expectations of a youth mental health care service. *Early Intervention in Psychiatry*, 7, 131–7.

Wei, Y., Hayden, J. A., Kutcher, S., Zygmunt, A. & McGrath, P. (2013). The effectiveness of school mental health literacy programs to address knowledge, attitudes and help seeking among youth. *Early Intervention in Psychiatry*, 7: 109–21.

Wilson, R. L. (2007). Out back and out-of-whack: Issues related to the experience of early psychosis in the New England region, New South Wales, Australia. *Rural and Remote Health*, 7(715): 1–6.

Wilson, R. L., Cruickshank, M. & Lea, J. (2012). Experiences of families who help young rural men with emergent mental health problems in a rural community in New South Wales, Australia. *Contemporary Nurse*, 42(2): 167–77.

Wilson, R. L., Ranse, J., Cashin, A. & McNamara, P. M. (in review). Health professions using social media, and why you should: The good, the bad, and the reluctant. *Collegian*.

Yung, A. (2013). Early intervention in psychosis: Evidence, evidence gaps, criticism and confusion. *Australian and New Zealand Journal of Psychiatry*, 46(1): 7–9.

12

Mental health of older people

Helen P. Hamer, Debra Lampshire and Sue Thomson

Introduction 263

Recovery 266

Culture of older people 267

Human connectedness 268

When things go wrong:
  Common mental illnesses 271

Cognitive decline, depression, delirium
  or dementia? Getting the diagnosis
  right 273

An ethical framework to underpin
  practice 277

The future of older people's
  mental health nursing 278

Chapter summary 281

Critical thinking/learning activities 281

Learning extension 281

Further reading 282

References 282

Learning objectives

At the completion of this chapter, you should be able to:

- Describe the process of positive ageing, life course and the changing cultural norms of older people.
- Identify the effects of ageism and multiple losses in older age on the mental health of older people and their carers.
- Demonstrate skills in detecting and assessing the major mental illnesses among older people and the nurse's role in facilitating care.
- Describe the medico-legal aspects related to collaborative care planning with older people.
- Discuss the future challenges for nursing in older people's mental health.

Introduction

This chapter discusses the process of positive ageing, the life course and the changing cultural norms of older people within contemporary society. The chapter aims to assist nurses to consider and understand how **ageism** and subsequent stigma and discrimination can affect the well-being of older people and their carers. The multiple losses and associated mental illness are also discussed, and specific approaches to nursing care required to support human connectedness with older people are explored. Common mental illnesses, associated risk factors and considerations for treatment embedded within a recovery approach are explained. The chapter concludes with an exploration of future issues for this area of specialty nursing practice.

> **ageism**
> an irrational prejudice on the basis of a person's age

Background

Getting older and doing more (Office for Senior Citizens, 2012) is a description that epitomises older people as an increasingly diverse and active group that continues to maintain its autonomy and well-being, even into later life. As the life expectancy of people in both New Zealand and Australia increases (Australian Bureau of Statistics, 2012; Office for Senior Citizens, 2012), older citizens are living longer than the previous generation. For example, demographic projections suggest that New Zealanders over the age of 65 years will exceed one million by 2030. Further, ageing citizens will live longer; in the year 2010, in New Zealand the male population in the 80 years and older age group increased by 5.1 per cent (2900) to reach 60 200, while the female population increased by 2.8 per cent (2500) to 93 200. Likewise, the Australian government has projected that the proportion of adults over 65 years will make up 25 per cent of the population by 2050. The majority of older Australians retain a reasonable standard of living; in 2009 only 7 per cent of older people were living below the low-income threshold, compared with 21 per cent of children (Pearson et al., 2012).

Importantly, by continuing to participate in society, older people maintain their status as full citizens (Brannelly, 2006; Hamer, 2012). Rather than being regarded as passive recipients of care, older people expect to continue to fulfil the same roles and responsibilities as others in society. These expectations, however, can be in contrast to the expectations of staff in some health care environments. Brannelly (2006) noted that the oldest 'olds' contemplated their rights as citizens in terms of having fought for their freedoms and are now wishing to realise their entitlements to health and social care. Furthermore, the 'baby boomers' (people born between 1946 and 1964) were well-established rights campaigners and willing to challenge what the welfare state had to offer if it was iniquitous with what other consumers received. Nurses, therefore, can expect to work alongside active, autonomous and informed older people who expect to participate in their care.

Social cohesion, inclusion and belonging within their community also provide the vital protective factors for older citizens' health and well-being. According to Bowling and Stafford (2007), being connected with one's neighbours and broader social support enables older people to cope with the challenges of illness and psychological distress. However, Lampshire and Latham (2000) reported that older people continue to encounter many barriers within society, particularly the obstacles of obtaining mental health care, problems with mobility, accessible transport and, for some, insufficient financial resources. Clearly, as this group continues to age, access to the latter resources that others in society take for granted is restricted because of the physical, psychological and sociological barriers derived from myths, stigma and discrimination directed towards older people.

The myths of ageing

Nurses must be mindful of the negative attitudes towards older people that proliferate within certain societies, including Australia and New Zealand. Ageism (Nelson, 2002) perpetuates the erroneous myths and stereotypes about older people: that they are weak, ill, unproductive, and even peculiar. These negative perceptions are often perpetuated in the popular media (for example, see Gillies, 2013). Older people and their families frequently experience prejudicial attitudes and discriminatory practices (Graham et al., 2003). Furthermore, older people with mental illness carry a double burden of stigma and discrimination. Negative attitudes held by health professionals towards older people with mental illness also mirror alarmist popular opinions about the 'burden' and cost of care for older people. Such negative attitudes can prevent older people seeking help from mental health and addiction services when needed. Not seeking help is also compounded by the older person's fear that he or she will be coerced into involuntary treatment and a rest or residential home, which further delays seeking treatment (Monahan et al., 1999).

Mental health professionals who provide care and treatment for older people also experience courtesy stigma; that is, being stigmatised as a result of working with older people (Angermeyer, Schulze & Dietrich, 2003; Parfene, Stewart & King, 2009) and are equally held in lower status by their professional peers. All mental health nurses are therefore required to reflect on their own attitudes and beliefs about older people (such as treating older people like children), and to act as advocates to assist in the elimination of ageism and promote opportunities for personal growth and community participation of older people in their care. Similarly, Adams and Collier (2009) have argued that

Reflective questions

- In pairs, write a list of some of the negative labels or words about older people that you have heard, in both your social and professional arenas.
- Briefly discuss how these labels and words are perpetuated through social media.
- What role do registered nurses have in changing these ageist assumptions?

nurses need to resist perpetuating the idea of a dichotomy between older and younger age groups, and the differential provision of health care that disadvantages older people with mental illness and addiction problems.

The life tasks

Cohen (2001; 2009) argued that evidence about the capacities and views of older people has led to a new theory about the life-tasks that characterise later life. Cohen proposed that, with increased longevity and due to better health and adequate resources, ageing is increasingly characterised by two potential phases in the final stages of the human life cycle: these are *retirement/liberation* and *summing up/swan song*. Contrary to myths about retirement and older age, Cohen asserted that most people fare well because retirement brings the liberating potential to explore new interests, activities and relationships. Subsequently, the older person experiences renewed feelings of freedom, courage and self-confidence. In short, this phase can be the springboard for creativity and improved mental and physical well-being.

The second of Cohen's (2001; 2009) life phases (summing up/swan song) relates to the inclination to appraise one's life work, ideas and discoveries, and to share them with family or society. The desire to 'sum-up' includes the need to complete one's life work, to 'give back' after receiving much in life, or the fear of time 'evaporating' before one has achieved all one would wish for in life. The swan song connotes the last act or final creative work of a person before retirement or death.

Cohen (2001; 2009) further argued that older people have a natural tendency to reminisce and relate their life stories. **Reminiscence therapy** is regarded as an approach that benefits older people (Jones & Beck-Little, 2002; McKee et al., 2005). Reminiscence therapy for health promotion and disease prevention is now commonly practised in some services for older people.

> **reminiscence therapy**
> the use of life stories – written, oral or both – to improve psychological well-being

Nurses can promote this approach to talking therapy as a platform by which to maintain the narrative in their practice, and as a record of the essence of the discussions within their nursing notes and care planning. Nurses need to feel confident that talking is equally as important as, for example, administering medication and other nursing tasks associated with the nursing care of an older person. Formally incorporating the narrative of the person's life story into everyday practice will strengthen the interpersonal alliance and preserve the dignity of the older person (Anderberg et al., 2007). Given that nurses make up the largest workforce within mental health services, they are ideally placed to formally incorporate the daily narrative, in the full confidence that the power of relating one's life story will increase the human connectedness that many older people long for in their daily lives.

> **ageing in place**
> when an older person continues to live in the facility of her or his choice for as long as the person is able to do so, and has the necessary services and supports in place to accommodate changing needs and circumstances

As the population ages and older people remain living in their own homes, it important for nurses to adapt their practice to bring the focus of care to a community setting and **ageing-in-place** initiatives

(Davies, 1995). Adoption of a community focus will support a sense of connection in the older person to her or his social structures and resources. Nurses will also be expected to ensure that older people feel safe and secure by offering a range of culturally appropriate services.

Recovery

The principles embedded within the **recovery** approach underpin mental health care within Australasia (Council of Australian Governments, n.d.; Mental Health Commission, 2001, 2012). The six guiding principles of recovery are hope, education, self-advocacy, personal responsibility, support and having meaning, purpose and direction (Lampshire & Hamer, 2012). The complex combinations of mental illness and addiction, disabilities, long-term health conditions and/or dementia must not be barriers to older people achieving the best quality of life. Having a life worth living is a core tenet of the recovery approach (Mental Health Commission, 2001). Recovery focused services are expected to deliver interventions and practices that promote recovery and reduce discrimination. Regaining and maintaining the major domains of one's life – housing, relationships, work and recreation – in order to live a satisfying, hopeful and contributing life are therefore essential for recovery (Deegan, 2005; Slade, 2009).

recovery
a deeply personal, unique process of changing one's attitudes, values, feelings, goals, skills and/or roles; it is a way of living a satisfying, hopeful and contributing life, even within the limitations caused by illness. Recovery involves the development of new meaning and purpose in one's life as one grows beyond the catastrophic effects of mental illness

Consumer narrative   Debra's story

As a consumer academic and advisor I have taught the recovery approach and the required competencies (Mental Health Commission, 2001) to many mental health professionals. It has become apparent in these workshop discussions that many participants believe that the concept of recovery does not apply to older people with mental illness. These assumptions are based on the view that older people are unable to recover from dementia and other organic brain changes.

I believe that these professionals are confusing 'cure' with recovery. Recovery, as a philosophy, equally applies to the older person. Older people have told me: 'We are not robbed of the ability to recover as we age; we rob ourselves when others hold the belief that it is not possible'. Recovery is not limited by age. Moments of hope are precious to the older person and should be celebrated. Any evidence of these moments tells us that recovery is entirely possible. Experiences of distress, despair and confusion are not

continued ›

Consumer narrative continued ›

exclusive to the older person, and neither, thank goodness, is recovery. Recovery happens when nurses harness the enduring strengths of the person so he or she can continue to thrive, even when the person has a limited number of life years left. Respect, love and being valued are universal imperatives required at any stage in the lifespan.

Culture of older people

Paying attention to the cultural aspects of nursing; that is, care that is congruent with the older person's cultural background and expectations (McBride, 2011) will influence and cultivate the development of human connectedness within the nurse–older person alliance. For example, cultural difference may be ethnicity or cultural identity, such as being lesbian or gay. Specific tasks of developing the alliance with the older person are concerned with **being-with** (Deegan, 2005; Randal et al., 2009). Being-with in each encounter helps to foster a genuine interest and conveys a sense of curiosity about the older person. Establishing the alliance helps the nurse discover who the person is, what kind of experiences she or he has had and who is significant in the person's life, both past and present. Joining with the older person in this spirit of cooperation fosters the human connectedness, trust and empathy that will privilege the person's life story or narrative in balance with the biomedical aspects of nursing care planning.

> **being-with** promotes deeper awareness of the meaning and dignity in human suffering

On a deeper level it is important that nurses pay attention to the more existential aspects of being human, and recognise the barriers to exploring specific areas of the lives of the older person. For example, we have noted that many nurses lack confidence in exploring aspects of the person's human experiences such as sexual orientation or spirituality. Further, nurses seem less confident in talking about sexual abuse and trauma (see Chapter 10), substance abuse and suicidal ideation. We call these the 'Five S' topics. The connection between sexual orientation and well-being is an important aspect to explore with older people. According to Bellamy and colleagues (2012), there are continuing reports of homophobia and prejudice against older lesbians and gays by staff in residential aged-care facilities, such as being refused a double room. Such prejudice not only affects their health care as they age; it is also a violation of the couples' human rights.

Older people wish to continue to be sexually active; however, Bodley-Tickell and colleagues (2008) have stated that an increasing number of older people were reported to be contracting sexually transmissible infections following unprotected sexual activity. This may be due to older people regarding the use of condoms, for instance, as a contraceptive rather than protection against infection. Nurses are able to support the recommendations by Bodley-Tickell and colleagues that sexual health programs should include preventative interventions, such as safe-sex messages aimed specifically at older people and that address societal and health care attitudes, and erroneous assumptions about sexual activity among older people.

Reflective activities

- In pairs, choose one of the five 'S' topics above and discuss your own emotional and behavioural reactions when planning to address this aspect with an older person in your care.
- Discuss the types of appropriate questions that maintain the human connectedness with the older person when discussing this aspect of nursing assessment and care planning.

Human connectedness

> Older people need nurses to have skills, not just pills.
>
> Lampshire & Latham, 2000, p. 6

In order to promote human connectedness in nursing practice, nurses can undercut ageist assumptions by paying attention to the narrative of the older person and his or her 'life before' the current mental illness. This requires the nurse to move beyond the primary focus on the biomedical understanding of the person's distress. Likewise, many older people focus on a biomedical understanding of their distress, and thus can be encouraged by the nurse to explore other factors, such as grief and loss. Older people have diverse life experiences that bring a unique and individual set of beliefs and values accumulated over years of having a life well-lived. Human connection is fostered by the respectful manner of the nurse. Taking the time to be-with the older person is also important.

Stebbins and colleagues (1999) reminded health professionals that giving people time to convey their answers to questions is important. For example, people with Parkinson's disease may have intact memory and recall, but due to impaired neurological functioning, such as bradyphrenia (Parkinson's Australia, 2010) or slowness of thinking, the time delay between hearing the question and providing a response is often misattributed to Parkinson's-related dementia. Allowing time for the person to answer requires patience, respectful listening and deference. The notion of *presencing* (Benner, Tanner & Chesla, 2009; Sandelowski, 2002) is the craft of being-with, rather than doing-to, and is equally important in the care of older people.

Human connectedness is also underpinned by the protection of the rights of older people and ensuring the provision of the range of services that promote their autonomy and well-being (Office for Senior Citizens, 2012). Older people are entitled to excellent care from qualified specialist nurses who are able to coordinate a range of options, such as psychosocial support, access to novel anti-psychotic and antidepressant medications, respite care, age-appropriate alcohol and other drugs treatment and, importantly, culturally appropriate services (Office for Senior Citizens, 2012).

The dignity of risk

According to Lord (2011), the term **dignity of risk** emerged from the disability sector and is increasingly being incorporated into the care of older people. Since de-institutionalisation of the large psychiatric hospitals, however, mental health services have progressively become risk-averse environments (Crowe & Carlyle, 2003; Hazelton, 1997, 1999; Rose, 1998; Sawyer, 2005). Likewise, the care of older people with mental illness is equally dominated by risk management, often at the expense of the therapeutic relationship (Sawyer, 2005).

> **dignity of risk**
> the right to choose to take some risks in your daily life, based on making an informed choice and accepting the possibility of harm or failure

While assessment of risk is concerned primarily with harm to self or to others, the nurse needs to assess specifically whether the older person is at risk *from others*. Balancing potential risk versus supporting the autonomy of the older person is a skill that develops as a nurse's practice advances and through experience in writing risk assessments that include the person's narrative in his or her treatment plans and clinical notes. The skill of assessing risk also requires that the nurse collaborate with the multidisciplinary team so that the nurse is not making such decisions alone. Restrictions on the older person's autonomy can also be minimised when incorporating the principles of professionally indicated risk-taking within nursing care planning (Krawitz et al., 2004).

Elder abuse

One of the most important aspects of the vulnerability of ageing is the risk of elder abuse. Fox (2012) provided a comprehensive review of the mostly unreported, poorly defined and researched, yet growing problem of elder abuse within older people's own homes; by family members, in wider society and by staff in residential care settings. Fox reported that five types of abuse are recognised: psychological, physical, sexual, financial and neglect (including self-neglect). Abuse of any kind is a violation of the person's human rights, yet as one of the sensitive topics described earlier, nurses often do not feel confident in detecting, exploring and reporting elder abuse. Nurses can, however, learn how to detect elder abuse and respond to disclosure in confidence when using effective skills in screening for abuse of any kind (Read, Hammersley & Rudegeair, 2007). Increasing the nurse's confidence in this area will maintain the human connectedness between the nurse and the older person. The nurse must never feel alone with this disclosure as the degree of moral distress experienced by the nurse can be overwhelming. Therefore, the nurse must always consult with a senior nurse or the multidisciplinary team to plan the next steps in care.

Medico-legal aspects

Nurses are both legally and ethically bound to ensure that older people are informed about their treatment and care options, and to support the person's participation in his or her health care or exercising of his or her right to refuse treatment (Health and Disability Commission, 1996; Nursing Council of New Zealand, 2012). Autonomous choices are voluntary and based on reasoning, and occur when people are adequately informed. If, due to dementia or other mental illness, a person cannot make autonomous choices he or she is said to lack decision-making capacity (Ganzini et al., 2005).

Capacity and competency

In the specialty area of older people's mental health, the question of whether people have decision-making capacity or competence is frequently tested. Nurses need to be aware of the differences between decision-making capacity and competency. Decision-making capacity is when a clinician assesses a person's ability to make decisions about health care, and is therefore a clinical assessment. In order to assess capacity, the clinician establishes whether the person is able to understand the information relevant to the decision and retain the information, even if only for short periods, and is able to use or weigh the relevant information in the decision-making process. This includes the capacity to see both sides of the argument and the ability to communicate his or her decision by talking, using sign language or another form of communication understood by others (Community Law Centre, 2013; Lai & Karlawish, 2007).

Competency is a legal definition and is determined by the Family Court, based on whether the older person has the capacity to reason and make decisions specific to the task, to appreciate her or his circumstances and understand the information being given (Chariand, 2001). It is important to note that capacity can fluctuate over time, and lengthy and ongoing medical procedures may require repeated assessments of the person's capacity.

In New Zealand, if a medical practitioner assesses that an older person no longer has capacity or competency to make these decisions, then the person's rights are protected through the *Protection of Personal Property Rights Act 1988* (3PR Act). The 3PR Act ensures that if the person has not nominated or appointed an Enduring Power of Attorney (EPA), and is now deemed to lack the capacity to do so, the Family Court will appoint both a property manager to protect and manage the person's property and financial matters, and a welfare guardian to protect future management of the person's health care and personal needs. It is important for nurses to ascertain, as part of the standard nursing assessment, whether the older person has an identified EPA, because the person's decision-making ability can alter dramatically within a short period of time.

In New Zealand, the *Mental Health (Compulsory Assessment and Treatment) Act, 1992* (Mental Health (CAT) Act) is invoked in situations in which the person is assessed to have a high degree of risk, or the person's safety is compromised due to an associated serious mental illness and where assessment and treatment without the older person's consent is required. In most cases, the Mental Health (CAT) Act can protect the older person who is extremely vulnerable and unable to adhere to psychiatric treatment as a result of cognitive impairment. However, an older person cannot be subject to the Mental Health (CAT) Act for reasons of competence alone. Regardless of the impairments, a person is entitled to have her or his wishes respected; hence, the importance of advance directives (Buchanan, 2004).

Advance directives

There are continuing debates about the effects of health law on the care of older people, particularly competence, capacity and assessment of the value-laden concept of insight (Diesfeld & Sjöström, 2007; Howorth & Saper, 2003). Such debates inform practitioners' decisions to use compulsory detention and treatment that suspends the rights and responsibilities of older citizens. In order to sustain older people's autonomy and preferences, the nurse can support the older person to complete an advance directive (Health and Disability Commission, n.d.; Wareham, McCallin & Diesfeld, 2005). An advance directive records the person's treatment preferences during an episode of illness when the person is unable to decide or communicate her or his preferences at that time. Advance directives, in part, protect the older person's right to choice of treatment; however, there is no law that specifically protects advance directives, which can be overridden if the person is subject to the Mental Health (CAT) Act.

So far, we have discussed the many sociopolitical, emotional and cognitive challenges that older people face as they age, and some of the protections that nurses need to be aware of to increase the human connection with older people. The following section focuses on the factors that contribute to common mental illnesses that bring older people to mental health services.

· ·

When things go wrong: Common mental illnesses

> Old age ain't no place for sissies.
>
> Actress Bette Davis (1908–89)

There are many challenges in growing older, such as increasing loneliness and isolation, the death of a partner or close friends, developing medical conditions and cognitive decline. These events may be barriers to older people adjusting to their new identity and roles, and their usual activities of socialising, housekeeping and/or driving. When these activities are curtailed this can lead to a sense of alienation, hopelessness and reduced self-esteem (Butterworth et al., 2006).

The prospect of having to endure years of emptiness and lack of purpose can raise levels of anxiety previously muted by the 'busyness' of everyday life. Stressful events and physical illness can increase anxiety and thus reduce the older person's capacity to ward off the trauma-related memories, images and feelings (Averill & Beck, 2000;

Hiskey et al., 2008). The power of the narrative and the telling of the life story can ameliorate such traumatic memories and increase the human connectedness with the nurse and other significant members of the older person's support network.

As well as risks of developing a depressive or anxiety illnesses, there is also an increase in the numbers of older people with psychotic illnesses (Oakley Browne et al., 2006). Manifestations of psychosis, such as hearing voices or talking to oneself can have an alternative explanation, as Margaret explains in her narrative.

Within the specialty practice of older people's mental health, the nurse can foster human connectedness by undertaking a collaborative and shared formulation of the person's presentation, based on both the narrative and the biomedical understanding of the older person's current problems.

Consumer narrative   Margaret's story

About seven months after my husband died I was out having lunch with my daughter. I came over all queer and demanded she take me home. I insisted she go home as I just needed to rest, I didn't want her there. I got out our photo albums and starting rummaging through it, taking out all the photos of my husband from different stages in our lives. You see, I had sat there with my daughter and I'd forgotten what he looked like. I just couldn't bring his face to mind and this terrified me. For 65 years he was my whole life, and suddenly I couldn't recall his face; I thought I'd really lost him then. I pasted his photos over everything: the cupboards, chairs, the toilet, everywhere I looked, so I wouldn't forget him. I started talking to him as if he was still around. I stopped going out. I just wanted to be with him and my memories. My kids thought I'd gone crazy. They came and took his photos down. I was furious and screamed at them to get out and never come into my house again. I had never in all their lives raised my voice to them; it must have been quite a shock when 'Mum blew her top'. Now, they really thought I was going mad. They sent someone round to see me from the mental health services. I thought they were trying to put me in a home or the looney bin and forget about me, like they were trying to forget about their father. The nurse was very patient and kind, though, and finally I agreed to talk to her. She was a lovely woman, very easy to talk to. She said she didn't think I was crazy, which was a relief; she thought I was lonely and sad, and grieving for my husband. She was absolutely right, and she got it. She helped me to cope with my loss and the enormity of it; she helped me link up with other widows and people with similar interests. She talked to my family and explained what was really going on for me. Everything is going well now. I have his photo by my bed and on the telly. His is the first face I see each morning and the last I see at night, just like it always was. I still talk to him about what's going on, but the nurse assured me that I am perfectly normal. So I sit at night and tell him all about my day and what's happening on *Coronation Street* and I feel content. You know, he's a much better listener since he died!

Reflective activities

- Write down a summary of the important aspects of Margaret's story that needs to be included in her clinical notes.
- Name three important elements of the communication style of the nurse in her interaction with Margaret.

Cognitive decline, depression, delirium or dementia? Getting the diagnosis right

It is particularly difficult for health professionals to recognise, identify and diagnose cognitive changes effectively in older people. For example, the *Diagnostic and Statistical Manual of Mental Disorders* (DSM-5, American Psychiatric Association, 2013) provides criteria in a new category to determine the appropriate diagnoses of mild and major neurocognitive disorders. In this chapter, we focus on how nurses can develop a clear understanding of the different presentations, or the 4Ds (Insel & Badger, 2002). Insel and Badger (2002) posited that cognitive decline is part of the ageing process. These changes are gradual; however, if the nurse notices a rapid decline, then the following diagnoses must be considered.

> **cognitive decline**
> changes in one's thinking and remembering, and difficulty in retaining new information or juggling multiple mental tasks

Depression

Unlike in other adults, depression in older people is often enduring in nature and associated with increased physical disability, cognitive impairment and mortality (Hybels et al., 2009). Depression is the most common mental illness, affecting 15–20 per cent of older people, with severe depression occurring in 3 per cent of older people (Oakley Browne et al., 2006). The similarity of symptoms between unresolved grief associated with multiple losses; for example, the loss of one's status, employment and/or home, and depression must also be considered and assessed. Pharmacological treatment of depression in older people places them at greater risk of injury as a result of adverse effects, such as postural hypotension, which can lead to falls and fractures (Peron, Gray & Hanlon, 2011). Psychological interventions for depression in either an individual or group format is often challenging because of age-related disabilities, in particular hearing loss and cognitive impairment. As discussed previously, nurses must work at a slower pace and be prepared to repeat conversations in all interactions with older people (Lenze & Loebach Wetherell, 2011).

Delirium

Insel and Badger (2002) reported that delirium, or acute confusion and behavioural change, is evident in 10 to 40 per cent of people over 65 years of age admitted to hospital. Of those admissions, 25 to 60 per cent of people are likely to develop delirium after discharge and, if left untreated, delirium effectively contributes to a mortality rate as high as 65 per cent of admissions. Of concern, Insel and Badger reported that even though the nursing notes contained information to diagnose delirium, only 5 per cent had an accurate diagnosis on discharge. Ryan and colleagues (2013) noted that nurses are more likely to detect delirium as they have more prolonged contact with older persons. The long-term consequences of less-than-optimal management of delirium result in falls, subsequent immobility and earlier admission to residential care (Fox et al., 2012). It is recommended that all nurses be alert to the complexity of such presentations and incorporate accurate diagnosis and treatment by using standardised assessment tools (Inouye et al., 1990; Insel & Badger, 2002; Milisen et al., 2006; National Institute for Health and Clinical Excellence, 2010; Neelon et al., 1996).

Consumer narrative   Helen's story

As an advanced practice nurse working in the liaison psychiatry team within a general hospital, I received a referral from a registered nurse on a medical ward, requesting an assessment of Tom, a 75-year-old man with diabetes. Tom was assessed as being psychotic and deluded, and had refused to leave his bed for the previous 24 hours. When I entered Tom's room he immediately shouted at me to 'Get down, they will shoot you!' I crouched down close to Tom's bed and at eye level with him. Maintaining a calm voice and gently probing Tom's reasons for his fear of harm to anyone who enters his room, I established that Tom was a war veteran who believed that he was back in the trenches and being shot at by snipers. The sudden onset of these beliefs, coupled with evidence of urinary incontinence and no prior history of mental illness, led me to conclude that Tom was delirious. I subsequently read the clinical notes to identify the tell-tale signs and symptoms of delirium, such as spiking temperatures above 38°C, frequency and discomfort on micturition, fluctuating blood sugar levels, inadequate hydration noted on the fluid balance chart and reversal of his sleep-wake cycle. I immediately explained to Tom the cause of his fear and confusion, and contacted and explained this to his family, who had been very distressed about his out-of-character behaviour. I wrote a medical and nursing delirium treatment plan in his clinical notes and briefed the nursing team at their handover. Once the delirium plan was in place Tom's confusion abated and he was able to start his activities of daily living again, and was soon discharged home.

Dementia

The numbers of people in New Zealand and Australia presenting with dementia are growing significantly due to the ageing of the baby-boomer population. Age is the most significant risk factor for the development of dementia. Of the people over 65 years of age, 5 per cent will develop dementia, while 20 per cent of people aged 80 years or older will develop dementia (Alzheimer's Disease International, 2011). However Bradford and colleagues (2009) have reported that at least two-thirds of this population attending primary and secondary health care providers will never receive the diagnosis of dementia and therefore are ineligible for support services and pharmaceutical interventions such as cognitive enhancers used to delay its progression. There are well-documented reasons for the sector's failure to diagnose dementia, including limited general practitioner time, lack of confidence in making the diagnosis, unwillingness to make the diagnosis because of a perception that no treatment is available and concern that providing the diagnosis will have an adverse effect on the person with dementia and his or her family (Ahmad et al., 2010). There is clear evidence that the diagnosis and long-term management of dementia may be a role for advanced practice nurses (Boustani, Schubert & Sennour, 2007).

Consumer narrative   Barbara's story

Barbara was a 77-year-old, gifted woman with a variety of interests and a busy social life. She owned her own home and was incredibly house-proud. She was about to be discharged from mental health services, having been involved with the services for a number of years.

Barbara had a history of childhood sexual abuse. She married an affluent but very violent man who regularly assaulted her, leading to many admissions to the emergency department. After the birth of her third child, Barbara experienced a psychotic episode and was admitted to a psychiatric institution. Subsequently, her husband left her for another woman and she lost custody of her children and was denied visitation rights.

Since that time, Barbara has been able to regain control of her life and to see her children again. Barbara developed a closer relationship with her youngest son, and was very careful not to burden him with discussion of the past. After a recent admission Barbara had an assessment at the memory clinic, as she had noticed a few memory lapses. More tests followed, and Barbara was told that she had Alzheimer's dementia. The health professional told her that she probably had about six months before she would be significantly impaired, and advised her to immediately sell her home, give up her volunteer work and arrange to live with her son. Barbara went home in a state of shock; she locked herself in her home and wept. She wouldn't answer the door or the phone. She stopped seeing her friends, gave up her volunteer job and stopped eating. Everything that had brought her any pleasure had now ceased. She spoke to her son, and

continued ›

Consumer narrative continued ›

while sympathetic, he was concerned about the burden of caring for her as he was just beginning a new marriage with young children.

Barbara then appeared to emerge from the state of shock; she put her house on the market, tidied everything up, packed her precious belongings away and made arrangements to go and visit her son. While a little thin, she seemed reasonably happy and content. Barbara died of heart failure six months after being given her diagnosis. Barbara had never had any heart problems prior to her diagnosis of Alzheimer's.

Reflective questions

- How would you explain the diagnosis of Alzheimer's dementia to Barbara and her family?
- Do you think there is a connection between Barbara's heart failure and the diagnosis of Alzheimer's dementia? Discuss.

Mental illness and intellectual disability

There is increasing evidence to suggest that intellectual disability is associated with a greater prevalence of mental illness (Lee et al., 2011). Dementia occurs in people with Down syndrome at a much higher rate than in the general population and at a much younger age, with the incidence estimated at 50 per cent in those over 50 years and 75 per cent for those 65 years and over (Lott et al., 2012). Diagnosis and management of dementia or other mental illness in people with intellectual disability is a complex process. Cardiovascular and respiratory conditions, and grief associated with residential relocation, often as a result of the death of older parent caregivers (Esbensen, Seltzer & Greenberg, 2007), also add to the complexity of the care. Because nurses have long-term relationships with people with intellectual disability they are often in the best position to notice subtle changes in the person's usual cognitive functioning (Stanton & Coetzee, 2004). Clearly, this is another opportunity for specialist input by advanced practice nurses.

Older people and suicide

Having depression is the most common cause of suicidal ideation in older people, with older men at higher risk than older women of completing suicide (Dwived, 2012). In Australia, suicide rates reach a second peak after the 25–44-year age groups, in men aged over 85 years. The highest age-specific death rate for Australian males in 2009 was observed in the age group of over 85 years and over (Department of Health and Ageing, 2010). When compared to other population groups, suicide in older people is often characterised by fewer warning or explicit cues, less history of previous attempts, physical illness and functional impairment (Deuter, Procter & Rogers, 2013). Recent New Zealand statistics for suicide (Ministry of Health, 2012) have indicated that people over 65 years of age have a suicide rate of 9.7 per 100 000 population. Males in all age groups have a higher suicide rate than females; however, the highest rate for males was seen in adults aged 85 years and older. Given the small numbers in this segment of the population, this figure should be treated with caution, as it represents only 0.2 per cent of all male deaths in that age group. However, suicide attempts by older people are more lethal because they tend to be physically frail, live alone and choose more lethal and planned modes of completing suicide (Beautrais et al., 2005). Beautrais and colleagues (2005) have further argued that only half of older people surveyed made a visit to a primary care physician for mental illness. Usually, older people attend with physical health concerns (Oakley Browne et al., 2006), and somatic illnesses appear to be the most important stressors in elderly suicides. This further supports the future role of the mental health nurse within primary care settings to support primary care professionals by undertaking opportunistic screening, referral and appropriate treatment for depression and suicidal ideation in older people (O'Connell et al., 2004).

An ethical framework to underpin practice

Hughes and colleagues (2002) reported that nurses working with older people lacked confidence in the ethical aspects of their practice; specifically, autonomy, consent, advance directives, truth-telling, research and end-of-life issues, including euthanasia and physician-assisted suicide. Brannelly (2006) suggested that nurses could integrate ethical aspects of their care within an **ethic of care** framework (Gilligan, 1982; Sevenhuijsen, 1998; Tronto, 1993, 1999). Further, Brannelly (2006) posited that this framework would assist nurses to provide care that fitted with the values and preferences of older people, particularly those with dementia and their carers.

> **ethic of care**
> a framework concerned with the principles of ethics; not only avoiding wrong-doing, but also reflection on and action towards affecting the conditions that make a good life possible

Brannelly (2006) briefly described the four elements of the ethic of care framework: *caring about* – seeing and recognising care needs, by paying attention to the person and developing strategies of action that are individually and culturally shaped; *taking care of* – taking responsibility for initiating caring activities that involve personal agency and responsibility; *care giving* – paying attention to the person's specific care needs, her or his routines as well as caring for others in the person's wider world so that she or he can live in that world as easily as possible; *care receiving* – the recipients of care will respond to the care given, or at times decline the type of care that is offered. This requires the nurse to pay attention and assess that these needs have been met, thus ensuring the quality of the care process.

In sum, Brannelly (2006) highlighted the notion of attentiveness by nurses as an empowering process that reaffirms personal agency and protects the older person's citizenship rights. The adoption of an ethic of care framework by nurses to underpin their practice will strengthen the opportunity for increased autonomy, participation and inclusion of older citizens.

The future of older people's mental health nursing

Given the increasing age of the population in Australia and New Zealand, a number of new areas of concern have developed within the arena of mental health services for older people, such as services for ageing offenders in prisons, support for families and carers and the recruitment and retention of nurses within this specialist field of mental health nursing.

Offenders and dementia

The most significant group to have an effect on both the aged residential care sector and the justice system are older offenders within the criminal justice system (Baidawi et al., 2011; Kingston et al., 2011). The 1970s saw changes to sentencing practices that resulted in offenders being sentenced for longer periods. There has also been an increase in the numbers of adult survivors of sexual abuse who have laid charges against their now-elderly, and predominantly male, caregivers resulting in an increasing number of older prisoners ageing and dying in prisons (Christodoulou, 2012).

Further, most offenders have a history of alcohol abuse, poor nutrition, often traumatic brain injury and the existence of a mental illness (Fazel et al., 2001; Fazel, McMillan & O'Donnell, 2002). Given the punitive prison environment, offenders' history of poor adherence or engagement with medical care results in this vulnerable population ageing 10 to 15 years sooner than the general population. Since age is the greatest risk factor for dementia, increasingly the numbers of offenders with dementia in prison are growing significantly (Maschi et al., 2012). Offenders often present with complex issues associated with dementia, such as coping with an enduring or terminal illness, fear of dying and pain management. Further risks to this vulnerable population are the cost of physical care, victimisation from other offenders and a prison environment and regime that is unsuited for the care of people with dementia. In a move to better serve this population, Rimutaka prison in New Zealand (APNZ, 2012) has opened a high-dependency unit for offenders who have dementia-related problems, so that they can end their detention in a dignified manner. In summary, this hidden population of older people with dementia challenges nurses working in the specialty of older people and forensic settings to consider the ethical implications of offenders' continuing detention. Less-than-adequate access to specialist nursing care and treatment will have major implications for offenders' basic rights.

The family and carers of older people

The in-home, 24-hour care of loved ones who have cognitive impairment and comorbid mental illness falls mainly to spouses and family members. Observing the decline of a loved one, described as a 'social death' (Sweeting & Gilhooly, 1997, p. 94), and loss of their personhood, begins the journey of grief for the carer. The carer will experience a range of emotions, such as confusion, anger and sadness at a time when her or his stamina, problem-solving abilities and resilience are being tested. It is important therefore that nurses maintain the human connectedness with carers to support and offer appropriate interventions that assist carers to maintain their own physical and mental health. Below are some recommendations for nurses to consider:

- Establish a good relationship with carers, such that they feel able to contact you when they have concerns of any kind (Marriot et al., 2000).
- Full-time caregiving can create emotional distress and fatigue (Turner & Findlay, 2012). Encourage caregivers to have a regular break from caregiving by, for example, exploring the use of day programs for their loved one or arranging respite care, either in-home or in a residential care facility (Alzheimer's New Zealand, 2012).
- Carers develop depression at higher rates than others in the general community (Livingston, Manela & Katona, 1996). The nurse can complete a carer's assessment when assessing the older person, and can continue to monitor the carer to ensure that her or his mood remains stable (Waite et al., 2004).
- The lack of coordinated services, both in the public and private sectors, has been an issue for carers. A designated key worker or a health navigator for an individual or family unit is highly desirable to assist in facilitating appropriate care (Hubert & Hollins, 2000).
- Facilitating or providing access to education and skills for carers is also recommended (Hayman, 2005).
- Facilitating access to home support enables carers to have regular breaks (Mast, 2013).
- A single point of entry with common eligibility, assessment and management processes ensures that resources are allocated appropriately and caregivers are not preoccupied with engaging services to seek their entitlements (Kietzman, Scharlach & Dal Santo, 2004).

The future nursing workforce

As far back as the 1980s, Butterworth (1988) argued that, traditionally, nurses working within mental health services for older people have been perceived as lacking the acumen to work within adult or youth mental health settings, or are there as a 'punishment' (p. 213). On the contrary, nurses in this specialist area are required to have a broad range of skills and knowledge to address the complexity associated with caring for the ageing. Retaining and recruiting specialist mental health nurses for this specialty in both Australia and New Zealand has been identified as a key area of government concern (Hamer et al., 2006; NSW Department of Health, 2006). However, negative attitudes within the nursing profession will have major implications for the recruitment and retention of nurses, given that the nursing workforce itself is also ageing. Working within older people's mental health care is a rewarding career option. The development of the advanced practice role for nurses, such as nurse practitioner status, continues to increase the job satisfaction for nurses and provides a clinical career pathway. Nurse practitioners can enhance the care of the older person, such as decreasing waiting times for assessments, poly pharmacy and improved mental and physical health as a result of early intervention and capacity to provide complex nursing interventions in the community (Langer, 2012).

Interprofessional connections — Sue's story

As a community mental health nurse, I am the care partner of Olivia, a 65-year-old Māori woman with a long history of bipolar affective disorder (BPAD). Olivia is about to be discharged from the acute in-patient unit for older people. She had been admitted once before with her first episode, over 30 years ago, and since that admission had managed her illness really well in the community with the support of her partner and her children. However, Olivia's partner had died six months prior to her recent admission, and all her children now live in Australia. In the past four weeks, Olivia has felt increasingly sad and alone, and quickly became unwell. She was unable to eat, stopped sleeping and stopped taking her medication regularly. Once in hospital, with 24-hour care Olivia stabilised quickly, once she began taking her regular medication and with support from staff. She began eating and exercising regularly and regained social contact with her extended *whānau* (family), who came from out of town to support her.

I reviewed Olivia's care at my multidisciplinary team meeting and advised the team of my plans for Olivia's discharge back into her community. First, by collaborating with the social worker Olivia will receive meals-on-wheels five days a week to support her nutritional requirements. I have arranged input from the community home help service to provide a support person to visit Olivia twice a week; this person will take her to the supermarket, undertake the heavier housework and provide some regular social contact and monitoring of Olivia's well-being. After gaining Olivia's consent, I have also arranged for a cultural support worker from Māori services to visit Olivia twice weekly. The cultural worker has invited Olivia to join the *kāumātua* (venerated older man) and *whāea* (venerated older woman) weekly support group so that Olivia could meet and converse in *te reo*, the language of Māori, with her peers. This support is vital for Olivia to nurture her spiritual needs and assist in grieving for her partner.

I have also rung her local pharmacy and arranged for Olivia's medication to be dispensed in a blister-pack, to support Olivia's regular medication regimen. Given that Olivia now lives alone, I have contacted the St John's Ambulance service and arranged for Olivia to have a monitored alarm bracelet so that she can feel safe in knowing that she can summon help in the event of a fall or an intruder in her home. Overall, reconnecting Olivia to the variety of support structures is paramount so that she can use her own resources and resilience to continue living as independently as possible within her community.

Chapter summary

This chapter has presented stories and information, supplemented by activities designed to deepen understanding of:

- contemporary issues in nursing care and approaches to the care of older people who experience the complexity of mental and physical illness;
- sociopolitical aspects of ageing and the prevailing cultural norms of older people;
- the multiple losses associated with older age that affect the mental health of older people and their carers;
- the role of the nurse in assessing the care requirements of older people, including the medico-legal and ethical aspects of care; and
- the future of the specialty practice of nursing the older person with mental illness.

Critical thinking/learning activities

1   What are some of the important priorities that you would need to consider in your plan of nursing care for a person experiencing cognitive decline?
2   What should be at the forefront of a nurse's mind when considering admitting an older person into an acute mental health unit?
3   An older person in your care tells you that he or she is worried about going home on weekend leave as the person feels frightened when his or her partner, who often is inebriated in the evenings, gets 'aggro' and starts yelling and shouting at him or her. On one occasion the partner has pushed the older person to the ground, resulting in a broken rib. You are concerned for the person's safety; what is your next step?
4   Unresolved grief is often not detected or may manifest as a depressive illness. It can have a profound effect on the older person. What are the contributing factors to unresolved grief?
5   The notion of recovery has been regarded as not having a place in the care of the older person with dementia. Hope is one of the guiding principles of recovery. How would you instil hope for an older person who is dementing and her or his carers?

Learning extension

In pairs, discuss and write a short paragraph on the following:

- Is an offender entitled to receive nursing care within a dementia unit located in a community health setting?
- What are some of the risk factors to both the offender and residents if the offender is to be nursed in the dementia unit?
- As the community mental health nurse for the offender, how might you assist and coach the registered nurses at this residential setting to plan effective care for the older offender?

Further reading

Fazel, S., Hope, T., O'Donnell, I. & Jacoby, R. (2001). Hidden psychiatric morbidity in elderly prisoners. *British Journal of Psychiatry*, *179*(6): 535–9.

Kingston, P., Le Mesurier, N., Yorston, G., Wardle, S. & Heath, L. (2011). Psychiatric morbidity in older prisoners: Unrecognized and undertreated. *International Psychogeriatrics*, *23*(8): 1354–60.

Maschi, T., Kwak, J., Ko, E. & Morrissey, M.B. (2012). Forget me not: Dementia in prison. *Gerontologist*, *52*(4): 441–51.

References

Adams, T. & Collier, E. (2009). Services for older people with mental health conditions. In P. Barker (ed.), *Psychiatric and Mental Health Nursing: The craft of caring*, 2nd edn. (pp. 486–92). London: Hodder Arnold.

Ahmad, S., Orrell, M., Iliffe, S. & Gracie, A. (2010). GPs' attitudes, awareness, and practice regarding early diagnosis of dementia. *British Journal of General Practice*, 60(578): 360–5.

Alzheimer's Disease International (2011). *World Alzheimer's Report 2011: The benefits of early diagnosis and intervention. Executive Summary*. Retrieved from www.alz.co.uk/research/WorldAlzheimerReport2011 ExecutiveSummary.pdf.

Alzheimer's New Zealand (2012). *How to Manage When Caring for Somebody with Dementia*. Retrieved from www.everybody.co.nz/page-fd486f24-f08b-40bb-91fa-7c1a11eab0e7.aspx.

American Psychiatric Association (2013). *Diagnostic and Statistical Manual of Mental Disorders: DSM-V*, 5th edn. Washington, DC: Author.

Anderberg, P., Lepp, M., Berglund, A.-L. & Segesten, K. (2007). Preserving dignity in caring for older adults: A concept analysis. *Journal of Advanced Nursing*, 59(6): 635–43.

Angermeyer, M.C., Schulze, B. & Dietrich, S. (2003). Courtesy stigma: A focus group study of relatives of schizophrenia patients. *Social Psychiatry and Psychiatric Epidemiology*, 38(10): 593–602.

APNZ (2012). Rimutaka prison to open first dementia unit. *New Zealand Herald*, 3 July. Retrieved from www.nzherald.co.nz/nz/news/article.cfm?c_id=1&objectid=10817081.

Australian Bureau of Statistics (2012). *Who Are Australia's Older People? Reflecting a nation: Stories from the 2011 census, 2012–2013*. Retrieved from www.abs.gov.au/ausstats/abs@.nsf/Lookup/2071.0main+features752012–2013.

Averill, P.M. & Beck, J.G. (2000). Posttraumatic stress disorder in older adults: A conceptual review. *Journal of Anxiety Disorders*, *14*(2): 133–56.

Baidawi, S., Turner, S., Trotter, C., Browning, C., Collier, P., O'Connor, D. & Sheehan, R. (2011). Older prisoners: A challenge for Australian corrections. *Trends and Issues in Crime and Criminal Justice No. 426*. Canberra: Australian Institute of Criminology. Retrieved from www.aic.gov.au/publications/current%20series/tandi.html.

Beautrais, A.L., Collings, S.C., Ehrhardt, P. & Henare, K. (2005). *Suicide Prevention: A review of evidence of risk and protective factors, and points of effective intervention*. Retrieved from www.health.govt.nz/publication/suicide-prevention-review-evidence-risk-and-protective-factors-and-points-effective-intervention.

Bellamy, G., Boyd, M., Neville, S., Neil, H., George, N., Meneses, V. & Karon, S. (2012). *Breaching the Chasm. Caring for ageing sexual minorities in residential aged care facilities: An exploratory study to inform practice*. Auckland: University of Auckland.

Benner, P.E., Tanner, C.A. & Chesla, C.A. (2009). *Expertise in Nursing Practice: Caring, clinical judgment and ethics*, 2nd edn. New York: Springer.

Bodley-Tickell, A.T., Olowokure, B., Bhaduri, S., White, D.J., Ward, D., Ross, J.D.C. & Goold, P. (2008). Trends in sexually transmitted infections (other than HIV) in older people: Analysis of data from an enhanced surveillance system. *Sexually Transmitted Infections*, *84*: 312–17.

Boustani, M., Schubert, C. & Sennour, Y. (2007). The challenge of supporting care for dementia in primary care. *Clinical Interventions in Aging*, 2(4): 631–6.

Bowling, A. & Stafford, M. (2007). How do objective and subjective assessments of neighbourhood influence social and physical functioning in older age? Findings from a British survey of ageing. *Social Science & Medicine*, 64(12): 2533–49.

Bradford, A., Kunik, M.E., Schulz, P., Williams, S.P. & Singh, H. (2009). Missed and delayed diagnosis of dementia in primary care: Prevalence and contributing factors. *Alzheimer Disease and Associated Disorders*, 23(4), 306–14.

Brannelly, T. (2006). Negotiating ethics in dementia care: An analysis of an ethic of care in practice. *Dementia*, 5(2): 197–212.

Buchanan, A. (2004). Mental capacity, legal competence and consent to treatment. *Journal of the Royal Society of Medicine*, 97(9): 415–20.

Butterworth, P., Gill, S.C., Rodgers, B., Anstey, K.J., Villamil, E. & Melzer, D. (2006). Retirement and mental health: Analysis of the Australian national survey of mental health and well-being. *Social Science & Medicine*, 62(5): 1179–91.

Butterworth, T. (1988). Breaking the boundaries: Community nursing. *Nursing Times*, 84(47): 36–9.

Chariand, L.C. (2001). Mental competence and value: The problem of normativity in the assessment of decision-making capacity. *Psychiatry, Psychology and Law*, 8(2): 135–45.

Christodoulou, M. (2012). Locked up and at risk of dementia. *Lancet Neurology*, 11(9): 750–1.

Cohen, G.D. (2001). The course of unfulfilled dreams and unfinished business with aging. *American Journal of Geriatric Psychiatry*, 9(1): 1–5.

Cohen, G. (2009). New theories and research findings on the positive influence of music and art on health with ageing. *Arts & Health*, 1(1): 48–62.

Community Law Centre (2013). *Orders Under the 3PR Act*. Retrieved from www.communitylaw.org.nz.

Council of Australian Governments (n.d.). *The Roadmap for National Mental Health Reform*: 2012–2022. Retrieved from www.coag.gov.au/sites/default/files/The%20Roadmap%20for%20National %20Mental%20Health%20Reform%202012–2022.pdf.pdf.

Crowe, M. & Carlyle, D. (2003). Deconstructing risk assessment and management in mental health nursing. *Journal of Advanced Nursing*, 43(1): 19–27.

Davies, S. (1995). Organization for Economic Co-operation and Development. Caring for frail elderly people: New directions in care. *Ageing & Society*, 15(2): 289–90.

Deegan, P.E. (2005). *Recovery as a Journey of the Heart*. Boston, MA: Center for Psychiatric Rehabilitation, Boston University.

Department of Health and Ageing (2010). *Commonwealth Response to The Hidden Toll: Suicide in Australia*. Report of the Senate Community Affairs Reference Committee. Canberra: Australian Government. Retrieved from www.health.gov.au/internet/main/publishing.nsf/Content/BB344E6E9F422A7FCA2577E5 0034118F/$File/toll3.pdf.

Deuter, K., Procter, N.G. & Rogers, J. (2013). The emergency telephone conversation in the context of the older person in suicidal crisis: Qualitative study. *Journal of Crisis Intervention and Suicide Prevention*, 34(4): 262–72.

Diesfeld, K. & Sjöström, S. (2007). Interpretive flexibility: Why doesn't insight incite controversy in mental health law? *Behavioral Sciences and the Law*, 25(1): 85–101.

Dwived, Y. (2012). *The Neurological Basis of Suicide*. Boca Raton, FL: CRC Press.

Esbensen, A.J., Seltzer, M.M. & Greenberg, J.S. (2007). Factors predicting mortality in midlife adults with and without Down syndrome living with family. *Journal of Intellectual Disability Research*, 51(12): 1039–50.

Fazel, S., Hope, T., O'Donnell, I. & Jacoby, R. (2001). Hidden psychiatric morbidity in elderly prisoners. *British Journal of Psychiatry*, 179(6): 535–9.

Fazel, S., McMillan, J. & O'Donnell, I. (2002). Dementia in prison: Ethical and legal implications. *Journal of Medical Ethics*, 28(3): 156–9.

Fox, A.W. (2012). Elder abuse. *Medical Science and Law*, 52, 128–36.

Fox, M.T., Persaud, M., Maimets, I., O'Brien, K., Brooks, D., Tregunno, D. & Schraa, E. (2012). Effectiveness of acute geriatric unit care using acute care for elders components: A systematic review and meta-analysis. *Journal of the American Geriatrics Society*, 60(12): 2237–45.

Ganzini, L., Volicer, L., Nelson, W.A., Fox, E. & Derse, A.R. (2005). Ten myths about decision-making capacity. *Journal of the American Medical Directors Association*, 6(3): S100–4.

Gillies, A. (2013). Karen Walker turns heads with ageless. *New Zealand Herald*, 9 February. Retrieved from www.nzherald.co.nz/lifestyle/news/article.cfm?c_id=6&objectid=10864307.

Gilligan, C. (1982). *In a Different Voice: Psychological theory and women's development*. Cambridge, MA: Harvard University Press.

Graham, N., Lindesay, J., Katona, C., Bertolote, J. M., Camus, V., Copeland, J. R. M. & Wancata, J. (2003). Reducing stigma and discrimination against older people with mental disorders: A technical consensus statement. *International Journal of Geriatric Psychiatry*, *18*(8): 670–8.

Hamer, H. P. (2012). Inside the City Walls: Mental health service users' journeys towards full citizenship. Unpublished PhD. University of Auckland.

Hamer, H. P., Finlayson, M., Thom, K., Hughes, F. & Tomkins, S. (2006). *Mental Health Nursing and its Future: A discussion framework*. Retrieved from www.health.govt.nz/publication/mental-health-nursing-and-its-future-discussion-framework.

Hayman, F. (2005). Helping carers care: An education programme for rural carers of people with a mental illness. *Australasian Psychiatry*, *13*(2): 148–53.

Hazelton, M. (1997). Reporting mental health: A discourse analysis of mental health-related news in two Australian newspapers. *Australian and New Zealand Journal of Mental Health Nursing*, *6*(2): 73–89.

Hazelton, M. (1999). Psychiatric personnel, risk management and the new institutionalism. *Nursing Inquiry*, *6*(4): 224–30.

Health and Disability Commission (n.d.). *Advance Directives in Mental Health Care and Treatment*. Retrieved from www.hdc.org.nz/publications/resources-to-order/leaflets-and-posters-for-download/advance-directives-in-mental-health-care-and-treatment-(leaflet).

Health and Disability Commission (1996). *Code of Health and Disability Services Consumers' Rights Regulation 1996*. Retrieved from www.legislation.govt.nz/regulation/public/1996/0078/latest/DLM209080.html.

Hiskey, S., Luckie, M., Davies, S. & Brewin, C. R. (2008). The phenomenology of reactivated trauma memories in older adults: A preliminary study. *Aging & Mental Health*, *12*(4): 494–8.

Howorth, P. & Saper, J. (2003). The dimensions of insight in people with dementia. *Aging & Mental Health*, *7*(2): 113–22.

Hubert, J. & Hollins, S. (2000). Working with elderly carers of people with learning disabilities and planning for the future. *Advances in Psychiatric Treatment*, *6*(1): 41–8.

Hughes, J. C., Hope, T., Savulescu, J. & Ziebland, S. (2002). Carers, ethics and dementia: A survey of the review of the literature. *International Journal of Geriatric Psychiatry*, *17*(1): 35–40.

Hybels, C. F., Blazer, D. G., Pieper, C. F., Landerman, L. R. & Steffens, D. C. (2009). Profiles of depressive symptoms in older adults diagnosed with major depression: Latent cluster analysis. *American Journal of Geriatric Psychiatry*, *17*(5): 387–96.

Inouye, S. K., Van Dyck, C. H., Alessi, C. A., Balkin, S., Siegal, A. P. & Horwitz, R. I. (1990). Clarifying confusion: The Confusion Assessment Method. A new method for detecting delirium. *Annals of Internal Medicine*, *113*(12): 941–8.

Insel, K. C. & Badger, T. A. (2002). Deciphering the 4Ds: Cognitive decline, delirium, depression and dementia – A review. *Journal of Advanced Nursing*, *38*(4): 360–8.

Jones, E. D. & Beck-Little, R. (2002). The use of reminiscence therapy for the treatment of depression in rural-dwelling older adults. *Issues in Mental Health Nursing*, *23*(3): 279–90.

Kietzman, K. G., Scharlach, A. E. & Dal Santo, T. S. (2004). Local needs assessment and planning efforts for family caregivers. *Journal of Gerontological Social Work*, *42*(3–4): 39–60.

Kingston, P., Le Mesurier, N., Yorston, G., Wardle, S. & Heath, L. (2011). Psychiatric morbidity in older prisoners: Unrecognized and undertreated. *International Psychogeriatrics*, *23*(8): 1354–60.

Krawitz, R., Jackson, W., Allen, R., Connell, A., Argyle, N., Bensemann, C. & Mileshkin, C. (2004). Professionally indicated short-term risk-taking in the treatment of borderline personality disorder. *Australasian Psychiatry*, *12*(1): 11–17.

Lai, J. M. & Karlawish, J. (2007). Assessing the capacity to make everyday decisions: A guide for clinicians and an agenda for future research. *American Journal of Geriatric Psychiatry*, *15*(2): 101–11.

Lampshire, D. & Hamer, H. P. (2012). The Recovery Approach in Mental Health Nursing: A one day workshop. Auckland: University of Auckland.

Lampshire, D. & Latham, L. (2000). *Combining Evidence, Recovery Principles, and Consumer and Provider Perspectives to Create a Strategic Plan for Older Adults with Mental Health Problems*. Auckland: District Health Board

Langer, L. (2012). *NP Older People's Mental Health, Southern DHB*. Retrieved from www.healthworkforce. govt.nz/tools-and-resources/for-employers-educators/nurse-practitioners-working-with-you-for-good-health/n-0.

Lee, L., Rianto, J., Raykar, V., Creasey, H., Waite, L., Berry, A. & Naganathan, V. (2011). Health and functional status of adults with intellectual disability referred to the specialist health care setting: A five-year experience. *International Journal of Family Medicine*, 1–9. Online doi: 10.1155/2011/312492.

Lenze, E. J. & Loebach Wetherell, J. (2011). State of the art: A lifespan view of anxiety disorders. *Dialogues in Clinical Neuroscience, 13*(4): 381–99.

Livingston, G., Manela, M. & Katona, C. (1996). Depression and other psychiatric morbidity in carers of elderly people living at home. *British Medical Journal, 312*(7024): 153–6.

Lord, J. (2011). Ageism is a Human Rights Issue: Equality reform law project. Retrieved from www. humanrightsactionplan.org.au/nhrap-blogs/ageism-is-a-human-rights-issue.

Lott, I. T., Doran, E., Nguyen, V. Q., Tournay, A., Movsesyan, N. & Gillen, D. L. (2012). Down syndrome and dementia: Seizures and cognitive decline. *Journal of Alzheimers Disease, 29*(1): 177–85.

Marriot, M., Donaldson, C., Tanner, N. & Burns, A. (2000). Effectiveness of cognitive-behavioural family intervention in reducing the burden of care in carers of patients with Alzheimer's disease. *British Journal of Psychiatry, 176*: 557–62.

Maschi, T., Kwak, J., Ko, E. & Morrissey, M. B. (2012). Forget me not: Dementia in prison. *Gerontologist, 52*(4): 441–51.

Mast, M. E. (2013). To use or not to use. A literature review of factors that influence family caregivers' use of support services. *Journal of Gerontological Nursing, 39*(1): 20–8.

McBride, M. (2011). *Ethnogeriatrics and Cultural Competence for Nursing Practice*. Retrieved from http://consultgerirn.org/topics/ethnogeriatrics_and_cultural_competence_for_nursing_practice/want_to_know_more.

McKee, K. J., Wilson, F., Chung, M. C., Hinchliff, S., Goudie, F., Elford, H. & Mitchell, C. (2005). Reminiscence, regrets and activity in older people in residential care: Associations with psychological health. *British Journal of Clinical Psychology, 44*(4): 543–61.

Mental Health Commission (2001). *Recovery Competencies for Mental Health Workers in New Zealand*. Retrieved from www.hdc.org.nz/publications/other-publications-from-hdc/mental-health-resources/recovery-competencies-for-new-zealand-mental-health-workers.

Mental Health Commission (2012). *Blueprint II: Improving mental health and wellbeing for all New Zealanders: How things need to be*. Retrieved from www.hdc.org.nz/media/207642/blueprint%20ii%20how%20things%20need%20to%20be.pdf.

Milisen, K., Braes, T., Fick, D. M. & Foreman, M. D. (2006). Cognitive assessment and differentiating the 3Ds (dementia, depression, delirium). *Nursing Clinics of North America, 41*(1): 1–22.

Ministry of Health (2012). *Suicide Facts: Deaths and intentional self-harm hospitalisations 2010*. Retrieved from www.health.govt.nz/publication/suicide-facts-deaths-and-intentional-self-harm-hospitalisations-2010.

Monahan, J., Lidz, C. W., Hoge, S. K., Mulvey, E. P., Eisenberg, M. M., Roth, L. H & Bennett, N. (1999). Coercion in the provision of mental health services: The MacArthur studies. In J. P. Morrissey & J. Monahan (eds), *Research in Community Mental Health. Coercion in mental health services. International perspectives*, vol. 10 (pp. 13–30). Stamford, CT: JAI Press.

National Institute for Health and Clinical Excellence (2010). *Delirium: Diagnosis, prevention and management*. Retrieved from www.nice.org.uk/nicemedia/live/13060/49909/49909.pdf.

Neelon, V. J., Champagne, M. T., Carlson, J. R. & Funk, S. G. (1996). The NEECHAM Confusion Scale: Construction, validation, and clinical testing. *Nursing Research, 45*(6): 324–30.

Nelson, T. D., (ed.) (2002). *Ageism: Stereotyping and prejudice against older persons*. Cambridge, MA: MIT Press.

NSW Department of Health (2006). *Specialist Mental Health Services for Older People (SMHSOP) – NSW Service Plan 2005–2015*. North Sydney: Author. Retrieved from www0.health.nsw.gov.au/policies/gl/2006/pdf/GL2006_013.pdf.

Nursing Council of New Zealand (2012). *Code of Conduct for Nurses*. Retrieved from http://nursingcouncil.org.nz/Nurses/Code-of-Conduct.

Oakley Browne, M. A., Wells, J., Scott, K. M. & McGee, M. A. (2006). Lifetime prevalence and projected lifetime risk of DSM-IV disorders in Te Rau Hinengaro: The New Zealand mental health survey. *Australian and New Zealand Journal of Psychiatry*, *40*(10): 865–74.

O'Connell, H., Chin, A.-V., Cunningham, C. & Lawlor, B. A. (2004). Recent developments: Suicide in older people. *British Medical Journal*, *329*(7471): 895–9.

Office for Senior Citizens (2012). *Briefing to the Incoming Minister. New Zealanders: Getting older, doing more*. Retrieved from www.msd.govt.nz/documents/about-msd-and-our-work/publications-resources/corporate/bims/osc-bim-2008.pdf.

Parfene, C., Stewart, T. L. & King, T. Z. (2009). Epilepsy stigma and stigma by association in the workplace. *Epilepsy & Behavior*, *15*(4): 461–6.

Parkinson's Australia (2010). *Dementia and Parkinson's: Parkinson's disease information sheet 2.10*: Retrieved from www.parkinsons.org.au/about-ps/pubs/InfoSheet_2.10.pdf.

Pearson, E. L., Windsor, T. D., Crisp, D. A., Butterworth, P. & Anstey, K. J. (2012). *Neighbourhood Characteristics: Shaping the wellbeing of older Australians. Monograph 2*. Retrieved from www.productiveageing.com.au/userfiles/file/NeighbourhoodCharacteristics.pdf.

Peron, E. P., Gray, S. L. & Hanlon, J. T. (2011). Medication use and functional status decline in older adults: A narrative review. *American Journal of Geriatric Pharmacotherapy*, *9*(6): 378–91.

Randal, P., Stewart, M. W., Proverbs, D., Lampshire, D., Symes, J. & Hamer, H. P. (2009). 'The re-covery model': An integrative developmental stress-vulnerability-strengths approach to mental health. *Psychosis: Psychological, Social and Integrative Approaches*, *1*(2): 122–33.

Read, J., Hammersley, P. & Rudegeair, T. (2007). Why, when and how to ask about childhood abuse. *Advances in Psychiatric Treatment*, *13*(2): 101–10.

Rose, N. (1998). Governing risky individuals: The role of psychiatry in new regimes of control. *Psychiatry, Psychology and Law*, *5*(2): 177–95.

Ryan, D. J., O'Regan, N. A., Caoimh, R. Ó., Clare, J., O'Connor, M., Leonard, M. & Timmons, S. (2013). Delirium in an adult acute hospital population: Predictors, prevalence and detection. *BMJ Open 3*(1).

Sandelowski, M. (2002). Visible humans, vanishing bodies, and virtual nursing: Complications of life, presence, place, and identity. *Advances in Nursing Science*, *24*(3): 58–70.

Sawyer, A.-M. (2005). From therapy to administration: Deinstitutionalisation and the ascendancy of psychiatric 'risk-thinking'. *Health Sociology Review*, *14*(3): 283–96.

Sevenhuijsen, S. (1998). *Citizenship and the Ethics of Care: Feminist considerations on justice, morality, and politics*. London, UK: Routledge.

Slade, M. (2009). *Personal Recovery and Mental Illness: A guide for mental health professionals*. Cambridge, UK: Cambridge University Press.

Stanton, L. R. & Coetzee, R. H. (2004). Down's syndrome and dementia. *Advances in Psychiatric Treatment*, *10*(1): 50–8.

Stebbins, G. T., Gabrieli, J. D. E., Masciari, F., Monti, L. & Geotz, C. G. (1999). Delayed recognition memory in Parkinson's disease: A role for working memory? *Neuropsychologia*, *37*(4): 503–10.

Sweeting, H. & Gilhooly, M. (1997). Dementia and the phenomenon of social death. *Sociology of Health & Illness*, *19*(1): 93–117.

Tronto, J. C. (1993). *Moral Boundaries: A political argument for an ethic of care*. New York: Routledge.

Tronto, J. C. (1999). Age-segregated housing as a moral problem: An exercise in re-thinking ethics. In M. Urban Walker (ed.), *Mother Time: Women, aging, and ethics* (pp. 261–77). Lanham, MD: Rowman & Littlefield Publishers.

Turner, A. & Findlay, L. (2012). Informal caregiving for seniors: Health matters. *Health Reports*, *23*(3): 1–5.

Waite, A., Bebbington, P., Skelton-Robinson, M. & Orrell, M. (2004). Social factors and depression in carers of people with dementia. *International Journal of Geriatric Psychiatry*, *19*(6): 582–7.

Wareham, P., McCallin, A. & Diesfeld, K. (2005). Advance directives: The New Zealand context. *Nursing Ethics*, *12*(4): 349–59.

13

Rural and regional mental health

Rhonda L. Wilson

Introduction 288

What is *rural*? 288

Overview of the rural and regional clinical context 291

Prevalence of mental health problems in rural and regional communities 294

Rural mental health promotion and prevention 297

Travel implications for rural people with mental health care needs 303

Natural disasters and rural implications 304

Agriculture, mining and itinerant workforces 305

Chapter summary 306

Critical thinking/learning activities 306

Learning extension 307

Acknowledgement 307

Further reading 307

References 308

Learning objectives

At the completion of this chapter, you should be able to:

- Describe the mental health needs of rural people.
- Identify and discuss rural vulnerability and resilience in regard to mental health and well-being.
- Understand the implications of travel, distance and access to mental health services for rural people.
- Recognise lifestyle practicalities of giving and receiving mental health care in a rural community, and how these relate to recovery.
- Identify some of the ways in which contemporary mental health services are delivered to people in rural communities.

Introduction

This chapter begins with an overview of the rural and regional clinical context, and explores the connections that rural mental health clinicians have within rural communities. Some models of mental health promotion and service delivery are discussed, such as community based services, visiting services, bed-based services, and e-mental health services. The nature of life in rural settings and the ways in which climate and geographical location affect the mental health of people are also considered in the context of mental health resilience and vulnerability. Attention is given to the effects of natural disasters, agribusiness, mining, itinerant rural workforce and under-employment, and the mental health consequences related to these matters. In addition, the story of a newly graduated registered nurse's experience in a rural hospital illustrates the real-life tensions between resourcing and helping rural people with mental illness. This chapter discusses some rural community benefits in regard to mental health promotion, such as a deeply felt sense of close social proximity despite significant geographical distances between rural people, and it explores aspects of rural stoicism. Rural and regional mental health promotion are considered and linked to key groups such as young people, and the agricultural and mining sectors. After reading this chapter, students will be able to reflect on, and critically think about, the ways in which mental health promotion, well-being and recovery can be enhanced among rural populations.

What is *rural*?

rural
a multi-dimensional concept that includes aspects of a person's culture, place, identity and geography, and the extent to which these align with standardised measures of rurality and remoteness

Rural is a multidimensional concept, which includes aspects of a person's culture, place, identity and geography, and the extent to which these align with standardised measures of rurality and remoteness. A range of perceptions and factors need to be considered when attempting to understand what it is to *be* a rural person. People who live in rural communities often identify closely with a deep sense of 'place'. The concept of place has a number of facets, which include psychological, emotional, socio-economic and geographical factors (Campbell, Manoff & Caffery, 2006). People in rural and regional communities may refer to themselves as being 'from the bush', or as a 'country person', or as 'rural', and all of these descriptions convey a sense of identity. People from within a similar geographical region usually share an interrelatedness that includes an inherent sense of connection and mutual support for each other, which can also be thought of as 'mateship'. It is important that mental health professionals strive to recognise the richness of rural identity and culture; that is, the real-life experiences of rural people in general, and to incorporate appropriate and uncontrived respect for this culture into their professional practice and therapeutic interactions.

In terms of mental health care, the rural person and the rural community are central to the concept of recovery for rural people. The cultural aspects underpinning what it is to be a rural person, and the places, people and interconnectedness that make up an individual's rural lifestyle, are critical to understanding the whole picture of a rural recovery system. Attention to these aspects of care will assist in developing a plan of mental health care that is realistic, achievable and person-focused rather than health service-focused. If we confine our thinking to a health service-focused perspective we will discover that there are perpetual health service shortcomings that we cannot hope to address sufficiently within the bounds of usual resources. However, if we consider the strengths that are inherent within rural communities and cultures, we will discover creative ways in which the mental health of rural people can be improved (Lourey, Holland & Green, 2012).

Government departments need to utilise pragmatic measures to define rurality, so that they can plan to distribute resources and services equitably. Rurality has been defined by the Department of Health and Ageing in Australia by using an equation that takes into account both the population size and the distance required to travel to services by road transport. The Accessibility Remoteness Index of Australia (ARIA) has been developed to describe the relative ease or difficulty that rural people are confronted with in regard to accessing services by road. This measure is used across five service sectors and is not limited to health services (Department of Health and Ageing, 2011). The ARIA scale rates from 0 (high accessibility) to a maximum of 15 (high remoteness), with five bands of remoteness identified in Australia (see Figure 13.1).

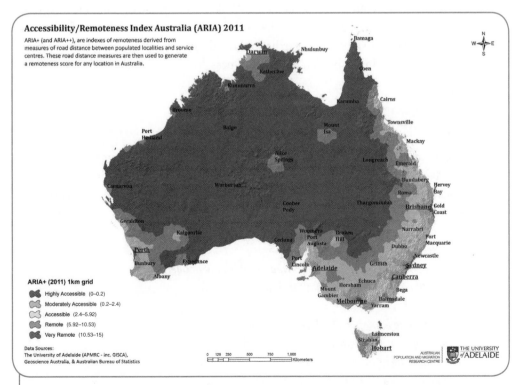

Figure 13.1. Remoteness zones in Australia

Source: Department of Health and Ageing, 2011.

Thus, rurality is not a straightforward concept, and care needs to taken by mental health clinicians, in both urban and rural clinical settings, to ensure that when planning for recovery in collaboration with the person who usually resides in a rural community, therapy is conducted with a positive regard to rural cultures and circumstances.

Waltzing Matilda

Perhaps nothing epitomises rural mental health, and rural context, as much as the Banjo Patterson poem, which has become the unofficial Australian national song: *Waltzing Matilda*. This song is popularly sung and played at many Australian community and sporting events, and it is even used as a cultural anthem to some extent. The irony is that the song is all about a rural itinerant worker; a man who travels alone, without wife, family or friends, in search of work and with his possessions carried in his backpack (swag). He has no transport and so he walks (waltzes) everywhere he needs to go. He fits a low socio-economic profile, and perhaps he is homeless, lonely and does not have enough good-quality food. He comes to the attention of the police because he has stolen a sheep for food. He feels that his circumstances are hopeless and his only option is to die by suicide, which he does by drowning himself in an oxbow dam (billabong). His experiences are a litany of mental health risk factors and vulnerabilities that continue to describe the hardship and struggles that many rural people face in contemporary times and, too frequently, with the same outcome. While we recognise the emotional pain that some rural people experience, it seems that Australian people – and culture – find it easier to sing about the hardships and make light of the difficulties in life, than to find ways to prevent the overwhelming burden of mental illness.

Reflective questions

Have you ever thought about the story behind this popular Australian song?
Read through the lyrics below and consider the effects this song, and perhaps the meaning of the lyrics, has in relation to Australian culture and how this aligns with mental health disadvantages today.

> Once a jolly swagman camped by a billabong
> Under the shade of a coolibah tree,
> And he sang as he watched and waited till his billy boiled:
> 'Who'll come a Waltzing Matilda with me?'
> ...
> Down came a jumbuck to drink at that billabong.
> Up jumped the swagman and grabbed him with glee.
> And he sang as he shoved that jumbuck in his tucker bag:
> 'You'll come a Waltzing Matilda with me.'
> ...

continued ›

Reflective questions continued ›

> Up rode the squatter, mounted on his thoroughbred.
> Down came the troopers, one, two and three.
> 'Whose is that jolly jumbuck you've got in your tucker bag?
> You'll come a Waltzing Matilda with me.'
>
> Up jumped the swagman and sprang into the billabong.
> 'You'll never catch me alive!' said he.
> And his ghost may be heard as you pass by that billabong:
> 'Who'll come a Waltzing Matilda with me?'

Overview of the rural and regional clinical context

Rural and regional communities vary in size, environment and public amenity. Geographical distance is often a factor in the isolation of people from a wide range of health and other services. The economic base is another significant factor that, for rural and regional communities, influences the social determinants of health (World Health Organization (WHO), 2013). There are benefits and limitations in residing in a rural community, and these will influence the health outcomes of people in those communities (Boyd & Parr, 2008). The challenges for rural and regional communities include promoting healthy conditions, opportunities and environments, and to provide people with sufficient resources so that rural and regional people are able to access mental health care that is equitably distributed as compared to that of their urban counterparts (WHO, 2013). Nevertheless, it is apparent that rural and regional people experience difficulties in accessing these services and this, in part, may explain why some rural young people experience lengthy durations of untreated mental illness compared to their urban counterparts (Wilson, Cruickshank & Lea, 2012).

The Council of Australian Governments (COAG) has prioritised mental health reform, with a focus on community participation and the promotion of good and resilient mental health and well-being for all people (COAG, 2012). There is a strong belief in the general population that good accessibility to health services is proportionate to the availability of adequate numbers and types of clinical services, and where there are more health services, this is perceived as demonstrating delivery of quality health care to community members (Young & McGrath, 2011).

In rural and regional communities, access to health services is problematic and is frequently raised as a matter of concern by rural citizens, health service managers and policy planners. Public opinion and political lobbying frequently demand a response by governments in providing improved access for rural citizens, with a view that more services will provide better mental health care for rural populations (Young & McGrath, 2011). A tension remains because there is disproportionate access to mental health services between urban and rural or regional populations, and this circumstance perpetuates inequities in mental health and well-being for rural people, generally (Young & McGrath, 2011). People with longer-term mental illnesses are more likely to find mental health service provision in rural and regional areas, while younger people with emerging mental illnesses are less likely to experience successful access to appropriate mental health services (Wilson et al., 2012).

Some studies have demonstrated that in communities and in age groups in which mental health problems are more prevalent, an increased physical comorbidity exists (Morgan et al., 2011). For example, increases in emergency department presentations, chronic pain, asthma, cardiac conditions, headache, diabetes and stroke have been shown to be higher among people with mental illness, and these problems are further exacerbated by rurality (Morgan, et al., 2011).

community participation
the involvement of local people in assessing their own needs, and planning strategies to address those needs

Governments, which fund public mental health services, have traditionally taken the view that **community participation** should be promoted as both an appropriate approach and an intervention to buffer rural health disadvantages (Preston et al., 2010; COAG, 2012). Community participation is defined as the involvement of local people in assessing their own needs, and planning their own strategies to address those needs. Despite widespread adoption of community participation models and techniques, there is scant evidence to support such an approach (Preston et al., 2010). Only a few studies have attempted to measure the success or evaluate the effectiveness of this approach, and more research about effective models of rural health care delivery are needed to advance rural and regional health care in the future.

A possible benefit of living in rural and regional settings is that strong community participation models contribute to the helpfulness and effectiveness of social and health or well-being capacities within the community. In small communities, health service clinicians represent a unique element of that social helpfulness, and they are able to develop informal linkages and intrinsically prompt well-being capacity because of their embedded close social proximity and shared social experiences with the rural people in their community, despite sometimes significant geographical distances separating each other (Boyd, Hayes, Wilson et al., 2008; Boyd & Parr, 2008).

Health professionals, simultaneously, hold dual roles as resident community members and health services providers, and both of these roles are thought to be important because community linkages are enhanced between health systems and the communities served by health professionals (Kilpatrick, 2009). This circumstance places clinicians in challenging situations at times as they seek to manage, and attempt to separate, their personal and professional relationships within rural and regional communities. It is inevitable in small communities that clinicians will be required to provide health care for people with whom they have a personal relationship (Endacott et al., 2006). Thus, mental health professionals in rural communities are adding value to the communities in which they live and work, across two domains: professional and personal, and these domains are interconnected to some extent. Therefore, maintaining ethical standards of care in such circumstances is of high importance for all health professionals (Australian Nursing and Midwifery Council, Royal College of Nursing Australia, & Australian Nursing Federation, 2008).

Reflective questions

- How difficult would you find separating the professional and personal aspects of your relationships in a clinical setting if you were a clinician in a small rural health service?
- List some of the people, or organisations, you could consult with to assist you to maintain ethical standards as a health care professional.

Consumer narrative
The story of Edwina, new graduate

Edwina is a newly graduated registered nurse. She completed her Bachelor of Nursing studies one month ago and, following registration, she was successful in gaining employment as a registered nurse in a small rural hospital. Filled with enthusiasm for her new role, in the first couple of weeks she met some people with mental illnesses and discovered that helping these people in the rural context is particularly challenging.

This is Edwina's story about two people she helped, and how it made her feel.

A 48-year-old woman and a 25-year-old man were admitted to the ward on the same day; both of them had overdosed. The woman had taken an overdose of benzodiazepines and paracetamol the previous night, with the intention of repeating her actions the next morning if she woke up. Luckily, her husband found her in the early morning and called the ambulance. The young man had overdosed on escitalopram, an antidepressant, and he had sent a text message to his wife, who was in Brisbane, telling her about what he was doing, and she rang the police. The man's wife and two children had recently moved from Brisbane, but not long afterwards his wife left him and took the two children back to Brisbane.

The woman was initially in the HDU (high dependency unit), and after she was moved onto the ward it was decided that she would be sent to the nearest mental health facility, about one-and-a-half hours away by road.

The man remained in hospital so his health could be monitored – his pupils were dilated to 9 millimetres! The biggest pupils I have *ever* seen. An appointment was made with the mental health team, but these mental health appointments are so scarce, and the waiting list is never-ending. An appointment was made for two-and-a-half weeks time, and he was sent home. I couldn't believe this! I expressed my concern to the nurse-in-charge, and she said that mental health appointments are so scarce and far away in this region that most people re-present to the emergency department before attending the appointment.

I had a lot of time for this young man. He was only a few years older than me, and I wanted to help him as much as I could, even if it was just getting him a bundle of magazines from the waiting room, because he had no belongings with him and the TVs weren't working. He needed something to take his mind off things!

continued ›

Consumer narrative continued ›

As predicted, the young man did re-present to the emergency department. This time he had taken a chainsaw to his leg. Apparently, his injuries weren't too severe but, as I was off duty at that time, from what I heard his injuries were treated and he was sent home … *again*! After that, I heard he got involved with the police (he had anger-management issues) and then, only then, was he sent to the nearest mental health facility.

To me, this was wrong, and I think more needs to be done about mental health in rural areas – it took *three* emergency admissions for this man to get the attention that he needed. That's *three* times this man was crying out for help. If this man had had an infection in his body with the potential to kill him, he would undoubtedly have been kept in hospital until it was cleared up, not sent home to simply hope for the best, and that he would be okay.

I remember being in university nursing classes and learning about how mental health was underfunded and that awareness of mental health needed to be improved in rural and regional areas. It is not until now, though, that I truly understand how essential it really is!

People can be so flippant and/or skeptical about mental health, and it frustrates me… My mental health clinical placement last year opened my eyes to the reality of mental health needs and how prevalent it really is, as did these experiences.

Reflective questions

Edwina found her first experiences in caring for people with mental illness in the hospital setting rather confronting.

- What emotions are stirred within you when you read Edwina's story?
- What strategies can you use to manage your own feelings about challenging situations you might experience in a rural setting?
- How can you participate positively in the wider health care team to facilitate timely and respectful help for people in general health settings who have mental illness?

Prevalence of mental health problems in rural and regional communities

People in rural communities self-report that they experience mental illness and behavioural problems at a rate of 16 per cent higher than their urban counterparts (Australian Bureau of Statistics (ABS), 2011). Idyllic notions about achieving a healthier lifestyle and greater well-being in rural communities may be based more on optimistic hopes than on actual facts (see Table 13.1). Unemployment and under-employment are higher in rural areas than in urban areas, and there are fewer senior positions available in most sectors, which limits career progression at an early stage and at lower remuneration for many people. Careers in rural communities are sometimes more vulnerable to the 'boom and bust' dynamics of the agricultural sector, and to related environmental changes such as drought, poor crop yields and the fluctuations of livestock sale prices and markets. These dynamics place stresses on the mental health and well-being of rural people, despite a widely held view that rural people are stoic and resilient (Boyd, Hayes, Sewell et al., 2008). Sometimes, the stoic expectation of rural people to endure hardship in itself becomes a barrier to rural people who may be reluctant to seek assistance for mental illness and related services, and rural men are particularly vulnerable in this regard. By contrast, rural women are more

Table 13.1 Benefits and limitations of rural lifestyles

Benefits	Limitations
Strong social connections and close social proximity	Higher proportions of mental illness and suicide prevalence, longer durations of untreated mental illness, persistent stigma and discrimination about mental health problems, and fewer mental health support services
Clean air to breath	Few and limited health services. Complex health diagnostics and interventions not available
Plenty of open space for work and play	Few and limited educational services, and a population with lower-than-average educational attainments
Fresh food and produce – sometimes at the farm gate	Less reliable public services, e.g. telecommunications (telephone, mobile and internet) and electricity or gas services.
Little time spent in travel on a local basis	Long distances to travel to urban commercial and service centres. Limited or no public transport options. Motor vehicle accident risk accentuated by variable road conditions, long distances and older manufacture dates of vehicles in rural communities
Space to grow own food (fruit, vegetables, meat, eggs and dairy), and capacity to exercise in the outdoors and natural environment	Few local consumer choice options in regard to retail and service sectors
More employment in the agricultural sector and in the mining sector	Higher levels of unemployment, under-employment and itinerant employment, and fewer prospects for middle to higher-income positions. Career pathways limited, with executive and management positions typically located in larger population centres
	Family disruptions as children, young people, adults and older people need to relocate to access services related to school, work, childbirth, or to ageing or death/palliative care
	High vulnerability to environmental irregularities and disasters, e.g. drought, fire, flood and with impacts felt across all rural sectors

likely to seek help for mental illness when they need it, and especially for problems such as depression and anxiety (Buikstra, Fallon & Eley, 2007).

Suicide rates among rural males, and especially young men aged 15–29 years, have been increasing over the past 20 years (Department of Health and Ageing, 2013) and at rates twice as high as young men who live in urban communities (ABS, 2011). Rural older men aged 85 years and over have been reported as having the highest rate of death by suicide, at 40 deaths per 100 000 men, and this is thought to be influenced by increased financial insecurity and agricultural stresses sometimes brought about by the experience of environmental events such as floods, droughts and bush fires (ABS, 2011). It has been suggested that people in rural communities often have access to more lethal means when they intend to harm themselves (ABS, 2011). Edwina's story demonstrates this to some extent; she said that the young man she had treated had later cut his leg with a chain saw, a situation that could have had a much worse outcome. In addition, loneliness and difficulty accessing mental health care are factors related to suicide (ABS, 2011), and these are also risk factors that can be identified in Edwina's account of the young man's experience.

The further people live away from an urban centre, the less they are likely to have access to general practitioner services, and the less likely they are to utilise national Medicare initiatives, such as the Better Access initiative (Department of Health and Ageing, 2013), which is promoted as a measure to ensure a more equitable share in mental health funding across the population (Lourey et al., 2012). Some risk factors in combination with rural residency have been noted as having an association with the prevalence of mental health illness, including:

- poverty;
- unemployment;
- female gender;
- unmarried;
- low socio-economic circumstances;
- alcohol abuse;
- history of childhood sexual abuse;
- poor social networks; and
- small size of primary support groups (Campbell et al., 2006).

However, the longer people reside in rural communities, if they are satisfied with their circumstances and feel that they have attained a quality of life in their place of residency, the greater the potential for mitigation of risk vulnerabilities and resilience against mental illness (Campbell et al., 2006).

Rural and regional mental health services vary in type and service mix across communities. Access to specialist mental health services, and specialist clinicians, are usually restricted to larger regional centres. Occasionally, however, these services send visiting teams to outlying rural and regional centres on semi-regular and ad hoc bases. In most cases, people seeking assistance for mental illness attend centre-based or bed-based mental health services, and usually in larger regional or metropolitan centres.

Rural mental health promotion and prevention

Mental health promotion and prevention services are most usually based in larger regional centres, and they often provide outreach or visiting services to smaller, outlying rural communities, using a **'hub and spoke' model** of service, whereby the hub represents the centralisation or home base of services and the spokes the outreach to specific communities or community events. Sometimes, major rural events such as agricultural field days are targeted for health promotion activities because they draw together large concentrations of rural people, and this makes it convenient and cost-effective for health services to provide mental health education and information to larger groups.

'hub and spoke' model of service, whereby the hub represents the centralisation or home base of services and the spokes the outreach to specific communities or community events

Partnerships between mental health services and other sectors contribute to building rural mental health and well-being capacity in innovative ways, such as in the example of a partnership between the Rural Adversity Mental Health Program and a national rural newspaper, *The Land* ('Glove box guide to mental health', 2012). This was a useful strategy because it conveniently placed mental health information where many rural people would have a chance encounter with the information, and this might trigger further personal investigation by people who could be helped by receiving such information. However, a limitation of this type of program is that they are often short-term in nature and are difficult to sustain beyond pilot stages because funds are frequently not available for replication or for more sustainable and long-term ventures, despite their success.

Rural early intervention mental health services

Early intervention services are needed, especially for young people, because most mental illnesses first develop in late adolescence and during early stages of adulthood. Specialist early intervention programs are very important, especially for treatment of early psychosis; recent evidence has suggested that early and ongoing intervention for up to five years are critical, and cost effective, in the reduction of the long-term effects of untreated psychosis (Yung, 2013). However, rural communities are often limited in the diversity of mental health services available. Generic mental health services are saturated with clinician caseloads predominated by people with long-term, and somewhat consolidated, mental illness. Access to mental health services for young people is especially challenging because few face-to-face local services are available in rural communities, and also because it is extremely difficult for the general public, and for non-mental health professionals, to determine whether the odd behaviours and 'not quite right' interactions that sometimes accompany emergent mental illnesses such as early psychosis and bipolar disorder are because a mental illness is developing or the changes observed are within a normal range for the personal developmental stage of a young person (Callaly et al., 2010; Rodd & Stewart, 2009). Rural young women are more likely than young men to access, or attempt to access, mental health services, especially for conditions such as depression. However, they sometimes have difficulty finding appropriate help because of the lack of services in their communities and because they sometimes experience long waiting periods prior to gaining help (Alston et al., 2006; Black, Roberts & Li-Leng, 2012). National mental health plans have recognised that more needs to be done to better address young people's mental health needs in rural communities; however, it remains to be seen what can be achieved with the funds available to rural mental health (COAG, 2012).

The *headspace* (www.headspace.org.au) model of care has been the Australian government's most determined recent initiative to address the mental health needs of young people. However, there are only 47 centres nationally in which face-to-face services may be accessed, and most of these are located in urban or large regional centres. Rural communities remain under-serviced in regard to young people's mental health, and there is an expectation that young people, and their families, should travel to major centres to attend to their mental health care needs. Headspace is advancing its e-mental health approach, because this is seen by the Australian government as a more inclusive and equitable approach for young people's mental health programs (Department of Health and Ageing, 2012).

An alternative for young people, their families and their general practitioners is to engage in telehealth and/or e-mental health linkages to specialist services based in metropolitan centres (for example, early psychosis services). It has been argued that small communities are unlikely to have sufficient quantities of people with early mental health problems to sustain the establishment of specialist face-to-face services (Early Psychosis Writing Group, 2010), and this highlights the compromises that are often required in the struggle for cost efficiencies and equity of service distribution, which rural communities continue to battle. Early mental health interventionists have noted that telehealth and e-mental health services should not be seen as a substitute for face-to-face, early intervention services, and some suggest that visiting services may be the next best alternative for rural communities (Early Psychosis Writing Group, 2010).

Community mental health and primary health services

Community mental health services are available in many rural communities, but not in all, and in some cases these are delivered in an outreach mode. A **case management** model is often used to manage the services delivered by a multidisciplinary team with combinations of mental health nurses, psychologists, occupational therapists, counsellors and psychiatrists, in the main. Case management models have a variety of subtypes, and it is beyond the scope of this book to outline them all, but they have in common the goals that mental health services should be provided in a coordinated way and that the outcomes of the services delivered should result in appropriate care (Purtell, Dowling & Fossey, 2008). There are four key phases to coordinated care: planning, implementation, monitoring and review, and they can be applied to all subtypes of case management models (Purtell et al., 2008). In general practical terms, teams of clinicians work together and meet regularly to consult about complex care planning for the people they help. Each team member is allocated a number of people for whom

case management
a key worker coordinates appropriate community care for people with mental illness, and plans, implements, monitors and reviews their progress, thereby promoting recovery and self-care

they will provide assessment, treatment and review, with a view to promoting recovery and well-being for their clients.

Mental health services are increasingly striving towards person-centred approaches for the delivery of care; however, the vocabulary used to describe service activities needs some modification, and 'case management' is one of these phrases that is becoming outdated, although a proposed alternative description is yet to emerge. It is no longer an acceptable practice to refer to people who require mental health care as 'cases to be managed'. Case manager roles in the future should bear a title that is person-centred, and should reflect activities that are more recovery-focused, such as enablers, and facilitators of well-being and functioning, and less orientated towards disease and disability (Purtell et al., 2008). There is a consistent call for reforms, so that people are increasingly enabled and encouraged to make informed decisions about their own recovery, rather than expected simply to comply with the directives of health professionals. Thus, it is appropriate that service delivery models should evolve further to better incorporate person-centred recovery models of care that reflect evidenced-based, good practice in the 21st century (Keen & Lakeman, 2009).

Bed-based mental health services

Bed-based units for mental health care in rural communities are extremely limited. Most bed-based units are both involuntary (following administration of a Mental Health Act), and voluntary units within regional or metropolitan hospital services. Bed-based units care for people who are experiencing an acute phase of mental illness and who are unable to cope at home or with the assistance of community mental health services alone. It is preferable that people are helped towards recovery prior to the acute need for bed-based care, but this is not always possible. Bed-based units require staffing levels that may not be possible to achieve in communities other than larger centres, because there may not be sufficient mental health nurses in smaller communities to resource a bed-based unit; traditionally, health services have experienced difficulty in recruiting mental health professionals to rural communities.

In regional communities, bed-based units are likely to service a wider-reaching rural community. It is important for these units to work closely with mental health clinicians in the home communities of their clients, because discharge poses multiple challenges, and careful consideration of medication, suicide risk, travel arrangements and future community or general practitioner appointments need to be planned so that there are no disruptions to the continuance of care. In addition, it is extremely important to collaborate with a team that includes the person receiving mental health care and any carers or family. The successful continuation of care, and the transition to home following discharge, is extremely important so that relapse can be minimised or prevented.

e-Mental health and telehealth

Over the past 10 years, telehealth has emerged as a cost-effective strategy to improve mental health service delivery in rural and regional communities. An example of how a telehealth service operates is described in a Queensland Health video: *Extending the Reach of Clinical Health Services Throughout Queensland* (Statewide Telehealth Services, 2013). Telehealth is usually conducted in a video-conference format whereby all parties are able to see each other in real time, using a video or TV screen, and they can participate in a synchronous clinical consultation during this time. In more recent times interactions have begun to develop within the Web 2 social media forum, especially in regard to mental health promotion, awareness and information discussions. An example of this is found on Facebook™, where Queensland Health has described its telehealth services (Queensland Health, 2013), thus demonstrating the potential for integration of social media into a more comprehensive and far-reaching **e-mental health** framework.

e-mental health
a variety of mental health interactions and interventions delivered using internet-connected devices such as computers, tablets and smartphones, or by using short message services (SMS) through mobile phone-based formats, and delivered in synchronous or asynchronous episodes

e-Mental health can be defined as interactions and interventions that can be delivered in a digital, electronic or telephone-based format and can take effect in synchronous or asynchronous episodes. e-Mental health is an evolving area of practice, and is an area that is likely to see significant development in the future (Rickwood, 2012). It will be impossible for Australia, or New Zealand, to develop adequate and equitable mental health plans for rural communities without also adopting e-mental health interventions, because the cost of placing specialist, face-to-face mental health services in all rural and regional communities would be cost prohibitive (Early Psychosis Writing Group, 2010; Rickwood, 2012; Smith, Skrbis & Western, 2012).

There are currently several examples of internet-based, or mobile phone-based, mental health interventions that might be applied to the rural context; for example, the self-care mood monitoring program myCompass (www.mycompass.org.au). There are both no-cost and low-cost options of programs such as this, and some of these have been rigorously evaluated and peer reviewed. In fact, there are so many open-source 'self-help' options available to the general public that the selection of quality e-mental health therapies needs particular attention before clinicians recommend them to consumers. The Centre for Mental Health Research at the Australian National University has developed a database (Beacon 2.0) of e-mental health programs reviewed and rated by health professionals, and this information can assist users and referrers to make informed decisions about the quality of online interventions, such as (for example) online cognitive behavioural therapy programs (Christenson, 2007; Griffiths & Christensen, 2007).

A shift towards e-mental health promotion can also be seen in the social media. Twitter™ and Facebook have been adopted by many rural mental health professionals as forums in which a great deal of discussion about rural mental health take place. While Twitter feeds lack the rigour of formal peer review and should not be considered sufficient evidence upon which to base professional practice, the mental health discourse in this social medium is certainly becoming increasingly influential and provides a mechanism by which rural people, carers and clinicians might develop supportive networks, exchange ideas, promote mental well-being and advocate for improved services to rural communities.

Mobile phones are increasingly being used to facilitate mental health awareness and health promotion, and to deliver some interventions. Mobile phones are used extensively in rural communities, and smartphones with internet connections are increasingly popular. Mobile phones are usually carried by individuals, and are usually turned on, so they are positioned helpfully (for example) in the pockets of people with mental illness, to be deployed in ways that can promote mental health, conduct some interventions and to prompt recovery (Proudfoot, 2013).

There is a growing capacity for e-mental health in all its guises to transform the delivery of rural mental health services. This is an important area of practice development, and mental health professionals will need to be aware of the changing e-mental health dynamic and be prepared to adapt to clinical changes in mental health service delivery, so that mental health and well-being can be promoted more effectively to rural people.

Recovery and rehabilitation

Recovery planning commences at first consultation wherever, and whenever, it takes place. A recovery focus will promote well-being and will engage people purposefully in their own decision-making about their future health, including the lifestyle changes they decide to make (Caldwell et al., 2010), and it will enable people to lead meaningful and contributing lives (Lourey et al., 2012). Some people living with complex long-term illnesses find coping with daily life extremely challenging, and they have to work hard to maintain a sufficient life balance in order to manage their own lives and to maximise their wellness. Community based recovery and rehabilitation centres and groups can be very helpful for these people. In rural communities, recovery services such as these, if they exist at all, are likely to be delivered by non-government organisations (NGOs) such as in the example provided here.

Billabong Clubhouse

Billabong Clubhouse, located in regional Tamworth, New South Wales, is a member of an international clubhouse movement (www.iccd.org). In Australia and New Zealand, it operates as an NGO. There are several other clubhouses in Australia and New Zealand, but what is most interesting about Billabong Clubhouse is that it is a community participation response, by local rural and regional people, to address the needs of people with long-term mental illness in their own community. The Tamworth community recognised that the needs of people with long-term mental illness in their midst were not being met, and that there were insufficient public health resources to meet this need, and so they formed an organisation to address the matter. Billabong Clubhouse

continued ›

Billabong Clubhouse continued >

has been operational for about 15 years, which is an outcome that many rural programs have been unable to achieve. The members of the Clubhouse are equally responsible for the management and day-to-day operations of the Clubhouse. Members gather on a daily basis to give support and encouragement to each other, to care for each other in practical ways, socialise, develop a routine, share or cook a meal together, and perhaps to undertake some work or vocational activities. The structure of the Clubhouse model fosters wellness, and many members report that it 'keeps them out of hospital', which is a very important personal outcome for each person. Initiatives such as this may be useful in other rural and regional communities that have similar populations and conditions as Tamworth.

Table 13.2 Rural mental health services

Type of health service	Description and examples
Rural multipurpose centres/ rural hospitals	• Multidisciplinary, clinic-based services that require people seeking help to attend either a scheduled individual appointment, or a group appointment or session. • Some bed-based services, mostly aged-care related, but some acute-care beds and first-response emergency services. These centres vary in size (e.g. 12–40 beds). • Visiting mental health services may be available on a regular or ad hoc basis, and the range of clinicians who attend includes several (e.g. 1–4) mental health nurses, psychiatrists, psychologists, social workers, occupational therapists and counsellors. • Other non-mental health services co-located in a service such as this might include child and family nurses, community nurses, aged care assistants, podiatrists, dietitians, sexual health and women's health nurses, drug and alcohol counselors and general practitioners. • More information about this service type: www0.health.nsw.gov.au/rural/rhhsp/index.asp • An example of a rural hospital: www0.health.qld.gov.au/services/darlingdowns/ddowns-goondiwind-hs.asp
Telehealth and e-mental health	• Video-conferencing, telephone-conferencing or internet-based services. Frequently, the clinicians providing mental health service are located in major metropolitan areas and the recipients of this care are situated in rural communities. Telehealth services help to reduce the barrier of poor access to specialist mental health services for rural people; however, they do rely on quality internet and telephone or data connectivity. An additional challenge for this type of service delivery is establishing trust and rapport at a distance, and with a fundamental difference in lifestyle and experiences.

continued >

Table 13.2 (continued ›)

Type of health service	Description and examples
Community health services	• Services available to ambulatory clients who are able to attend a community health centre for regular health appointments, or clients who are able to remain at home with the support of a visiting clinician to provide in-home care. • An example of services provided by a community health service: www.dhhs.tas.gov.au/mentalhealth/mhs_tas/gvt_mhs/adult_community_mental_health_services
Case management	• Occurs at large regional centres and requires a team for optimum functionality. • Sometimes, outreach versions of case management apply to outlying rural communities.
Indigenous emotional and social well-being or mental health services	• Indigenous people have a significantly higher propensity for mental illness. This video describes how one community was able to positively address some of the mental illnesses encountered in their Bathurst Island community and to focus further on promoting mental well-being: www.youtube.com/watch?v=jQWqBWy8HRE • Medicare Local centres are involved in developing care connections and facilitating mental health and social health and well-being support for Aboriginal and Torres Strait Islander people in Australia. An example of this service type is found at New England Medicare Local (www.neml.org.au/Aboriginal-Health-Services-19/). • A further example of mental health care in remote Aboriginal communities can be found in Purdie, Dudgeon & Walker, 2010.

'A guideline for interdisciplinary telehealth': Jakowenko, 2012.

Travel implications for rural people with mental health care needs

A challenge for people seeking mental health care, and their clinicians alike, is that often rural people need to travel many hours to attend mental health appointments, and this means that other personal, vocational and educational activities are disrupted. Significant personal expenses may also be incurred because fuel in rural areas is usually more expensive to purchase than it is in metropolitan areas. In addition, maintaining roadworthy vehicles for long-distance travel, paying for away-from-home meals and sometimes the need for accommodation away from home add further financial burdens to people who are experiencing mental illness. Managing these travel requirements can be very difficult for people with mental illness and their carers, because frequently people with mental illness also experience symptoms that affect their logical thinking processes, motivation and planning. There is not an abundance of public transport systems for rural communities, and if people do not have access to a personal vehicle, or they are not able to drive (because sometimes the medications they take to address their mental illness cause them to be drowsy and unsafe to drive a car), they are further isolated and have to rely on the goodwill and kindness of others to assist them with transport needs. Thus, any therapy that is dependent upon rural or regional people being required to invest significant personal resources is a factor for consideration by clinicians when they are planning short-term and long-term recovery goals.

Natural disasters and rural implications

Australia and New Zealand are prone to natural disasters, and over the past few years it seems there have been many different major disasters. The climate and environment in rural Australia make rural communities especially vulnerable to the effects of bush fires, heat waves, storms or cyclones, floods and droughts, while New Zealand has had devastating earthquakes. There has been a great deal of development in Australia to improve preparation and early warning systems to assist rural people to cope with these adverse conditions (Jones, 2013). For example, population-wide emergency alert messages have been sent to mobile phones to warn people within the geographical surrounds of impending natural disaster events; rural residents have been informed about developing self-plans to improve their survival of storms and bush fires; and water storage and timing of releases have been improved. All of these examples represent improvements that are of great importance to rural communities.

The mental health impacts of disasters for rural people are also significant, with vulnerabilities well recognised for poorer rural people, farmers and rural men in particular (Saniotis & Irvine, 2010). The immediate crisis that accompanies a natural disaster can be traumatic for some people, and this requires monitoring and intervention of individuals and, sometimes, the entire population. However, the longer-term effects of disaster-related trauma can result in the mental health decline of some people and can include serious and/or longer-term consequences; this, then, becomes the focus of targeted mental health assessment and intervention in those communities. Mental health professionals in rural communities have to address unique health and well-being problems, and especially with regard to natural and other disasters. A recent story broadcast on Australian national radio recounted the experiences of nurses in the rural town of Moree, New South Wales, where their response to flood conditions provide an example of the roles of health professionals in times of natural disaster: www.abc.net.au/local/stories/2012/02/10/3428111.htm?site=newengland.

The prevalence of mental illness following natural and other disasters is not well known, and this is a field in which more research is needed. The robust nature of rural communities and the close social connections within them are thought to be protective in regard to mental health, and so there is capacity to strengthen resilience (Boyd, Hayes, Sewell et al., 2008) through mental health promotion and awareness before, during and after these events.

Reflective questions

Can you imagine what it would be like to experience first-hand flood conditions? (Or perhaps you have done so in your own life?)

- Imagine (or recall) the feelings and emotions of uncertainty, anxiety, worry, fear, loss and the pressure of having to make a quick decision.
- What could others do to help you cope with these types of challenges?
- Now, imagine that you are person doing the helping (a nurse, paramedic or social worker).
- List some of the ways you think you may be able to help others to cope with the emotional and practical difficulties people may face in this situation.

Agriculture, mining and itinerant workforces

Rural communities are shaped by some unique vocational groups: the agricultural workforce, the itinerant and seasonal rural workforces (for example, in fruit harvesting), and the mining workforce. The uncertainty and seasonality of these industries have population-wide effects that, in turn, influence the mental health of these groups, and the wider rural community. The mining industry has developed significantly in recent times in rural Australia, and this has implications for community health and well-being for both new mining residents and long-term residents in rural communities. The mining workforce has to contend with shift work and fly-in, fly-out (FIFO) conditions, both of which affect families and the personal connections people have with places and people in their lives. These circumstances may predispose vulnerable individuals towards mental illness on occasion, and this is emerging as an area of concern to health services in those communities. Relative shifts in population sizes, and especially sudden increases in populations, place additional demands on current health services and other rural amenities, such as housing and employment. An example is in Mt Isa, Queensland, where local people and services have noticed an increased need for mental health services as the mining industry has expanded.

Chapter summary

- The mental health needs of rural people are diverse and unique. Rural people identify and are identified both by their connection to rural people and places and according to standardised measures of rurality. Respect should be afforded to rural culture in promoting mental health recovery. There is disparity in access to mental health services between rural and metropolitan regions, and this disparity presents many challenges.
- There are many mental health vulnerabilities and risk factors that can be identified in rural communities, such as rural industry dynamics, occurrence of natural disasters, difficulties in accessing services, distances from specialist mental health services, loneliness, unemployment, poverty, transport difficulties and having fewer local retail and service choices. However, resilience can be fostered and mental health and well-being nurtured by the close social connections rural people have with each other, and the contentment and satisfaction that people have socially and in their personal circumstance. Rural communities have social strengths that can help to mitigate some mental health risks.
- Travel implications and mental health service utilisation are profound challenges for rural people, and consideration to travel distance and disruptions in other areas of lifestyle are important in planning.
- Recovery in rural communities entails understanding the unique rural culture, geography and opportunities. e-Mental health is showing promise in relation to overcoming some of the practical barriers to accessing specialist services, and minimising the burden of travel for some people.
- Mental health services are delivered using a variety of service models. The service dynamics between communities often differ; however, some similarities have been addressed in this chapter, such as the use of outreach services, community services and bed-based services. Models of service continue to be adapted in an effort to improve equitable mental health care delivery for all people, with e-mental health care showing promise for the future.

Critical thinking/learning activities

1 Describe some benefits and some vulnerabilities for mental health that may be experienced by rural people.
2 How can rural people and communities participate in rural mental health promotion?
3 Is a rural lifestyle a healthy lifestyle? Why? Or, why not?
4 What are some of the strengths and limitations of e-mental health strategies? Who might be best suited to receiving e-mental health interventions?
5 Describe how a person-centred recovery could be achieved in a rural community.

Learning extension

Activity One

First: Watch the news report about the experiences of young people in Mt Isa and their need for mental health support: www.youtube.com/watch?v=MsjYhKjBlX4 ('Rural mining town battles mental health issues').

Second: Think about the following questions. What types of mental health care might be suitable for use with rural young people to help reduce the burden of mental illness and suicide in rural communities? Why do you think those you have chosen would be useful? How can talking about mental health be initiated when it seems as though it is too hard to talk about?

Third: Reflect on your own experiences, using these questions as a guide. What issues (if any) strike a chord for you personally in this video? What is it about your past and current experiences or beliefs that help to bring this issue to the fore of your thinking? Do you need to discuss your reflection with a trusted colleague, clinical supervisor or counsellor?

Activity Two

Review some examples of rural mental health promotion and information using social media, including these Facebook open groups and Twitter streams and handles:

- **Rural Mental Health Australia:** www.facebook.com/RuralMH/info and #RuralMH
- **Rural Mental Health:** http://anzmh.asn.au/rrmh/ and #RuralMental_Hth
- **MentalHealthAUST:** http://anzmh.asn.au/conference and #MentalHealth_AU
- **Schizophrenia Fellowship of NSW Inc.:** www.facebook.com/SFNSW
- **Australian College of Mental Health Nurses:** www.facebook.com/AustCollMHNs and #ACMHN
- **International Journal of Mental Health Nursing:** www.facebook.com/pages/International-Journal-of-Mental-Health-Nursing/451215961599310?ref=ts&fref=ts

Acknowledgement

Thanks to Edwina Casey RN BN, who shared her story and contributed to this chapter to provide a perspective from a recent graduate nurse.

Further reading

ABC News. Mental health clients feel stigmatised. (2011). *7:30 Report*. Retrieved from www.youtube.com/watch?v=xqlQS3IANdQ.
Centre for Mental Health Research, Australian National University. Beacon 2.0: https://beacon.anu.edu.au/
Fairfax Agricultural Media (2012). *Glove Box Guide to Mental Health*. Retrieved from www.theland.com.au/theland/magazines/mentalhealth.

Fairfax Agricultural Media (2012). *The Land*. Retrieved from www.theland.com.au/news/agriculture/agribusiness/general-news/mental-health-resources-for-the-bush/2632004.aspx.

Lourey, C., Holland, C. & **Green, R.** (2012). *A Contributing Life: The 2012 national report card on mental health and suicide prevention*. Sydney: National Mental Health Commission Retrieved from www.mentalhealthcommission.gov.au.

Purdie, N., Dudgeon, P. & **Walker, R.** (eds). (2010). *Working Together: Aboriginal and Torres Strait Islander mental health and wellbeing principles and practice*. Canberra: Commonwealth of Australia.

References

ABC News. (2011), Rural mining town battles mental health issues. *Lateline*. Retrieved from www.youtube.com/watch?v=MsjYhKjBlX4.

Alston, M., Allan, J., Dietsch, E., Wilkinson, J., Shankar, J., Osborn, L. et al. (2006). Brutal neglect: Australian rural women's access to health services. *Rural and Remote Health, 6*(475): 1–19.

Australian Bureau of Statistics (ABS) (2011). *Australian Social Trends, March 2011. Health outside major cities*. Canberra: Author.

Australian Nursing and Midwifery Council, Royal College of Nursing Australia & Australian Nursing Federation (2008). *Code of Ethics for Nurses in Australia*. Dickson, ACT: Australian Nursing and Midwifery Council.

Black, C., Roberts, R.M. & **Li-Leng, T.** (2012). Depression in rural adolescents: Relationships with gender and availability of mental health services. *Rural and Remote Health, 12*(2092): 1–11.

Boyd, C.P., Hayes, L., Sewell, J., Caldwell, K., Kemp, E., Harvie, L. et al. (2008). Mental health problems in rural contexts: A broader perspective. *Australian Psychologist, 43*(1): 2–6.

Boyd, C.P., Hayes, L., Wilson, R.L. & **Bearsley-Smith, C.** (2008). Harnessing the social capital of rural communities for youth mental health: An asset-based community development framework. *Australian Journal of Rural Health, 16*: 189–93.

Boyd, C.P. & **Parr, H.** (2008). Social geography and rural mental health research. *Rural and Remote Health, 8*(804): 1–5.

Buikstra, E., Fallon, A.B. & **Eley, R.** (2007). Psychological services in five south-west Queensland communities – supply and demand. *Rural and Remote Health, 7*(543): 1–11.

Caldwell, B.A., Sclafani, M., Swarbrick, M. & **Piren, K.** (2010). Psychiatric nursing practice and the recovery model of care. *Journal of Psychosocial Nursing, 48*(7): 42–8.

Callaly, T., Ackerly, C.A., Hyland, M.E., Dodd, S., O'Shea, M. & **Berk, M.** (2010). A qualitative evaluation of a regional early psychosis service 3 years after its commencement. *Australian Health Review, 34*: 382–5.

Campbell, A., Manoff, T. & **Caffery, J.** (2006). Rurality and mental health: An Australian primary care study. *Rural and Remote Health* (online), 6(595).

Christenson, H. (2007). Internet Based Mental Health Interventions for Young Australians. Paper presented at the New South Wales Early Psychosis Forum, Westmead Hospital, Sydney.

Council of Australian Governments (COAG) (2012). *Roadmap for National Mental Health Reform 2012–2022*. Retrieved from www.coag.gov.au/node/482.

Department of Health (2011). *Victorian Health Priorities Framework 2012–2022: Rural and regional health plan*. Retrieved from http://docs.health.vic.gov.au/docs/doc/E9DF1F9EF227FF09CA2579680004BC2B/$FILE/1108032_Rural%20and%20Regional%20Health%20Plan%20WEB.pdf.

Department of Health and Ageing (2011). *Accessibility Remoteness Index of Australia (ARIA) Review Analysis of Areas of Concern – Final Report*. Retrieved from www.health.gov.au/internet/publications/publishing.nsf/Content/ARIA-Review-Report-2011.

Department of Health and Ageing (2012). *e-Mental Health Strategy for Australia*. Canberra: Australian Government. Retrieved from www.health.gov.au/internet/main/publishing.nsf/Content/D67E137E77F0CE90CA257A2F0007736A/$File/emstrat.pdf.

Department of Health and Ageing (2013). *Better Access to Psychiatrists, Psychologists and General Practitioners through the MBS (Better Access) initiative.* Retrieved from www.health.gov.au/internet/main/publishing.nsf/content/mental-ba.

Early Psychosis Writing Group (2010). *Australian Clinical Guidelines for Early Psychosis*, 2nd edn. Melbourne: ORYGEN Youth Health.

Endacott, R., Wood, A., Judd, F., Hulbert, C., Thomas, B. & Grigg, M. (2006). Impact and management of dual relationships in metropolitan, regional and rural mental health practice. *Australian and New Zealand College of Psychiatry, 40*: 987–94.

Glove box guide to mental health. (2012, 1 November 2012). *The Land.* Retrieved from www.theland.com.au/news/agriculture/agribusiness/general-news/mental-health-resources-for-the-bush/2632004.aspx.

Griffiths, K. M. & Christensen, H. (2007). Internet-based mental health programs: A powerful tool in the rural medical kit. *Australian Journal Rural Health, 15*: 81–7.

Jakowenko, J. (2012). Implementation guidelines for video consultations in general practice. In S. Benson, C. Preeston, C. Ryan, V. Wade, M. Civil & N. Pinskier (eds), 3rd edn. East Melbourne: Royal Australian College of General Practitioners.

Jones, R. (2013). In search of the 'prepared community': The way ahead for Australia? *Australian Journal of Emergency Management, 28*(1): 15–18.

Keen, T. & Lakeman, R. (2009). Collaboration with patients and families. In P. Barker (ed.), *Psychiatric and Mental Health Nursing. The craft of caring*, 2nd edn.(pp. 149–61)). London: Hodder Education.

Kilpatrick, S. (2009). Multi-level rural community engagement in health. *Rural and Remote Health, 17*: 39–44.

Lourey, C., Holland, C. & Green, R. (2012). *A Contributing Life: The 2012 national report card on mental health and suicide prevention.* Sydney: National Mental Health Commission. Retrieved from www.mentalhealthcommission.gov.au.

Morgan, V. A., Waterreus, A., Jablensky, A., Mackinnon, A., Mcgrath, J. J., Carr, V. J. et al. (2011). *People Living with Psychotic Illness 2010. Report on the second Australian national survey.* Canberra: Department of Health and Ageing.

New England Medicare Local (Producer). (2013). Aboriginal Health Services. Retrieved from www.neml.org.au/Aboriginal-Health-Services-19.

Preston, R., Waugh, H., Larkins, S. & Taylor, J. (2010). Community participation in rural primary health care: Intervention or approach? *Australian Journal of Primary Health, 16*: 4–16.

Proudfoot, J. (2013). The future is in our hands: The role of mobile phones in the prevention and management of mental disorders. *Australian and New Zealand Journal of Psychiatry, 47*(2): 111–13.

Purdie, N., Dudgeon, P. & Walker, R. (eds). (2010). *Working Together: Aboriginal and Torres Strait Islander mental health and wellbeing principles and practice.* Canberra: Commonwealth of Australia.

Purtell, C., Dowling, R.-M. & Fossey, E. (2008). Case management. Case management models: similarities and differences. In G. Meadows, B. Singh & M. Grigg (eds), *Mental Health in Australia: Collaborative practice*, 2nd edn. (pp. 343–5). Melbourne: Oxford University Press.

Queensland Health (2013). *Telehealth* (posted on 5 March). Retrieved from www.facebook.com/notes/queensland-health/telehealth/379845328790222.

Rickwood, D. J. (2012). Entering the e-spectrum: An examination of new interventions for youth mental health. *Youth Studies Australia, 31*(4): 18–27.

Rodd, H. & Stewart, H. (2009). The glue that holds our work together. The role and nature of relationships in youth work. *Youth Studies Australia, 28*(4): 4–10.

Saniotis, A. & Irvine, R. (2010). Climate change and the possible health effects on older Australians. *Australian Journal of Primary Health, 16*: 217–20.

Smith, J., Skrbis, Z. & Western, M. (2012). Beneath the 'digital native' myth. *Journal of Sociology, 49*(1): 97–118.

Statewide Telehealth Services (2013). *Extending the Reach of Clinical Health Services Throughout Queensland* [video www.youtube.com/watch?v=Hfl3iPk6t2o]. Brisbane: Queensland Health. Retrieved from www.health.qld.gov.au/telehealth/docs/testimonial_vid_text.pdf.

Wilson, R.L., Cruickshank, M. & Lea, J. (2012). Experiences of families who help young rural men with emergent mental health problems in a rural community in New South Wales, Australia. *Contemporary Nurse, 42*(2): 167–77.

World Health Organization (WHO) (2013). *Social Determinants of Health*. Retrieved from www.who.int/social_determinants/en.

Young, J. & McGrath, R. (2011). Exploring discourses of equity, social justice and social determinants in Australian health care policy and planning documents. *Australian Journal of Primary Health, 17*: 369–77.

Yung, A. (2013). Early intervention in psychosis: Evidence, evidence gaps, criticism and confusion. *Australian and New Zealand Journal of Psychiatry, 46*(1): 7–9.

14

Mental health in the interprofessional context

Denise McGarry and Anne Storey

Introduction 312
Historical professional precedents 312
Arguments for an interprofessional mental
   health workforce 313
The composition of the mental health
   workforce: Preparation and scope of
   practice 314
Regulation of the mental health
   workforce 321

Effectiveness of interprofessional
   workforces 323
Looking after yourself 326
Chapter summary 333
Critical thinking/learning activities 333
Learning extension 333
Further reading 333
References 334

Learning objectives

At the completion of this chapter, you should be able to:

- Describe the roles of traditional and emerging members of the interprofessional health care team.
- Identify different roles of the nurse.
- Discuss the changing nature of professionals contributing to mental health care.
- Recognise the preparation and expertise brought to mental health care by different professions.
- Understand regulation and standards governing the mental health workforce.
- Appreciate the strengths and weaknesses of the interprofessional team in mental health care.
- Recognise and appreciate the contribution of clinical supervision to the professional outcomes of mental health nursing.

Introduction

interprofessional
of, relating to, or
involving two or more
academic disciplines that
are usually considered
distinct to undertake a
task together

multidisciplinary
combining or involving
several academic
disciplines or professional
specialisations in an
approach to a topic or
problem

Regardless of the setting of mental health care, an **interprofessional** or **multidisciplinary** approach is a sound response to the multifaceted problems faced by people with mental illness. Different staff may contribute different expertise. Through collaboration with consumers, the needs of the person experiencing mental illness can be comprehensively met.

Such extensive engagement of an interprofessional model of care delivery does have some drawbacks. At times, the extent of overlap may result in the blurring of roles. Responsibilities may be uncertain or unclear. Consumers and their carers may find it difficult to identify whom to approach, especially if care is delivered across service organisations. Mental health services have responded with the development of a number of roles based on the function performed rather than the preparation for practice undertaken. Team leaders and case managers are examples of such roles.

An interprofessional workforce involves a range of professions and other staff with different preparatory backgrounds. These are broadening, increasingly, from the traditional professions employed in mental health services – medical, nursing, social work, psychology and occupational therapy – to embrace other workers with skills to contribute. These may be drawn from increasingly diverse educational backgrounds. Some of these groups are subject to regulation through their professional bodies and national regulatory authorities. Other groups working with the mental health workforce are not subject to such authority or regulation. This has supported the development of standards for the mental health workforce in Australia and New Zealand, in order to provide uniform and consistent guidelines to govern everyone delivering services to people experiencing mental illness.

This chapter reviews the range of workers who contribute to mental health care. It examines the differing programs of preparation undertaken by participants to support their expertise. The roles of traditional mental health care disciplines – psychiatry, nursing, social work, occupational therapy and psychology – are explored, as are those of emerging disciplines now entering the mental health workforce in greater numbers.

Historical professional precedents

Until the late 19th century, care for people experiencing mental illness was usually delivered outside of the medical paradigm. Families, religious and criminal justice systems played significant roles at different times. Today, their roles continue under various guises and to differing extents, and their influence continues to be felt. It is not infrequent that these out-dated models are perpetuated in the popular media, particularly in film.

It was late in the 19th century that care for the mentally ill was assumed by the medical profession. The medical profession was experiencing marked growth in expertise across a range of clinical areas, in part as a result of its adoption of the scientific model. It was hoped that advances in medical science would also apply to the problems of mental health. Luminaries in the field, including Sigmund Freud, did much to promote the notion of mental illness being amenable to medical intervention.

The two great wars of the 20th century also can be argued to have been instrumental in the alignment of mental health care with a medical paradigm. Large numbers of the young people from many of the nations of the world experienced mental illness following their exposure to these events.

The nursing workforce traditionally working in mental health services have evolved from the role of 'attendants'. During the early 20th century, localised training programs became increasingly formalised and by the mid-20th century had developed into a separate but equal nursing certificate, subject to regulation and professional nursing standards.

Social workers, occupational therapists and psychologists were later additions to the mental health workforce, becoming established during the middle of the 20th century. It would be negligent to fail to acknowledge the continuing role of religious institutions, whether formalised or not. Some services continue to be delivered by religious orders that have a long history of supporting the mentally ill, such as St John of God. Pharmacy is another professional group that has contributed to mental health care. The absolute numbers have been small, belying the importance of pharmacology in mental health care. However, it has been unusual to have staff from this profession solely focused on mental health care. Pharmacy services have often been sourced as needed by other health services.

Arguments for an interprofessional mental health workforce

Under the auspices of the World Health Organization, a committee was convened to consider issues of interprofessional education and workforce collaboration (Health Professions Networks, Nursing & Midwifery & Human Resources for Health, 2010). This committee is testament to the recognition given to the notion of interprofessional work, and its report was titled in part, 'A framework for action'. The message of this report was to promote an interprofessional workforce as a key response to an impeding global crisis in the health workforce. Further, the committee asserted that a health workforce characterised by interprofessional education and collaboration could deliver improved health outcomes for consumers, but concluded that this would represent a challenging cultural change for health services.

··

The composition of the mental health workforce: Preparation and scope of practice

Consumer narrative   Sal's story

scope of practice
in the health context, this refers to the range of work practices and activities undertaken by health professionals, according to the competence of the practitioners, education and training of the practitioners and regulatory authorities, and health-related legislation overseeing the practitioners; a 'scope of practice' is neither a job description nor a list of tasks or set of procedures

One of the questions you are routinely asked when attending a job interview is 'Have you worked in a multidisciplinary/ interdisciplinary team?' My answer is always a firm and resounding 'Yes', in spite of the lack of consensus in definitions of these terms. Yes to all definitions. I have always worked as part of a collaborative team; I work with people, and people are unique and complex. I would argue that you cannot work within health care and not be a part of a team, whether it be a formal or informal collaboration. How else do you meet all the unique and complex needs of the individual who has invited us in to assist her or him on the journey to recovery? The team structure and dynamics have differed depending on the environment, but the answer is always, 'Yes'. When I worked within the hospital environment, the teams were multidisciplinary, led by a medical professional and taking a coordinated (but biomedical and linear) approach to consumer care. Consumers were not involved in the decision-making process but were required to abide by the decisions the team made. In contrast, when I have worked within community environments, the collaborative team would be led by a team member who was not necessarily a medical professional. The client was actively involved in the decision-making process. So, I am always curious when I am part of an interview panel and the question is asked: 'Have you worked in a multidisciplinary/interdisciplinary team?' and the respondent answers 'No'.

Reflective questions

Sal describes two environments that involve multidisciplinary work in providing mental health services.

- What different needs would be better served by a different discipline?
- If team leaders had different professional preparation, how would this affect the service offered to people with mental illness and their carers? Consider issues such as client-centred care, intervention-offered leadership and family and carer concerns.

Traditional professions

Medicine

A range of medical professionals works within mental health services, including doctors, psychiatrists and registrars. Career medical officers are doctors whose preparation does not include advanced studies in psychiatry beyond their initial medical qualification. Their contribution is broad and somewhat akin to that of the general practitioner in the community setting. Registrars are enrolled in postgraduate medical studies in psychiatry. They progress through a number of placements in different mental health services as part of this education program. Their placement incorporates significant contribution to the services offered to consumers, under supervision of a qualified psychiatrist. Psychiatrists have completed their postgraduate studies and are registered as a separate division of medicine by the regulatory authority. Their professional body, the Royal Australian & New Zealand College of Psychiatrists, plays a central role in their regulation, standards and delivery of training.

Nursing

Nursing is a traditional part of the mental health workforce and has a dominant position in terms of numbers (Australian Institute of Health and Welfare (AIHW), 2012). One in 20 nurses works in mental health services (see Figure 14.1) – an estimated 15 557 nurses (registered and enrolled) of a total nursing workforce of 276 751, across Australia (AIHW, 2012).

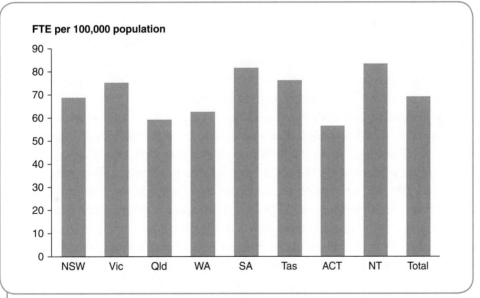

Figure 14.1 Mental health nurses, FTE per 100 000 population, states and territories, 2009.
Note: State and territory mental health nurses estimates should be treated with caution due to low response rates in some jurisdictions.
Source: AIHW, *Nursing and Midwifery Labour Force Survey, 2009.*

The preparation of and composition of nurses have changed significantly over the past 30 years in Australia. The First Division regulated nurse, or registered nurse (RN), became the standardised initial nursing preparation for employment in the mental health workforce from 2010. This is a comprehensive undergraduate nursing degree delivered through 41 Australian and New Zealand universities; it qualifies graduates for practice as a beginning health practitioner across all clinical environments. All courses include mandated theoretical subjects in mental health nursing and clinical placements in mental health services. The extent of this component is quite varied between different universities, in part due to difficulty in securing sufficient numbers of high-quality clinical placements and mental health nursing academics (Mental Health Nurse Education Taskforce, 2008).

Mental health nursing remains a contested specialty in nursing. The professional bodies, the Australian College of Mental Health Nursing, Inc. (ACMHN) and the New Zealand College of Mental Health Nursing, Inc. (NZCMHN) provide a credentialled award that recognises nurses with advanced qualifications in mental health nursing. The Australian government recognises the professional credentialling award of the ACMHN for employment in certain positions, notably those falling under the Mental Health Incentive Program. However, it is not a required award for working in other areas of this field.

Postgraduate courses are run by a number of tertiary education providers in mental health nursing. These courses do not bestow a different professional award as they do in medicine. Instead, the qualifications can support promotion to positions such as Clinical Nurse Specialist or Clinical Nurse Consultant. Nurse practitioners have a scope of practice regulated by the Australian Nurses & Midwifery Accreditation Council (ANMAC) and the Australian Health Practitioners Regulation Authority (AHPRA) following completion of a specific postgraduate program of study and successful application for a designated nurse practitioner position within a mental health service. The nurse practitioner (NP) was a new scope of practice launched by the Ministry of Health and the Nursing Council of New Zealand in May 2001. It is an advanced nursing role that is a unique blend of nursing and medical knowledge, clinical leadership, scholarship, research, planning and advocacy. NP positions in mental health nursing exist in child and adolescent services and emergency departments, but could be established in a range of other areas.

Second Division, or enrolled nurses (ENs), have been employed in small numbers across mental health services for many years. Their scope of practice must be supervised by a RN, and now includes administration of medication. Educational preparation for this role is ordinarily at an undergraduate diploma level, obtained through the Tertiary and Further Education (TAFE) sector. These courses do not include mandated mental health nursing curricula or clinical placement, although many individual institutions do include this preparation. ENs are now a required proportion of the skill mix in mental health services in some Australian state and territory health services, such as in New South Wales, where it is around 20 per cent.

Although not strictly part of the nursing workforce, Assistants-in-Nursing (AINs) is a recent inclusion in the mental health workforce. Some people employed in this role may be engaged in current studies for a Bachelor of Nursing (BN). Completion of two years of a BN and enrolment in the third year enables employment as an AIN. Alternatively, a formal qualification as an AIN can be obtained. This qualification can be obtained in the TAFE sector or from registered training organisations (RTOs) that include health services and other groups. This form of training is limited to around three to four weeks of formal education. The focus has been on aged care services, but some courses are now training students for work in acute medical and surgical health services. There is not as yet a dedicated preparation for work in mental health services, but this does not preclude employment in these services.

Social work

In mental health care, social work is a specialised field of practice that focuses on the social context and consequences of mental illness. The purpose of social work practice in mental health is to promote recovery, restore individual, family and community well-being, enhance development of each individual's power and control over his or her life and advance principles of social justice. Social workers are employed in treatment and rehabilitation services across the public, private and non-government mental health service sectors, as well as in primary health care (Australian Association of Social Workers (AASW), 2006). Social workers are not currently regulated under AHPRA.

Occupational therapy

Occupational therapists work to improve the functional performance of a person in order to achieve maximum independence. Their work is with people of all ages, aiming to overcome barriers to participation in the occupations and activities. Occupational therapists work in a wide range of mental health services, including in-patient and out-patient settings, in government and non-government organisations. Most occupational therapists work in community based positions. Their roles predominantly involve case management. Mental health occupational therapists primarily work with consumers, assessing the effects of mental illness on the person's ability to function in everyday occupations and roles. They also focus on how a person's lifestyle can support mental health and improve quality of life (Department of Human Services, 2006; Hayes et al., 2008).

Occupational therapists typically complete a four-year undergraduate program accredited by the Australian Association of Occupational Therapists (OT Australia). These degrees do not always require placement in a clinical in mental health services as a mandatory component of education. Occupational therapists have only recently become a regulated health practitioner workforce.

Psychology

Clinical psychologists are frequently the type of psychologist employed in mental health services. They have specialist training in treatment of mental illness. Clinical psychologists have a minimum of four years' university education, and usually including placements in mental health services. Clinical psychologists complete all the same basic training as other specialist psychologists (there are eight other specialist areas) but undertake a masters or doctorate program in clinical psychology in order to be eligible for membership of the Australian Psychological Society's (APS) College of Clinical Psychologists. Psychologists are regulated health practitioners under AHPRA.

Emerging professions

Aboriginal mental health workers

These members of the mental health workforce are university prepared through a three-year undergraduate program. They are not regulated health practitioners with AHPRA.

Consumer narrative — The teacher is the student: Cindi's story about a service's first trainee Aboriginal mental health worker

Three years ago I was fortunate to meet Kim, our service's first trainee Aboriginal mental health worker (TAMHW). I was immediately interested in being part of Kim's training program, and quickly became her clinical mentor and supervisor.

I worked with Kim to develop her skills in mental health care and provided support during her clinical placements, university education residencies and her transition into our workplace and organisation. During this time Kim had a comprehensive program requiring significant academic education combined with workplace learning and clinical placements throughout the sector. Having Kim in our service brought us the opportunity to review our cultural awareness practice and to offer Aboriginal clients an opportunity to be supported by a TAMHW.

Throughout this period I learned about Aboriginal mental health issues, culture and, ultimately, how a willingness to step beyond my own experience and comfort welcomed a new richness to my practice. Kim graduated last year, and that remains one of my proudest professional contributing accomplishments. Recently, I realised that initially I believed I was the teacher in our relationship; however, as Kim's graduation neared I realise that it was I who had been the student. I was able to learn new ways of thinking about my practice, about how I engaged with consumers and my personal and professional growth.

Reflective questions

- How might different professions maintain their disciplinary knowledge while working in interprofessional teams?
- How might consumers and carers maximise the benefits of interprofessional teams for their recovery?
- How do consumer and carer requirements of the interprofessional team differ?

Peer support and consumer consultants

Since the 1970s, the involvement of users of health services, in both policy development and service delivery, has been witnessed in Australia and New Zealand (Barnes & Cotterell, 2012). This has not been a development without controversy. At the heart of the debate is the conflict engendered by the 'insider–outsider' status of such workers.

This development can be understood by an overall rise in consumer movements, which in health services was in part implemented by the separation of providers and purchasers of services, in an effort to improve consumer choice. Another manifestation could be argued as being embedded in the development of service and organisational charters of patient rights and the like.

Mental health services have actively participated in engagement of service users and have faced similar challenges. In some small way the range of terminology employed and the debates surrounding accepted nomenclature are representative of some of the dilemmas that have been faced in the sector. These dilemmas also include the claim for representativeness that can be sustained by such workers. It is quite clear that no single worker, or indeed small group, could claim to represent the entire range of mental health service users.

Dietitians

A small but growing part of the mental health workforce, dietitians are making contributions to help with preventative and treatment approaches to the lives of people who experience mental illness. This is particularly important in addressing the metabolic syndrome that is increasingly experienced by this group. Dietitians are part of an unregulated workforce, prepared by a university program with a strong scientific framework. Mental health is not a compulsory component of this bachelor degree, although some students may undertake a mental-health specific clinical placement.

Speech pathologists

Expertise in swallowing and speech provide skills of particular usefulness for people experiencing mental illness. Dysphagia is a common experience of consumers being treated with anti-psychotic medications. Speech disorders are also prevalent. Speech pathologists undertake preparation at university through an undergraduate program with a strong scientific component. All students do not undertake mental health placements, but mental health theory is covered in most of these courses. Speech pathology is not a regulated profession in the health workforce.

Clergy

As historical providers of mental health services, the religious or clergy are perhaps not correctly designated an emerging part of the workforce in mental health. However, there is some resurgence in engagement by clergy, now utilising a multi-denominational model that more accurately reflects the spiritual allegiances of consumers of mental health services.

Police

The police force has held a critical role in mental health services as the first point of contact of many people experiencing distress. Under the mental health legislation of many jurisdictions, police officers are frequently given power to transport people involuntarily to designated places for assessment of their mental health. Police officers are educated through a mix of training provided within the police force in the community and at university level. Education about mental illness is variable, both across time and jurisdiction, but mental illness is always addressed as a topic. This is because of the special powers of police and also because of their pivotal role at times of crisis for people experiencing mental illness.

Paramedics

The education of the paramedic workforce is currently transitioning from training within the ambulance service, to education within a university structure. As first responders in the health workforce, paramedics also perform this role in mental health services. Special powers are increasingly being conferred upon paramedics under mental health legislation to transport people involuntarily to mental health services for assessment (see, for example, Section 20 of the *Mental Health Act 2007* (NSW)). Paramedics are currently unregulated in the Australian health workforce.

Hospital and community pharmacists

Specialist mental health pharmacy professionals are not commonly employed in the mental health sector. This regulated health practitioner workforce makes critical contributions to interventions in mental health care. Within the hospital environment, it could probably be argued that the contribution of pharmacists is more specialised, due to the extensive role of psycho-pharmacology in helping consumers attain recovery. However, community pharmacists have an important collaborative role to help maintain a consumer's well-being in the community. Pharmacists are prepared with an undergraduate bachelor degree.

Technical and further education (TAFE) preparation

TAFE institutions are the providers of education preparation for both ENs and a range of other participants in the mental health workforce. These educational programs are increasing the range and diversity of workers providing mental health care. Such programs include courses such as counselling, community welfare work and the like. Many of the graduates of these programs are more highly represented in non-government organisations than in the public health system.

Counsellor

This part of the mental health workforce is an unregulated group whose educational training can be extremely varied. Some undertake formal, assessed programs, but essentially this is not a requirement to be self-described as a counsellor. Approaches and interventions can widely vary. Employment is primarily within non-government organisations.

Welfare worker

This non-regulated health practitioner has a similar role to counsellors, with varied educational preparation. The non-government organisation sector is the primary employer for these workers in the mental health services.

Regulation of the mental health workforce

New Zealand has health regulatory authorities under the *Health Practitioners Competence Assurance Act 2003* that are responsible for the registration and oversight of practitioners in specified health professions. Each of the regulatory authorities describes scopes of practice for its profession, prescribes necessary qualifications, registers practitioners and issues annual practising certificates. These authorities also set standards of competence. The regulatory authorities, through professional conduct committees, can investigate individual practitioners' competence and conduct.

Australia commenced a national registration scheme for the pre-existing 14 registered health professions in 2010, and announced the intention to extend registration to include others progressively. The new body created to coordinate this scheme is AHPRA. Each profession has a national board that is supported by AHPRA and is charged with the primary role of protection of the public. AHPRA manages the registration of health professionals and of students around Australia. It is the body to which any member of the public may make a **notification** about a health professional or student. On behalf of the national boards, except in New South Wales, where the Health Professional Councils and Authority and the Health Care Complaints Commission perform the role, AHPRA manages investigations into professional conduct, performance and the health of registered health professionals. It also publishes national registers of health professionals in a manner accessible to the public. AHPRA works with the individual boards in development of registration standards, codes and guidelines.

notification conveying facts with the intention to apprise a person of a proceeding in which his or her interests are involved, or informing of some fact which the informer has a legal duty to communicate

Registered health professionals are those legally able to practise, within the scope of their registration. The current regulated health professions are Aboriginal and Torres Strait Islander health practitioners, Chinese medicine practitioners, chiropractors, dental practitioners, medical practitioners, medical radiation practitioners, nurses, midwives, occupational therapists, optometrists, osteopaths, pharmacists, physiotherapists, podiatrists and psychologists.

Some of these professions, including dental practitioners, medical practitioners and nurses have divisions into which are grouped specialties or health practitioners with different scopes of practice or preparation. Nursing has two divisions: First Division, or RNs with a bachelor degree in nursing, and Second Division, or ENs, whose preparation is at an undergraduate diploma level provided by the TAFE sector.

Employment within mental health services is not defined by registration. There is no specific group whose scope of practice is exclusively mental health services. However, medical practice includes the specialty of psychiatry, which has extended preparation to equip these health practitioners for work in mental health services.

Clearly, the mental health workforce includes more than registered health practitioners. Primary among these are social workers, who have long been part of the mental health workforce. But many of the professions who have more recently joined the mental health workforce, such as speech pathologists, dietitians and AINs, are not regulated through AHPRA.

Professional bodies

Professional bodies are also called professional associations or societies. They are groupings of professionals organised by the professionals themselves to further the interests of that profession and the individuals engaged in the profession, and to protect the public. The roles of these bodies are multifaceted, but share as a central tenet the self-regulation of the professions' scope of practice. This control of the profession is powerful and closely linked with the professional bodies' role in protection of the public. In some ways these aspects of professional bodies are in conflict. Protection of the public is addressed by standards of practice, ethics and education. However, professional bodies also have characteristics of trade unions in their roles to promote the interests of their members and profession. In this way, professional bodies can be charged with promoting self-interest and control of the profession.

In mental health nursing, the professional bodies in Australia and New Zealand (ACMHN and NZCMHN) can be seen as embodying this contradiction. They are involved in protection of the public by developing standards for practice in this specialist field. They are also involved in policy development to establish the educational preparation standards recognised for practice in this field. Although intertwined with protection of the public, such argument can also be interpreted as an effort to control this part of the health workforce.

Professional standards for practice

Mental health nursing in Australia has a set of practice standards devised by its professional body (Australian College of Mental Health Nurses Inc. (ACMHN), 2010). However, these standards are voluntarily adopted by nurses practising in mental health, and have no formal regulatory authority. Nursing practice in the field is also guided by competency standards administered by the Nursing and Midwifery Board of Australia, which are recognised by AHPRA (Australian Nursing and Midwifery Council, 2006). Overarching standards for the mental health workforce have been developed by the Australian government to guide all health practitioners, irrespective of their profession (Commonwealth of Australia, 2010). As with the mental health nursing practice standards, the national standards do not have formal regulatory status, but carry much informal weight in circumstances in which professional practice is called to account.

The substance of the national standards for the mental health workforce is to provide guidelines for the development and implementation of appropriate practices and to promote continuous improvements in services. The standards are constructed for application across the breadth of services. Many of the standards are designed to allow assessment and measurement. The revised standards of 2010 included a recovery standard – a new addition that reflected in some part the active involvement of people with mental illness and carers in the development and revision of these standards.

The consumer standard addresses the rights, responsibilities and expectations that may be held for services available to those with mental illness. Implementation of the standards is monitored in part through service accreditation systems.

The Ministry of Health in New Zealand is the government agency concerned with health policy, regulation and monitoring, among other functions. TePou o TeWhakaaro Nui is the National Centre for Mental Health Research, Information and Workforce Development. The development of the first national mental health strategy in New Zealand was fundamental to the growth and quality improvement seen up to 2005. *Te Tahuhu – Improving Mental Health 2005–2015: The second New Zealand mental health and addiction plan* (Ministry of Health, 2005) augments the plan, *Looking Forward and Moving Forward Together with TeKokiri: The mental health and addiction action plan 2006–2015* (Ministry of Health, 2006).

'Let's get real' is the mandated governmental framework from the *Te Tahuhu – Improving Mental Health 2005–2015* plan (Ministry of Health, 2005). It sets out the standards expected of people working within mental health services, irrespective of the type of organisation, profession or consumer group. 'Let's get real' comprises seven 'real skills' that are interrelated. The development of 'Let's get real' and the 'real skills' emerged from competency frameworks for mental health and addiction treatment services within New Zealand.

Effectiveness of interprofessional workforces

Historically, consumers of mental health services have been passive recipients of care, with minimal say about how care was decided or delivered. Recovery based care emerged from a growing consumer movement in the 1970s–80s, designed to increase consumer involvement in care planning and treatment (Deegan, 1988). In the literature, recovery is depicted as a movement, paradigm, model and philosophy (Clearly & Dowling, 2009). Recovery is difficult to define, and every individual's journey is self-defined and unique, with the consumer considered an expert on his or her own needs. All journeys of recovery are highly individual, but the recovery model of mental health has as its underpinning a philosophy of empowerment, hope and therapeutic optimism.

Within the National Standards for a Mental Health 2010, a recovery based approach to service delivery is emphasised (Commonwealth of Australia, 2010), with recovery stated as a sense of hope, meaning and purpose in life, and an understanding of one's abilities and disabilities alongside with a personal and social identity. The term 'consumer' refers to a person who has experienced some form of mental illness that has involved use of mental health services. Implicit in the notion of recovery is the position that the consumer is active in her or his treatment plan, and that the treatment is an equal partnership between the consumer and the interprofessional team (IPT).

The concept of recovery has changed the ways in which mental health services are now structured within Australia and New Zealand. Consumer and carer participation has been an important aspect of government policy for approximately 20 years, requiring consumer input into mental health service planning and delivery. An underpinning principle of the National Standards for a Mental Health Workforce 2010 states that consumers should educate mental health professionals while also having an active role in planning, implementation and evaluation of mental health services (Commonwealth of Australia, 2010). While this can be seen as a positive move for inclusive, recovery based mental health services, it could be seen conversely as tokenistic, given that of the 208 specialised mental health service organisations in Australia in 2010–11, only 46.6 per cent employed mental health consumer workers (AIHW, 2012). Policies to promote recovery are often vague and have no clearly articulated guidelines for implementation into practice (Happell, 2008b). Lack of training and inadequate training for consumers in requisite skills reduce their confidence and capacity to participate effectively within the IPT.

The recovery model emphasises hope, empowerment and connectedness with life while also acknowledging the difficulties of living with a mental illness. Recovery is viewed as a process, a way of life in approaching life's challenges. The main focus is on strengths of the consumer and not simply management of the symptoms of the illness or medications (Camann, 2010; Deegan, 1996; Warner, 2009) Empowerment of consumers through goal setting and participation in their care is central to the recovery model. (Happell, 2008a; Camann, 2010). It has been stated that a new concept of wellness or well-being has superseded the recovery movement. The focus of well-being is to move away from the biomedical model of diagnosis and treatment to a model of resilience, social inclusion, growth and participation (Ning, 2010). Whether the term 'recovery' or 'well-being' is used, the challenge remains for mental health professionals within the IPT to expand and grow in a very different paradigm.

Teamwork

Teams matter in mental health, given the increasingly complex, knowledge-rich environment in which mental health professionals work. The IPT comprises a range of professionals from different agencies or organisations, working together to deliver comprehensive, consumer-centred care. This care is delivered under the umbrella of the IPT and can convey benefits to the consumer with specialised expert advice while also providing efficient use of resources. As the consumer's circumstances change, the IPT needs to adjust recovery plans and perhaps also its composition as it relates to that individual to reflect the consumer's changing requirements.

New, evidence-based therapies are constantly emerging; pharmaceuticals are changing while changes in policies can have a direct effect on a consumer's finances or ability to work. No single professional group can be versed in all areas of a consumer's recovery. For a team to work effectively there needs to be collaboration along with respect; shared leadership including sharing of power. This can be on the basis of knowledge and experience, not necessarily of roles. For an IPT to function effectively, the team needs to work together and independently, relying on each other's knowledge and expertise to carry out tasks required to achieve the desired goal.

This method of working can be daunting for many members of the IPT, as it challenges the traditional, biomedical model of mental health care in which the doctor has been the team leader. The recovery model requires a shift in IPT values and attitudes, but mostly it requires a fundamental shift in the power base. Recovery shifts power to the consumer, thereby challenging all IPT members' roles. Recovery challenges the IPT to develop practices that are less formal, allows a consumer to take risks and encourages independence, not **co-dependence**. This requires the function and values of the IPT to change: with more discussion than direction, strengths-based, not psychopathology and autonomous rather than paternalistic values. Empowerment of the consumer represents the civil right to autonomy and addresses power inequalities.

> **co-dependence**
> a psychological condition or a relationship in which a person is controlled or manipulated by another who is affected with a pathological condition (such as an addiction to alcohol or other substances); broadly, dependence on the needs of or control by another

Barriers to implementation of IPT

Barriers to implementation of a recovery based IPT stem from the biomedical approach to mental health. Traditionally, many mental health professionals have worked within the custodial form of mental health, with the biomedical approach being the dominant model of care. This has led inadvertently to dependence on the biomedical approach to care, with many consumers only receiving care within a hospital setting. Unfortunately, this directly affects the effectiveness of the recovery model and needs to be addressed if the recovery approach is to be authentically engaged.

With a blurring of roles within the IPT, mental health nurses are at times unclear about the role they are to perform. It can be challenging for members of the IPT to have a thorough understanding of each team member's role. The consumer can find it even more difficult to know who is responsible for his or her housing concerns, or medication issues, for example. Lack of role clarity extends to many mental health nurses who are unsure of their roles and have difficulty describing mental health nursing.

Nurses' stigmatising attitudes towards mental illness can directly affect the functioning of the IPT when nurses are unable to acknowledge the person behind the mental illness (Storm, Hausken & Mikkelson, 2010). Some mental health nurses nominate caring, counselling and alleviation of distress as their main roles within the IPT, whereas others talk of maintaining control and administering medications (O'Brien & Cole, 2004). Nurses risk playing a very limited role within the IPT if they do not clarify and define their own roles.

Individuals who need to work collaboratively need to temper their independence. Reciprocal interdependence is defined as individuals working together while actively coordinating care in collaboration with the consumer (Bharwani, Harris & Southwick, 2012). This can only occur if the team members have appropriate expertise and are able to speak safely, freely, openly and meaningfully with each other. Recovery for any consumer requires a well-functioning IPT, yet skills required for the team to work together are rarely addressed. These challenges need to be communicated, acknowledged, discussed and explored if the IPT is to work in the true sense of the recovery model.

With the increasing drive for IPT, new problems have arisen regarding who should be the team leader, how responsibility is to be shared, how the role of the doctor has changed and whether all members of the team are ready for this change. IPT models encourage partnership and collaboration and, with this, trust and respect for each team member along with the most appropriate skills mix for the consumer. Mental health nurses working within the IPT can take on the role of facilitator of individual consumer journeys, which is a much more comprehensive and consumer-centred approach to care than the traditional custodial approach. With their broad educational backgrounds and therapeutic experience with consumers, mental health nurses are in a perfect position to champion this role.

Each IPT will have a different approach, although every team should be based on sharing roles, power and knowledge. Leadership has emerged as a dominant theme in studies of IPTs (Lingard et al., 2012). Due to the structures of many medical models within the Australian and New Zealand health care systems, consumers may only be referred to another professional by a medical doctor, and many diagnostic tests may only be ordered by doctors. Therefore, regardless of the model that defines an IPT, it will still operate within a larger system in which a doctor's authority is required for certain procedures, such as involuntary admission, seclusion, discharge, ordering tests and referring consumers. This confers a special position upon doctors, with rights and responsibilities in the health system in part due to insurance arrangements. Although this may not be problematic, it does create a tension and a power imbalance on the IPT team. Due to their medico-legal responsibilities, doctors may be obliged to take control or be responsible for the team. With each health care worker expected to be part of the team, ultimately doctors may bear the responsibility and accountability in greater measure.

Looking after yourself

In personal terms, health care work can be one of the most stressful and costly for workers. Support systems such as mentoring, clinical supervision and preceptorship are essential for all health care workers. Mental health nursing is reliant on therapeutic communication skills, humanistic philosophy and knowledge of psychological therapies; therefore, traditional models of mentoring and preceptorship may not be adequate to address these needs. The development of clinical supervision (CS) is ideally suited to mental health nursing staff whose primary goal is caring for consumers with a mental illness. Clinical supervision incorporates a skills-based approach (reflection), which is often lacking in other forms of mentoring. CS is a formal mentoring arrangement that enables nurses to discuss their work.

Clinical supervision

The term 'clinical supervision' is used to describe regular, planned periods of time between a supervisor and supervisee. The time period is usually one hour per month during working hours, at a mutually convenient time and place. Supervision provides a safe, confidential and supportive forum for the nurse to reflect on past clinical experiences.

The phrase 'professional supervision' is used in New Zealand in place of CS. CS is an implied expectation of the legislative and regulatory requirements for nurses working in New Zealand in the mental health and addiction sector. All professional bodies for mental health nursing in New Zealand, including the Nursing Council of New Zealand, TeAoMaramatanga New Zealand College of Mental Health Nurses, along with the Drug and Alcohol Practitioners Association of Aotearoa New Zealand, support CS. Through CS nurses have an opportunity to embed 'Let's get real' into their organisational culture.

Although there is no agreed single definition of CS in the nursing literature (Lynch, Happell & Sharrock, 2008), in general CS can be defined as a process of reflection upon practice. The aim of this reflection is to improve clinical practice and hence consumer outcomes while supporting and encouraging the supervisee. Yegdich (1999) asserted that the nature of CS has as its narrative the patient's human suffering. What is examined in supervision is the effect of the consumer's suffering on the nurse's ability to respond, interact and think. It can be seen as identifying solutions to problems and increasing understanding of professional issues. CS is a process of learning and professional support, in which nurses are assisted in developing their practice through reflective discussions with knowledgeable and experienced supervisors. The aim of CS is to focus on the moment and to facilitate awareness of feelings and behaviours with an appropriate response to these feelings, allowing the nurse to return to the consumer with an increase in confidence. The purpose of CS is to improve nursing practice, and the focus is always on the nurse–patient interaction and relationship.

Nurses who engage therapeutically in a helping relationship find it is both demanding and complicated. In this relationship both the nurse and consumer need to be understood. The consumer cannot be understood independently of the nurse. The nurse has her or his own unique nature, which will inevitably interact with the consumer; the nurse contributes to what transpires during therapy. Emotion can take precedence over logic in decision-making. CS helps the nurse to reflect on feelings as well as thinking, which can be a catalyst for positive behavioural change. Therefore, what is examined and reflected upon in CS is the nurse's ability to think, respond and interact.

CS improves the nurse's ability to confirm the consumer as a unique individual. It also increases the nurse's ability to support the consumer and to be in a relationship with the consumer. While providing an opportunity for the nurse to consider his or her contribution to the therapeutic relationship, CS provides a safe forum in which nurses might contemplate their own emotional reactions.

The framework of CS is commonly built on Bridget Proctor's Interactive Framework of Clinical Supervision (cited in Sood & Driscoll, 2004). The three interactive elements of CS present a clear framework for training. These elements are, first, the formative function (learning) in which the clinical supervisor encourages the supervisee to reflect on practice, and second, the restorative function (support) in which the supervisor is concerned with how the supervisee responds emotionally to the stresses and demands of mental health nursing. The third element is the normative (accountability) function in which the supervisor is concerned with maintaining and monitoring the effectiveness of the supervisee's everyday work.

Although these three elements were intended to be applied equally, they tend to compete or overlap. The tool, although useful, may not necessarily be the best construct for experienced mental health nurses. According to Driscoll (2007), Proctor's framework is useful for a beginning supervisee, although with increasing experience other frameworks can be incorporated.

The framework for CS can also be guided by two main categories of supervision models, depending on the skill and background of the supervisor. The supervision-specific models and the psychotherapy-based models. The psychotherapy-based models use the distinct methods and orientation of psychotherapy to guide CS, which could be in the form of role therapy or psychodynamic approaches. The second category includes cognitive therapy supervision, guided by Heron's six-category intervention analysis, and solution-focused supervision (Heron, 1989; Driscoll 2007).

CS was implemented as a mandatory tool following clinical governance problems years ago in many jurisdictions both in Australia and New Zealand as well as, notably, the United Kingdom. The misperception that CS is a management tool for governance has coloured some health practitioners' beliefs about the purpose of CS. The emphasis needs to be very clear to all staff that CS is not managerial supervision, mandatory counselling or management scrutiny (Yegdich & Cushing 1998). Confusion remains about the function of CS, with many nurses suspicious of managerial involvement. Workplace culture can also be a barrier to implementing CS in organisations that do not acknowledge, encourage or provide time for staff members to attend CS. Nurses need constant reassurance that CS is confidential and not managerial scrutiny. Supervisors and management encouraging CS need to be above the suspicion, tokenism and resistance that has plagued CS, and should demonstrate a robust evidence base for CS (Cottrell, 2002).

Managerial support and collaboration, including upper and middle management and educators, are important for successful implementation of CS. Nursing has struggled with CS due to its association with failure and professional frailty. This suspicion can be reduced by holding sessions away from the workplace, allowing supervisees to choose their supervisors based on their own needs and the skills of the supervisor (Edwards, Burnard & Hannigan, 2006; Mullarkey, Keeley & Playle, 2001).

Unless the purpose and benefits of CS are clearly defined, it is unlikely that CS will ever become an embedded universal practice for nurses (Clearly & Freeman, 2005).

Clinical supervisors need to be trained and competent, especially in group dynamics and interpersonal communication. Supervisors need to be competent in dealing with the interpersonal anxieties that can so often emerge within supervision. When CS is implemented it is essential that it is continuous and consistent, with clear aims and benefits specified, along with the model of CS clearly articulated. Inconsistent supervision leads to supervisees feeling that CS is not important or relevant. Nurses have reported that it is often difficult to prioritise time for CS (Cottrel, 2002). This may be a cultural aspect of nursing; another perspective is that the human pain nurses see on a daily basis necessitates quarantined, prioritised time for CS, which is when management support is essential (Cottrell, 2002).

Models for CS include group supervision, open or closed groups, one-to-one supervision with a supervisor from the same discipline or a different discipline, one-to-one peer supervision and networking supervision (Butterworth, Bishop & Carson 1996). Group supervision is the most common model and the most cost-effective, involving a supervisor facilitating a group of nurses. This provides a rich environment for learning and feedback regarding consumer care. Rotating rosters often necessitate open-group CS, which unfortunately also adds the burden of constantly changing participants and potential problems with confidentiality and group cohesion.

In South Australia, a group of mental health nurses met monthly for peer CS, facilitated by a different group leader each month. Every group member participated as the supervisor, and the results demonstrated a strong sense of cohesion (Walsh et al., 2003).

Telephone CS has also been used as a one-to-one supervision method, and it has been expanded to include group CS. Group CS by telephone or video-conferencing provides an excellent medium for short-term CS, particularly for remote area nurses (Rosenfield, 2003). With various forms of technology available today, CS can be offered within various rural and remote regions of Australia and New Zealand.

A Finnish study found that models of CS varied depending on the different phases of a nurse's career. The changing models and demands of CS are important characteristics to be highlighted when considering implementation (Sirola-Karvinen & Hyrkas, 2008). Reflective skills in nursing take time to develop and to be utilised appropriately. Therefore, an effort to support nurses in CS should be a constructive and collaborative experience, while also providing an opportunity for safe professional development that ultimately leads to improvement in consumer-centred care.

It is clear that a one-size-fits-all approach is definitely not the desired way to implement CS. Management needs to be directly involved at all levels in supporting and encouraging all mental health nurses to attend CS. Nurses need to be involved in the decision-making and the desired framework of CS that suits their individual needs at their specific stage of their career. Supervisees must be freely able to choose their supervisor, one who has had formal training in CS, and should feel comfortable in changing their supervisor if required, without management scrutiny.

Consumer narrative

Raining blood: James's reflection on an emergency application of team training

You would have heard many stories of how someone can go into 'auto pilot' when faced with an emergency. This emergency happened in the afternoon. The ward I was working in was settled and I was walking to the kitchen to get a coffee. An alarm went off. I asked a colleague what the alarm was, and he responded that it was a push-button in a remote part of a campus we were close to, so I put down my coffee and started to run.

Running in response to an alarm was generally enjoyable as a large majority of the alarms on this side of campus were either false or easily managed with the extra clinical staff numbers. Attending alarms is a social occasion; you get to talk to those you have worked with previously and get some fresh air at the same time. While running towards the sound of the alarm, a sense of urgency fell on us as we saw a nurse standing at the front of the building. I sprinted ahead and thought the nurse was laughing. I felt silly when I realised she was in hysterics, with blood all over her hands.

This moment, however bizarre it may sound, I remember as a movie, where the background went out of focus, sounds other than the nurse's voice become dull. I asked her what had happened, wanting to know what I was running into. Her colleague had been stabbed in the chest. While she was telling me this I looked at her wounds; they looked defensive, inflected by a blade. She did not appear to be in immediate danger, but she was still potentially in harm's way. She continued to incoherently and rapidly tell me aspects of the situation. Without thinking I loudly and firmly ordered her to wait on the other side of the road, further down from where cars would be coming from. I called 000 for ambulance assistance and while on the phone ran to the building where the event had occurred. The clearest image I remember is of drops of blood, 5 centimetres in diameter, spreading after hitting concrete wet from previous rain. I had never seen so much blood.

I wasn't experienced in emergency responses and I had never been in a situation like this. I have never experienced an adrenaline rush such as this. However, I was able to assess the nurse's wound, and to function in a way completely out of character – taking on an authoritarian role – and to prioritise to safely and quickly manage the situation. This situation of 'autopilot' is actually an example of training and education coming into effect.

Reflective questions

The contrast James describes between his expectation of a social team response and the reality of this particular emergency call is stark.

- What feelings could arise? Does this disparity occur in other areas of nursing?
- Is it important to resolve the feelings engendered by this event?
- How could this be achieved?

Consumer narrative

Kristen's story: Billy returns to country

Billy is a 50-year-old Aboriginal man, born and bred in Collarenebri, also known as Kamilaroi country. Billy has a diagnosis of paranoid schizophrenia and is currently being treated under the Forensic Mental Health Act. He has been a client of a local community mental health team in Sydney. Over two years ago, Billy relapsed and severely injured himself. The result was brutal damage to the bottom half of both his legs, particularly his heels. Billy was confined to a wheelchair and progressed to crutches over time.

As I was new to the service I started working with Billy after his accident. Over the two years that Billy lived in Sydney and waited for his heels to heal, as the Aboriginal Mental Health Clinician I worked very closely with Billy while thoroughly monitoring his mental state to prevent any relapses. Further investigating into Billy's past I found that he had a history of extreme drug and alcohol misuse, and this I learned had contributed to Billy's illness. Billy has since been abstinent from all drugs and alcohol.

From the time I began to work with Billy, I noticed the lack of a culturally appropriate practice by all services in Sydney that had contributed to Billy's care. As an Aboriginal person myself, I knew that an Aboriginal man from the outback needed cultural contact in order to feel safe and comfortable. This is when I stepped in. I would meet with Billy on a regular basis, and I escorted him to the Ku-Ring-Gai National Park to meet with the Aboriginal Ranger, Les. Les would take us on tours comfortable enough for Billy to enjoy and relax. Billy would also comment to me, 'I feel recharged'. This happened a fair few times during the two years. During a home visit to Billy the home care nurse dressing his wounds noticed that there had been no change in the healing of his left heel. This concerned me.

After visiting the specialist at St. Vincent's Hospital, it was decided that Billy could either wait longer and see if the heel would repair, or his leg could be amputated. Billy knew it would not heal, so made the brave decision to have it amputated. I have never known a person to be so patient during such a tremendously stressful time. Billy's bottom left leg was amputated. He received a prosthesis and took to rehabilitation. Soon enough, Billy was walking around like he had two healthy legs.

This is where the other challenge comes in. I wanted to return Billy to his country, Kamilaroi country. I wanted to return Billy to his family, return him to where he belongs. I knew Billy needed to return home to continue to heal his spirit. This was then my mission. With Billy's case managers I liaised with the services near his home town to take over Billy's care. The final challenge was the Forensic Mental Health Tribunal. We put up a fair case of Billy's progress over the years and his recovery since the incident. Billy was allowed to return home. This was when I saw the biggest smile on Billy's face in the two years I had worked alongside him. It was my great pleasure to have met Billy and to have had such a positive outcome.

Reflective questions

Consider Kristen's story about Billy's return to country. List the different professions that had contributed to this outcome.

- What particular expertise might they have lent to it?

Kristen's story addresses the importance of country to Aboriginal mental health.

- Investigate the means by which Aboriginal mental health clinicians can be contacted and involved in the care of Aboriginal people experiencing mental illness.
- What policies are there to guide work of Aboriginal and Torres Strait Islander peoples?

Chapter summary

- The roles of the traditional members of the interprofessional health care team and different roles of the nurse were identified.
- Changing professionals or skills mix contributing to mental health care were explored against an evaluation of their different preparations for practice in mental health services and that of the traditional mental health workforce.
- Regulation and standards governing the mental health workforce were discussed against the preparation and education of the different professions.
- Strengths and weaknesses of the IPT were explored as they exist in mental health care.
- The contribution of clinical supervision to the professional outcomes of mental health nursing was described and different models analysed.

Critical thinking/learning activities

1 Is goodwill sufficient preparation to work in the mental health workforce?
2 What minimal levels of educational preparation should be required for the (specialist) mental health workforce?
3 What constitutes a mental health environment for clinical placement purposes in undergraduate preparation?

Learning extension

When does a peer support worker's allegiance to consumer advocacy change to organisational loyalty? Does payment, the nature of the employment body or participation in policy development influence this?

Prepare a class debate to explore these issues, addressing the proposition:

The concept of peer support workers is doomed to failure as peer support workers cannot serve two masters.

Further reading

Australian College of Mental Health Nurses Inc. (2010). *Standards for Mental Health Nursing in Australia 2010*. Retrieved from www.mhtlc.gov.au/sites/default/files/ACMHN_Standards_2010.pdf.

Commonwealth of Australia (2010). *National Standards for Mental Health Services 2010*. Retrieved from www.health.gov.au/internet/main/publishing.nsf/Content/DA71C0838BA6411BCA2577A0001AAC32/$File/servst10v2.pdf.

....

References

Australian Association of Social Workers (AASW) (2006). *Social Work in Mental Health Care*. Retrieved from www.aasw.asn.au/document/item/2061.

Australian College of Mental Health Nurses Inc. (ACMHN) (2010). *Standards of Practice for Australian Mental Health Nurses 2010*. Canberra: Author.

Australian Institute of Health and Welfare (AIHW) (2009). *Nursing and Midwifery Labour Force Survey, 2009*. Canberra: Australian Government.

AIHW (2012). *Mental Health Services in Australia*. Canberra: Australian Government.

Australian Nursing and Midwifery Council (2006). *National Competency Standards for Registered Nurses*, 4th edn. Dickson, ACT: Author.

Barnes, **M.** & **Cotterell**, **P.** (eds). (2012). *Critical Perspectives on User Involvement*. Bristol, UK: The Policy Press.

Bharwarni, **A.**, **Harris**, **C.** & **Southwick**, **S.** (2012). A business school view of medical interprofessional rounds: Transforming rounding groups into rounding teams. *Academic Medicine, 87*: 1768–71.

Butterworth, **T.**, **Bishop**, **V.** & **Carson**, **J.** (1996). First steps towards evaluating clinical supervision in nursing. Theory, policy and practice development A review. *Journal of Clinical Nursing, 24*(1): 32–4.

Camann, **M.A.** (2010). The psychiatric nurse's role in application of recovery and decision-making models to integrate health behaviours in the recovery process. *Issues in Mental Health Nursing, 31*: 532–6.

Clearly, **A.** & **Dowling**, **M.** (2009). Knowlege and attitudes of mental health professionals in Ireland to the concept of recovery in mental health: A questionnaire survey. *Journal of Psychiatric and Mental Health Nursing, 16*: 539–45.

Clearly, **A.** & **Freeman**, **A** (2005). The realities of clinical supervision in an acute inpatient mental health setting. *Issues in Mental health Nursing, 26* (5): 489–505.

Commonwealth of Australia (2010). *National Standards for a Mental Health Workforce 2010*. Canberra: Author.

Cottrell, **S.** (2002). Suspicion, resisitance, tokenism and mutiny: Problematic dynamics relevant to the implementation of clinical supervision in nursing. *Journal of Psychiatric and Mental health Nursing, 9* (6): 667–71.

Deegan, **P.** (1988). Recovery: The lived experience of rehabilitation. *Psychosocial Rehabiitation Journal, 11*(4): 11–18.

Deegan, **P.** (1996). Recovery and the Conspiracy of Hope. Paper presented to the Sixth Annual Mental Health Services Conference of Australia and New Zealand, Brisbane.

Department of Human Services (2006). *Occupational Therapy Labour Force Survey: Victoria 2003–04*. Melbourne: State Government of Victoria.

Driscoll, **J.** (ed.) (2007). *Practicing Clinical Supervision. A reflective approach for healthcare professionals*, 2nd edn. Edinburgh: Elsevier.

Edwards, **D.**, **Burnard**, **P.** & **Hannigan**, **B.** (2006). Clinical supervision and burnout. The influence of clinical supervision for community mental health nurses. *Journal of Clinical Nursing, 15*(8): 1007–15.

Happell, **B.** (2008a). Determining the effectiveness of mental health services from a consumer perspective. Part 1: Enhancing recovery. *International Journal of Mental Health Nursing, 17*(2): 116–22.

Happell, **B.** (2008b). Determining the effectiveness of mental health services from a consumer perspective: Part 2: Barriers to recovery and principles for evaluation. *International Journal of Mental Health Nursing, 17*(2): 123–30.

Hayes, **R.**, **Bull**, **B.**, **Hargreaves**, **K.** & **Shakespeare**, **K.** (2008). A survey of the recruitment and retention issues for occupational therapists working clinically in mental health. *Australian Occupational Therapy Journal, 55*: 12–22.

Health Professions Networks, Nursing & Midwifery & Human Resources for Health (2010). *Framework for Action on Interprofessional Education & Collaborative Practice*. Geneva: World Health Organization.

Heron, **J.** (1989). *Six Category Intervention Analysis*, 3rd edn. Surrey, UK. Human Potential Resource Group, University of Surrey.

Lingard, **M.**, **Durrant**, **M.**, **Fleming-Caroll**, **B.**, **Lowe**, **M.**, **Rahotte**, **J.**, **Sinclair**, **L.** & **Tallett**, **S.** (2012). Conflicting messages: Examining the dynamics of leadership on interprofessional teams. *Academic Medicine, 87*(12): 1762–7.

Lynch, L., Happell, B. & Sharrock, J. (2008). Clinical supervision: An exploration of its origins and definitions. *International Journal of Psychiatric Nursing Research, 13*(2): 1–19.

Mental Health Nurse Education Taskforce (2008). *Final Report. Mental Health in Pre-Registration Nursing Courses*. Melbourne: Mental Health Workforce Advisory Committee.

Ministry of Health (2005). *Te Tahuhu: Improving Mental Health 2005–2015: The second New Zealand mental health and addiction plan*. Wellington: Author

Ministry of Health (2006). *Looking Forward and Moving Forward Together with TeKokiri: The Mental Health and Addiction Action Plan 2006–2015*. Wellington: Author.

Mullarkey, K., Keeley, P. & Playle, J. F. (2001). Multiprofessional clinical supervision: Challenges for mental health nurses. *Journal of Psychiatric and Mental health Nursing, 8*: 205–11.

Ning L. (2010). Building a 'user driven' mental health system. *Advances in Mental Health, 9*: 112–15.

O'Brien L. & Cole R. (2004). Mental health nursing practice in acute psychiatric close observation areas. *International Journal of Mental Health Nursing, 13*: 89–99.

Reeves, S., Lewin, S., Espin, S., & Zwarenstien, M. (2010). *Interprofessional Teamwork for Health and Social Care*. Iowa: Blackwell Publishing.

Rosenfield, M. (2003). Telephone counseling and psychotherapy in practice. In S. Goss & K. Anthony (eds), *Technology in Counseling and Psychotherapy: A practitioner's guide*. Great Britain: Palgrave Macmillan.

Sirola-Karvinen, P. & Hyrkas, K. (2008) Administrative clinical supervision as evaluated by the first line managers in one health care organization district. *Journal of Nursing Management, 16*: 588–600.

Sood, A. & Driscoll, J. (2004) Clinical supervision in practice: A working model. *Macmillan Voice Sharing Good Practice, 29 (Spring)*. Retrieved from www.supervisionandcoaching.com/pdf/page2/CS%20&%20 Radiography%20%28Driscoll%20&%20Sood%202004%29.pdf.

Storm M., Hausken K. & Mikkelson A. (2010). User involvement in in-patient mental health services: Operationalisation, empirical testing and validation. *Journal of Clinical Nursing, 19*: 1897–1907.

Walsh, K., Nicholson, J., Keough, C., Pridham, R., Kramer, M. & Jeffrey, J. (2003). Development of a group model of clinical supervision to meet the needs of a community mental health nursing team. *International Journal of Nursing Practice, 9*: 33–9.

Warner, R. (2009). Recovery from schizophrenia and the recovery model. *Current Opinion in Psychiatry, 22*: 374–80.

Yegdich, T. (1999). Clinical supervision and managerial supervision: Some historical and conceptual considerations. *Journal of Advanced Nursing 30*(5): 1195–1204.

Yegdich, T. & Cushing, A. (1998). An historical perspective on clinical supervision in nursing. *Australian and New Zealand Journal of Mental Health Nursing, 7*: 3–24.

15

Conclusions: Looking to practice

Nicholas Procter

Introduction 337
A message of leadership 337
The need to self-question 337

Clinical mentoring and empowerment 338
References 340

Introduction

By now readers of this book would have been thinking quite deeply about the topic of mental health and the practical ways in which they might collaborate with and support people with a mental illness, their families and carers. The preceding chapters have given considerable emphasis to a narrative approach. This final chapter is orientated towards a discussion of leadership – particularly for new entrants into mental health settings.

Effective clinical care requires consideration being given to the lives and needs of consumers, carers and families, and having all of this richness combined with evidence-based practice. At the heart of the decision to take this approach in this book has been the fundamental belief in human connectedness. Each of the chapters contained within this book has set about encouraging discovery and learning by making sensitive revisions regarding the ways in which nursing, health and human services practices can be made more meaningful in the lives of those who need them.

By working through each of the chapters, readers will have been challenged to think about how and when to move in new ways when working with resilient and vulnerable people, which might be helpful across a range of practice settings when seeking to make a difference in the lives of people experiencing a mental illness. And while this is important in providing a theoretical and practical basis for care, it is at the point of care that effective leadership is required.

A message of leadership

What we say, do, think and feel as nurses and health professionals can be an expression of leadership. This approach speaks directly to the process of making sense of what people around us are doing together and how best to understand, engage and, as far as possible, be committed to support each other (Holm & Severinsson, 2010). Why is this important? Because there have been and continue to be reports of people with a mental illness not accessing any kind of mental health care. Some are being turned away. Others are being left behind. Many in the sector advocate that change is urgently needed, and that simply to continue with the current inadequate pace of reform, to perpetuate the same fragmented resource base, utilise the same governance structures and fail to invest in innovation is to condemn many of the most disadvantaged of our community to many more years of poor mental and physical health.

The need to self-question

Leadership in mental health is across all levels of practice, education and service delivery. While national governments set about committing to monetary investment, coordinated national leadership and accountability to design and build services, it will be the current and future generation of mental health professionals who will be called upon to respond. There will be, among many things, the need to self-question (Rozuel & Ketola, 2012). Leaders at all levels can begin by reflecting upon what it is they do and to what extent it is in the best interest of consumers, their families and clinical colleagues. Is he or she primarily a leader or a manager? Does she or he make long-term decisions about her or his own development, or does the employer? Does the leader have the *opportunity* to challenge? The *right* to challenge? Does he or she have the *obligation* to challenge what is happening within the practice setting (adapted from Goldsmith, 2003)?

For people entering the profession of mental health nursing, what might be the best way to influence and lead? Perhaps the answer begins with communicating respect and warmth, because 'Warmth is the conduit to influence: It facilitates trust and the communication and absorption of ideas. Prioritising warmth helps you connect immediately with those around you, demonstrating that you hear them, understand them, and can be trusted by them' (Cuddy, Kohut & Neffinger, 2013, p. 56).

Also important will be positive working relationships, healthy resolution of conflict, debriefing, support and discussion. This involves focusing on what practitioners say, do, think and feel, for leadership growth and capacity building. Empowerment for new and emerging leaders is, in this sense, more than 'being able to simply voice and opinion (although clearly that is important too); it gives a broad range of people the authority to make decisions and express points of view that matter' (Kets de Vries, 2001, p. 272).

Empowerment also contributes to the positive workplace culture required in an interdisciplinary world that is marked by potential collaborative failures across nursing and allied health care disciplines (see Freshwater, Cahill & Essen, 2013). The cultivation of positive workplace cultures can also be a platform for delivery of evidence-based practices and to foster a collaborative and supportive work environment (Clearly et al., 2011).

Clinical mentoring and empowerment

Clinical leadership and mentoring opportunities for beginning practitioners in mental health can also be seen as a reciprocal process whereby people learn from each other the clinical, professional and personal dynamics at play in order to recognise areas for personal and professional growth and further development. The idea being advanced here is that personal and professional leadership development in mental health practice can be inclusive of personal and professional goal setting and feedback to help identify best practices and provide a pathway to understanding of how to grow and move in new ways.

When workplace mentoring and support are done well, they can be greatly empowering, improving self-awareness and self-expression, facilitating self-discovery and the creation of new learning about emotional well-being (Kets de Vries, 2013).

Having a trusted advisor (for example) to facilitate practice-based mentoring can be an effective way to encourage and develop emerging leaders, with particular emphasis upon their creativity and imagination. This, in turn, facilitates depth of thinking and encourages mutual benefit as it allows those working in mental health to learn about how self-motivation and drive can assist in abandoning ineffective practices, attitudes and beliefs. Moreover, effective mentoring becomes a crucial means through which to help maintain a sense of purpose, commitment and ethical comportment in practice.

Expressed in this way, leadership in mental health draws upon formal and informal networks and supports, which are mutually beneficial and incentive building. In meeting these challenges Procter (2003) identified the following enabling objectives:

- Remain accessible to consumers and carers as well as clinical colleagues and clinical mentors, for ongoing development and learning, encouragement and support.
- Generate through negotiation and consultation a professionally appropriate feedback loop for professional practice to freely present views and experiences.
- Ensure development of initiatives aimed at targeting areas for future growth and development for optimal service delivery to consumers and their families.
- In consultation with fellow clinical staff, seek out opportunities for interprofessional exchange and support in the workplace.
- Demonstrate emotional intelligence. Emerging leaders know how to manage their own emotions and read the emotions of others. Possessed of a good sense of reality, they are aware of their strengths and weaknesses, know what they stand for and know how to establish and maintain relationships for the better (Kets de Vries, 2001).
- Make time for confidential debriefing with managers and/or mentors about the nature and scope of your involvement with clients, their families and other mental health professionals.
- Be actively involved in what is happening in the workplace without feeling the need for rigid control.

This approach is, therefore, a reflective and dynamic one with scope and potential for autobiographical connections to be made between clinical practice, mentors and mental health service reform. Importantly, the personal and professional development opportunities engaged in are made more relevant and meaningful, rather than far removed from the day-to-day realities of professional practice (Procter, 2003).

Viewed in this way, your journey as an emerging leader is marked by personal and professional growth. At the outset of this process, mentors and other trusted guides are central to discussion of professional and personal goals. These initial discussions – later to be incorporated into an individualised professional development process – are designed to explore the range of various perceived needs *before* planning any specific learning objectives. In addition, there should be scope and freedom to review goals and re-think direction in light of feedback from colleagues and others. The main purpose is to create learning opportunities in the context of a cohesive, dynamic team in which people feel valued and involved without the burden of unrealistic expectations – either self-imposed or originating from an external source. Mentoring and career support in mental health settings is, in this sense, a means by which to identify personal characteristics, enhance inherent skills and improve individual development. In addition to this, leadership growth and development for emerging leaders in mental health within one discipline may facilitate the development of new leadership attributes in another (Jenkins, 2012).

References

Clearly, M., Horsfall, J., Deacon, M. & Jackson, D. (2011). Leadership and mental health nursing. *Issues in Mental Health Nursing*, 32: 632–639.

Cuddy, A.J.C., Kohut, M. & Neffinger, J. (2013). Connect, then lead. *Harvard Business Review*, July–August: 55–61.

Freshwater, D., Cahill, J. & Essen, C. (2013). Discourses of collaborative failure: Identity, role and discourse in an interdisciplinary world. *Nursing Inquiry*. First online, DOI:10.1111/nin.1203.

Goldsmith, M. (2003). The changing role of leadership. In L. Segil, M. Goldsmith & J. Belasco (eds). *Partnering: The new face of leadership*. New York: American Management Association.

Holm, A.L. & Severinsson, E. (2010). The role of mental health nursing leadership. *Journal of Nursing Management*, 18: 463–71.

Jenkins, D.M. (2012). Exploring signature pedagogies in undergraduate leadership education. *Journal of Leadership Education*, 11: 1–27.

Kets de Vries, M. (2001). *The Leadership Mystique: A user's manual for the human enterprise*. London: Prentice Hall.

Kets de Vries, M.F.R. (2013). Coaching's 'good hour': Creating tipping points. *Coaching: An International Journal of Theory, Research and Practice*. First online, DOI: 10.1080/17521882.2013.806944.

Procter, N.G. (2003). Leadership and mentoring for mental health service reform. Editorial. *Contemporary Nurse*, 14: 223–6.

Rozuel, C. & Ketola, T. (2012). A view from within: Exploring the psychology of responsible leadership. Guest editorial. *Journal of Management Development*, 31: 444–8.

Index

Aboriginal and Torres Strait Islander Healing
        Foundation Development Team, 53, 64
Aboriginal mental health workers, 318
Aboriginal people
    Aboriginal identity, 60–62
    Aboriginal worldviews, 55
    alcoholism, 63
    assimilation policy, 52
    biomedical model of health, 53
    child removal policy, 52
    cigarette smoking, 150
    colonisation, 52, 54–55
    cultural bias, 68
    culture, 53–54
    cumulative trauma, 63
    ecological trauma, 62
    fair-skinned issue, 61
    government policies, 56–62
        assimilation, 56–57
        BTH Report recommendations, 57
        child removals, 52
        formal apology, 58–59
    healing, 65–67
    historical and contemporary circumstances, 53
    identity, 55
    identity loss, 62
    intergenerational trauma, 63
    kinship, 55
    mental health assessment, 107
    mental health examination, 167
    monoculturalism, 68
    resilience, 52
    situational trauma, 62
    social and emotional well-being, 52–53
    terra nullius, 54
    trauma, 62–64
    trauma-informed practice, 64
Accessibility Remoteness Index of Australia, 289
ACMHN. *See* Australian College of Mental
        Health Nursing Inc.
ageism
    advance directives, 271–72
    being-with, 267
    bradyphrenia, 268

capacity, 270–71
care giving, 277
care receiving, 277
careers of older people, 279–79
cognitive decline, 273
competency, 270–71
courtesy stigma, 264
culture of, 267–68
definition, 263
delirium, 274
dementia, 275–76, 278
depression, 273
dignity of risk, 269
elder abuse, 269
ethic of care framework, 277
future of, 278–80
guiding principles, 266
homophobia, 267
human connectedness, 268–71
intellectual disability, 276
interprofessional connections, 280
life tasks, 265–66
medico-legal aspects, 270
mental health problems, 271–72
mental illness, 276
myths of, 264–65
negative attitudes, 264
nursing workforce, 279–80
Parkinson's disease, 288
reasonable standard of living, 263
recovery, 266
reminiscence therapy, 265
safe-sex messages, 267
sexual abuse, 267
social cohesion, 264
suicidal ideation, 267
suicide and, 276–77
AHPRA. *See* Australian Health Practitioners
        Regulation Authority
alcohol, 140
    binge drinking, 140
    depressant drug, 140
    explanation for use, 145–46
    long-term consumption, 140

low-risk drinking, 140
mental health, 158–61
mood disorders, 74
motivational interviewing, 159
solution-focused therapy, 159–60
stages of change, 159
withdrawal from, 140
alcohol abuse, 64
Alcohol Tobacco Other Drug Services, 66
alcoholism, 63
American Psychiatric Association, 110
amphetamines, 142
ANMAC. *See* Australian Nurses & Midwifery
    Accreditation Council
antenatal clinic, 189
antidepressant, 45, 180, 181
anti-psychotics, 181, 183
anxiety
    benzodiazepine use, 143
    comorbidity, 4
    co-occurrence, 4
    incidence, 4
    Māori population, 74
    mental illness, 5
    nicotine use, 144
    obsessions, 100
    pregnancy, 223
    raised level, 271
    refugee and asylum seeker, 201
    young people, 257
APA. *See* American Psychiatric Association
APS. *See* Australian Psychological Society
ARIA. *See* Accessibility Remoteness Index of
    Australia
assessment
    Aboriginal mental health, 107
    CANFOR–S, 108–9
    forensic psychiatry, 107–8
    in custody, 108
    physical health, 189
    risk-based, 103–4
    standard tools, 182
    strengths-based, 104–5
assimilation, 52
assimilation policy, 52
Assistants in Nursing, 316
ATODS. *See* Alcohol Tobacco Other Drug
    Services

Australaian Human Rights Commissions, 218
Australian Association of Occupational
    Therapists, 317
Australian College of Mental Health Nursing,
    Inc., 316
Australian Health Practitioners Regulation
    Authority, 316
Australian Health Professions Registration
    Authority, 321
Australian Nurses & Midwifery Accreditation
    Council, 316
Australian Psychological Society, 317

baby boomers, 263, 275
behavioural risk, 8
benzodiazapine, 143–44
Billabong Clubhouse, 301–2
biomedical model of psychiatry, 12
bipolar disorder, 74
BMI. *See* body mass index
body mass index, 176
bradyphrenia, 268
Bringing Them Home, 57, 60, 61
BTH. *See Bringing Them Home*

caffeine, 140–1
Camberwell Assessment of Need, 108, 109
CAN. *See* Camberwell Assessment of Need
cancers, 178–79
CANFOR–S assessment, 108–9
cannabis, 141
cardiovascular disease, 7, 168, 176
    Framingham risk equation, 176
    lifestyle factors, 176
    prevalence of, 176
'Care without Coercion' principles, 131
case management model, 298–99
caste system, 73
Catholicism, 12
causative factors, 63
CCHC. *See* culturally competent human
    connectedness
central obesity, 174
cerebrovascular disease, 8
child removal policy, 52, 58, 60
Children of Parents with a Mental
    Illness, 258
chronic respiratory disease, 8

cis-normativity, 219
nursing context, 219
clang association, 100
clergy, 319
clinical facilitator, 30
clinical mentoring, 338–40
confidential debriefing with
superiors, 339
consumer accessibility, 339
emotional intelligence demonstration, 339
fellow staff consultation, 339
initiative development, 339
negotiation and consultation, 339
workplace mentoring, 338
clinical nurse specialist, 316
clinical placement
features, 39
interactions record, 20
objectives, 38–40
pragmatic strategies, 42–43
clinical reasoning cycle, 35
clinical supervision, 35–37, 327–30
aim of, 327
benefits of, 328
cognitive therapy supervision, 328
definition, 327
effectiveness of, 37
form of, 37
formative function, 37
framework, 328
group, 329
innovative means, 36
interactive elements of, 328
managerial connotation, 36
models for, 329
nature of, 327
normative (accountability) function, 328
participation in, 37
psychotherapy-based model, 328
purpose of, 327
rates of, 37
reflective skills, 329
restorative function, 37, 328
solution-focused supervision, 328
supervision specific model, 328
supportive relationship, 36
telephone, 329
workplace culture, 328

clinical supervision for novice
nurses, 35–38
clinical supervision, 36–37
mentorship, 35–36
preceptorship, 35
Clubhouse model, 302
CoAG. See Council of Australian
Governments
cocaine, 142
cognitive behavioural therapy program, 300
cognitive brain activity, 148
cognitive decline, 273
cognitive therapy (CT) supervision, 328
collaboration, 29
collaborative practice, 18–20
colonisation
Aboriginal people, 52, 54–55
alienation, 82
definition, 52
impact of, 52, 60, 68
intergenerational trauma, 10
communication skills, 39
community participation, 292
community participation models, 292
community treatment order, 121, 172
comorbidities, 166, 168–73
cardiovascular disease, 168
diagnostic overshadowing, 168
high blood pressure, 168
metabolic syndrome, 168
obesity, 168
psychosis or crisis experiences, 173
recovery oriented medication, 173
smoking, 168
type 2 diabetes, 168
consumer-centred care, 324, 329
Convention on the Rights of Persons with
Disabilities, 122, 123, 166, 172
coping skills, development of, 17
COPMI. See Children of Parents with a
Mental Illness
coronary heart disease, 8
Council of Australian Governments, 291
counter-transference, 30
critical thinking process, 34–35
CTO. See community treatment order
cultural backgrounds, 74
cultural competency/responsiveness, 198

cultural safety
    historical component, 75
    Māori population, 76
culturally competent human connectedness, 224
culture
    Aboriginal and Torres Strait Islander,
        53–54, 151
    definition, 53
    diversity, 150
    explanatory models, 203–6
    influence, 150
    kava, 150
    older people, 267–68
    workplace, 328, 338
    young people's, 246

debriefing, 31
delirium
    ageism, 273–74
    diagnosis, 110
    management, 274
    mortality, 274
    symptoms, 274
dementia
    ageism, 275
    alcohol related, 140
    Alzheimer's, 275
    baby-boomers, 275
    diagnosis of, 275
    Down syndrome, 276
    language loss, 207
    management, 275, 276
    offenders and, 278
    Parkinson's related, 268
    risk factor, 278
dental health, 182–84
    periodontal disease, 183
    prevalence of comorbidities, 183
    psychotropic medications, 183
    xerostomia, 183
depressants, 139
depression
    ageism, 273
    alcohol, 140
    cannabis, 141
    cocaine, 142
    depressed mood, 5
    diabetes, 175
    low self-esteem, 5

    neuro-vegetative feature, 45
    pregnancy, 223
    prevalence of, 175
    psychological interventions, 273
    psychotic, 45
    reduced energy, 5
    refugee and asylum seeker, 201
    respiratory, 143
    young people, 257
    young psychotic, 45
developmental milestones, 83
diabetes, 8, 175
    delay in diagnosis, 175
    eye damage and blindness, 175
    kidney impairment, 175
    occurrence of, 175
    rate of, 175
    type 2, 168, 174
diabetes educator, 189
Diagnostic and Statistical Manual of Mental
        Disorders, 110, 222, 273
diagnostic criteria, 45, 90, 111
diagnostic overshadowing, 168
dialectical behaviour therapy, 235
dietitians, 319
dignity of risk, 269
Disorders of Sex Development, 220
Drug and Alcohol Practitioners Association of
        Aotearoa, 327
drugs
    explanation for use, 145–47
    holistic framework for misuse, 146–47
    model of care, 158–61
    motivational interviewing, 159
    solution-focused therapy, 159–60
    stages of the change, 159
dry mouth. See xeriostomia
DSD. See Disorders of Sex Development
DSM. See Diagnostic and Statistical Manual of
        Mental Disorders
Duluth model, 231, 239
dyslipidaemia, 174
dysphagia, 184–85
    behavioural factors, 185
    fast-eating syndrome, 185

elder abuse, 269
electroconvulsive therapy, 119
e-mental health, 252–56

cognitive behavioural therapy interventions, 252

smiling mind application, 252

SMS, 252

social media, 252

young people, 252–53

emerging professions, 318–20

Aboriginal mental health workers, 318–19

clergy, 319

consumer consultants, 318–19

counsellor, 310

dietitians, 319

hospital and community pharmacists, 320

paramedics, 320

peer support, 318–19

police, 319–20

speech pathologists, 319

Technical and Further Education (TAFE) preparation, 320

welfare worker, 321

emotional competence, 34

ability to respond, 34

development of, 26

emotional intelligence, 34

interpretation ability, 34

recognising ability, 34

emotional exhaustion, 44

empathy, 28–29

endocrinologist, 170, 171, 172, 189, 221, 226, 227, 228

Enduring Power of Attorney (EPA), 270

ethical framework, 118–19

electroconvulsive therapy, 119

human rights, 119

principles, 119

ethical influences, 41

explanatory model of mental health, 203

Facebook, 252, 300

face-to-face early intervention, 298

family violence, 9, 64, 223

family/partner violence, 231

internal homo-negativity, 231

minority-group stress, 231

sexual terrorism, 231

fast-eating syndrome, 185

FIFO. See fly-in/fly-out

flight of ideas, 100

fly-in/fly-out, 305

Forensic Mental Health Act, 331

forensic psychiatry, 107

CANFOR–S, 108

HoNOS, 108

HoNOS – secure, 108

formative function, 37

gay and lesbian activism, 222

gender

continuums of, 218–19

cultural framework, 219

fluidity, 221

gender and sexual diversity, 219

gender identities, 218

health and, 223–24

child birth, 223

distress during the perinatal period, 224

pregnancy, 223

role of nurses, 223

sexual violence, 224

human connectedness, 224

intersex, 220

LGBTTIQ, 219

pathologising, 222

power and, 223

rights-based approach, 120

self-identification, 220

transgender, 218

gender identities, 218

genetic factors, 12

Guardianship Board, 122

half-castes, 57, 60

hallucinogens, 139

harm minimisation, 138

definition, 138

demand reduction, 138

stakeholder partnerships, 138

supply reduction, 138

headspace, 245

headspace model, 298

healing

Aboriginal people, 65–67

definition, 58

painful part, 60

Healing Forum Working Group, 62

Health Consumer Treatment Act, 131

Health Improvement Profile, 187

health insurance scheme, 182

Health of the Nation Outcome Scales, 108
Health Practitioners Competence Assurance
        Act, 321
hepatitis, 143, 179, 203
hetero-normativity, 219, 222
hetero-sexism, 222
high blood pressure, 168
HIV/AIDS, 143, 179
homelessness, 9, 41
homophobia, 228
Homosexual Law Reform Act, 222
homosexuality, 222
        bio-medical views, 226
HoNOS. *See* Health of the Nation Outcome
        Scales
hospital and community pharmacists, 320
hub and spoke model, 297
human connectedness, 128
hyperglycaemia, 8, 174–75
hyperlipidaemia, 8, 175, 176
hypertension, 8, 176

ICD. *See* International Classification of Diseases
institutional racism, 74, 76
Interactive Framework of Clinical
        Supervision, 328
International Classification of Diseases, 110
International Diabetes Federation, 175
International Hearing Voices Movement, 173
interpersonal abuse, 229–31
interpersonal skills, 31
        courteous curiosity, 31
        feedback request, 31
        learning opportunity, 30
        manner and methods, 31
interpersonal trauma, 231–33
        betrayal, 231
        childhood abuse, 233
        organised sexual exploitation, 233
        powerlessness, 231
        stigmatisation, 231
        traumatic effects, 232
        traumatic sexualisation, 231
interprofessional approach, 312
interprofessional connections, 20–21, 46
        importance of, 20
        initial contact with consumers, 20
interprofessional workforce, 323–26
        composition of, 324

effectiveness of, 323–26
        recovery model, 323
        symptom management, 324
intimacy, notion of, 223
involuntary treatment, 124–25
IPT implementation, barriers, 325–26
        reciprocal interdependence, 325
        teamwork, 324–25

kava, 150
Kawa whakaruruhau, cultural safety, 75–78

leadership message, 337
        positive relationship, 338
        warmth prioritising, 338
Learning Circles program, 65
legal framework
        advance directives, 121, 130
        alternatives to, 130
        compulsory treatment, 120
        crisis plans, 130
        dangerousness standard, 121
        human rights, and, 122–23
        involuntary treatment, 124–25
        mental health law, 122–23
        mental health legislation, 130–32
        nature of the power, 33
        need for treatment standard, 121
        police rationale, 121
        police role, 121
        procedural justice, 126–29
        reciprocity and recovery, 123–24
        right to voluntary treatment, 120
life expectancy, 7–8
        mental illness, 211
lifestyle clinics, 187
lifestyle factors, 176

Madhouses Act 1774 (UK), 120
manaakitanga, 81
Māori model, 87
Māori population
        access to mental health, 75
        anxiety, 74
        background, 74–75
        bipolar disorder, 74
        colonisation, 75
        cultural safety, 75
        Hapū, 75

Hauora, 75, 78–80
initial nursing assessment, 86
institutional racism, 76
Iwi, 76
Kaumatua, 77
Kawa whakaruruhau (cultural safety),
    75–78
Kuia, 77
levels of engagement, 81
manaakitanga, 81
mood disorder, 74
oranga (wellness), 78–80
Rangatiratanga, 76
re-traumatisation, 82
schizophernia, 74
sense of belonging, 85
social structures, 77
socio-economic need, 74
storytelling, 81
suicide rate, 75
Tamariki, 77
Taonga, 76
Te Taha Hinengaro (thoughts and emotions),
    80
Te Whare Tapa Wha (the four sided house),
    79–80
Ten Commitments, 80–82
Tikanga Maori, 76
trauma-informed care, 82
Treaty of Waitangi, 75–76
Whakaruruhau, 76
Whanau ora, 76
whanaungatanga, 76
Māori-specific programs, 77
Marriage Amendment Bill, 222
Medicare, 189
mental disorders
    classification, 110
    diagnosis of, 110–12
    mental state examination, 111
    psychiatric diagnoses, 111
    symptoms classification, 110
mental health
    Aboriginal mental health assessment, 107
    alcohol model of care, 158–61
    assessment, 90
    assessment process, 93, 95–97
    BATOMI PJR, 98
    conditions, 90

    definition, 90
    diagnosis, 90
    drug model of care, 158–61
    evidence-based approaches, 90
    explanatory model, 203
    forensic psychiatry, 107–8
    listening to understand, 93–94
    meaning of, 90–91
    mental status examination, 98–104
    motivational interviewing, 159
    neurological dysfunction, 91
    nursing assessment, 90, 91, 95, 97
    person-environment approach, 97
    professional boundaries of nurse, 94
    sensitive topics, 94
    solution-focused therapy, 159–60
    stages of the change, 159
    strengths-based assessment, 104–6
    substance use and, 158
    therapeutic communication, 92–95
    Tidal Model, 106
    WHO definition, 91
*Mental Health (Compulsory Assessment
    and Treatment) Act 1992*, 120, 123,
    124, 128, 270
Mental Health Act 1990 (NSW), 33
Mental Health Act 2009 (SA), 6
Mental Health Incentive Program, 316
mental health legislation, 130–32
Mental Health Nurses Incentive
    Program, 295
mental health nursing, 13–14, 38
    caring and compassion, 13
    collaborative practice, 18–20
    encouraging, 15
    interprofessional connections, 20
    practice standards, 37
    proactive in care, 15
    as a specialist field, 15–16
    supporting and advocating, 15
    therapeutic, 13
    trust, importance of, 15
mental health workforce regulation, 321–23
    *Health Practitioners Competence Assurance
    Act 2003*, 321
    national registration scheme, 321
    regulated health professions, 321
mental illness, 4–6
    affective condition, 5

anxiety, 5
assessment, 90
beliefs, 11–13
community, 6
community awareness, 11
contemporary approach, 6
homelessness, 9
life expectancy, 7–8
organisation, 7
perpetual discrimination, 10
risk, 9
social determinants, 6–7
stigma, 10–11
stress, and, 10
substance misuse, 5–6
violence, 9
whole society, 7
mental state assessment, 16
mental status examination, 98–104
    affect, 99–100
    behaviour and appearance, 98–99
    dress, 98
    facial expression, 99
    insight, 102
    judgement, 103
    mood, 101
    motor activity, 99
    orientation, 101
    perception, 102
    physical characteristics, 99
    posture, 99
    risk assessment, 103–4
    speech, 99
    thought content, 100
    thought content disturbances, 100–1
    thought form, 100
mentorship, 30, 35–36
metabolic syndrome, 168, 174–75
    cardiometabolic measures and, 174
    incidence of, 7
    prevalence of, 8, 174
    risk factors, 174
    social factors, 174
methamphetamine, 142
MetS. See metabolic syndrome
MHNIP. See Mental Health Nurses Incentive
        Program
Midwifery Board of Australia, 322

Mihi, 73
misogyny, 223
monoculturalism, 68
mood disorder, 74
MSE. See mental status examination
multidisciplinary approach, 312
myCompass, 300

N-acetylcysteine infusion, 145
narrative approach, 3–4
    mechanistic style of engagement, 3
    special meaning, 3
    storytelling, 3
National Aboriginal and Torres Strait Islander
        Health Council, 52
National Mental Health Commission, 260
National Mental Health Working Group, 52
national registration scheme, 321
National Standards for Mental Health Services,
        333
NCD. See non-communicable disease
New Zealand College of Mental Health Nursing,
        Inc., 316
nicotine, 144
non-aspiration choking, 185
non-communicable disease, 8, 166
non-suicidal self-injury, 256
noradrenalin, 148
normative functions, 37
novice nurses
    challenges for, 37
    clinical supervision, 35–38
    development of, 35
    preceptorship, 36
NSWNMA. See Nursing Midwifery Association
nurse–patient relations, 32
nursing assessment, 90
Nursing Council of New Zealand, 75, 316, 327
nursing education, 26–28
    clinical application, 27
    communication skills, 27
    community, 27
    education curricula, 27
    forensic, 27
    non-government, 27
    stereotypes, 27
    stigma, 27
    theoretical component, 27

theoretical instruction, 27
Nursing Midwifery Association, 314
nursing placements, 46, 47
nutritional patterns, 178

obesity, 7, 168, 174, 175, 176–78
    anti-psychotic medications, and, 177
    psychotropic drugs, and, 177
    psychotropic medications, 177
    reduced income/poverty, 177
opioids, 142–43
over-the-counter medications, 145

paracetemol, 145
paracetamol toxicity nomograph tool, 145
paramedics, 320
Parkinson's disease, 268
pathologising, 32
person-centred approach, 299
personal awareness, 76
personal disclosure, level of, 83
personal problem solving, 40
personal skills, development of, 11
petrol sniffing, 66, 144
physical health assessment, 188
physical ill health, prevalence of, 166
physical illnesses, 174–80
    cancers, 178–79
    cardiovascular disease, 176
    diabetes, 175
    hyperglycaemia, 175
    hyperlipidaemia, 175–76
    nutritional patterns, 178
    obesity, 176–78
physiology courses, 46
piper methysticum. See kava
police, 319–20
political influences, 41
post-traumatic stress disorder, 232
Power and Control Wheel, 230
pragmatic strategies, 42–44
    communication, 42–43
    looking after, 43
    preparation, 42
preceptorship, 30, 36
premature death, 167
problem-solving skills, development of, 17
procedural delivery model, 28

procedural justice, 126–28
professional associations, 322
professional bodies, 322
    role of, 322
professional boundaries, 30–31
    maintenance of, 32
    transgression of, 30
professional precedents, historical, 312–13
Protection of Personal Property Rights Act 1988,
        270
psychological trauma, 229–31
psychosis, 257
psychosomatic component, 45
PTSD. See post-traumatic stress disorder

recovery, 17
recovery model, 324, 325
Recovery orientated prescribing and medicines
        management, 173
reform agenda, 41
refugee camps, 203
Refugee Convention, 201
refugees and asylum seekers
    anxiety, 201
    clinical assessment, 207
    cultural models, 203–5
    culturally and linguistically diverse (CALD), 207
    definitions, 198
    depression, 201
    explanatory models, 203–4
    helping strategies, 207
    isolation, 206–7
    lack of English proficiency, 207
    mainstream mental health services, 207–8
    meaning, 200–1
    mental health, 201
    monocultural business as usual approach,
        208
    older people, 211–12
    physical ill-health, 169
    post-traumatic stress, 201
    protective factors, 202
    risk, 202
    therapeutic sensitivity, 207
    traumatic stress, 208–10
    urban sprawl, 207
    Western medical model, 204
registered training organisations, 316

reminiscence therapy, 265
remoteness zones, 289
resilience
    development of, 103, 258
    meaning of, 52
    strengthening capacity, 304
    treatment model, 324
restorative function
    clinical supervision, 37
    elements of, 328
Right to Treatment order, 131
risk-based assessment, 103
RTO. See Right to Treatment order
RUOK Day, 245
Rural Adversity Mental Health Program, 297
rural and regional communities
    agriculture, 305
    bed-based mental health services, 299
    benefits of, 296
    careers, 295
    community-based recovery, 301
    community mental health, 298–99
    early intervention, 297–98
    e-mental health, 299–301
    hub and spoke model, 297
    itinerant workforces, 305
    limitations of, 296
    mental health promotion and prevention,
        297–303
    mental health services, 296
    mining, 305
    natural disasters, 304
    prevalence, 294–96
    prevalence of mental health problems, 294
    primary health services, 298–99
    recovery and rehabilitation, 301–3
    rural implications, 304–5
    rural mental health services, 301
    rural residency risk, 295
    self-care mood monitoring program, 300
    suicide rates, 295
    telehealth, 299–301
    travel implications, 303
rural recovery system, 289
rural residency, risk factors, 295
rural stoicism, 288

same-sex couples, 222
schizophrenia

    comorbidity, 4
    diagnosis of, 8, 12, 108, 178, 185
    family violence, 9
    low life expectancy, 7
    Māori population, 74
    mortality ratio, 8
    perpetual discrimination, 10
    prevalence of, 175
    smoking, 181
score-based assessment, 103
screening interventions, 187
screening tools, 187
selective serotonin re-uptake inhibitors, 180
self-assessment, 40
self-care, 229
SEWB. See social and emotional well-being
sexual abuse, 82, 149
sexual assault, 12
sexual dysfunction, 172, 179–80
sexual orientations, 218
sexual terrorism, 231
sexual violence, 224
sexuality
    cis-normativity, 219
    continuums of, 218–19
    cultural framework, 219
    definition, 218–19
    gender and sexual diversity, 219
    hetero-normativity, 219, 222–23
    hetero-sexism, 222–23
    human connectedness, 224–25
    intersex, 220
    LGBTTIQ, 219
    pathologising, 222
    power and, 223
    rights-based approach, 226
    self-identification, 220
    sexual orientations, 218
sexually transmitted diseases, 179
    hepatitis, 179
    HIV/AIDS, 179
    sexual disinhibition, 179
    sexual dysfunction, 179–80
SHRG. See Social Health Reference Group
significant mental illness, 166
smoking, 180–81
    anti-psychotic medication, 181
    cessation of, 181
    cognitive deficits, 181

multifactorial reasons, 182
social and emotional well-being, 52–53, 66
social determinants, 6–7
    individual, 6
Social Health Reference Group, 52
social helpfulness, elements of, 292
social well-being, 91
solution-focused (SF) supervision, 328
solvents, 144
speech pathologists, 319
speech pathology courses, 46
SSRIs. See selective serotonin re-uptake
        inhibitors
St John of God, 313
standards, 322–23
    Improving Mental Health, 323
    recovery standard, 322
    service accreditation, 323
stereotypes, 27
stigma, 27
stimulants, 139
Stolen Generations, 57
    Aboriginal identity, 60
    formal apology, 58
    survivor of the, 58
strengths-based assessment, 104–6
    benefit, 105
    Strengths Model, 104
    Tidal Model, 104
Strengths Model, 104
stress
    coping strategies, 149
    drug use, 149
    financial, 256
    impacts of, 97
    levels of, 11
    marriage patterns, 55
    mental condition, 90
    nicotine use, 144
    therapeutic addressal, 143
    traumatic, 208–10
substance misuse, 5–6
substance use
    alcohol, 139, 140
    amphetamines, 142
    benzodiazapine, 143–44
    biological influences, 147
    caffeine, 140–41
    cannabis, 141

chocolate, biological impact, 147–48
cocaine, 142
cultural influences, 150–51
depressants, 139
developmental influences, 151
drugs, 139
drugs groups, 139
ecological influences, 151
hallucinogens, 139
holistic care model, 146
mental health and, 158–59
methamphetamine, 142
nicotine, 144
opioids, 142–43
paracetemol, 145
psychological influences, 148–49
social influences, 149–50
solvents, 144
spiritual influences, 151
stimulants, 139
synthetic drugs, 141
suicidal ideation, 44, 45, 267, 276, 277
synthetic drugs, 141
TAFE. See Tertiary and Further Education sector
Tangata whaii te ora, 74
team work, 24–25
    biomedical models, 235
    co-dependence, 325
    evidence-based therapies, 324
    recovery model, 324
Technical and Further Education (TAFE)
        preparation, 580
telehealth, 298, 299–301
Temporary Protection Visas 201
Tertiary and Further Education sector, 316
therapeutic alliance, 29
    between person and nurse, 108
    mental state assessment, 16
    therapist contributions, 29
therapeutic communication, 92–95
therapeutic interaction model, 47
therapeutic optimism, 11, 17, 323
therapeutic relationship
    critical elements, 28, 29
    development, 229
    expense of, 131
    foundational component, 28
    foundational expense of, 269
    foundational foundations of, 238

importance of, 28
power relations, 31–33
TIC. *See* trauma-informed care
Tidal Model, 74, 81, 86, 106
traditional profession, 314–17
    medicine, 314–15
    nursing, 315–16
    occupational therapy, 317
    psychology, 317
    social work, 317
transference, 30
transphobia, 228
trauma
    Aboriginal people, 62–64
    brain injury, 278
    cumulative, 63
    definition, 58
    ecological, 62
    effects of, 232
    incidence of, 62–64
    informed care, 233–38
    intergenerational, 10, 63
    interpersonal, 231–33
    multiple layers, 62
    physical, 101
    psychological, 149, 229
    recovery stages, 234
    situational, 62
    types of, 62
    young people, 249–50
trauma-informed care, 208–10
    biomedical paradigm, 233
    collaborative investigation, 236
    dialectical behaviour therapy, 235
    medications, 235
    nurse's role, 233–38
    safety and stabilisation, 234–37
    self-soothing skills, 235
    social reconnection, 237
    trauma resolution, 237
traumatic stress, 208–10
    access and engagement, 210
    barriers to talking about trauma, 209–10
    principles of trauma-informed services, 209
    trauma-informed care, 208–9
    trust and human connectedness, 211
traumatising seclusion, 84
Treaty of Waitangi, 75–76, 86
Twitter, 252, 300

UK clinical supervision, 37
UK Physical Health Checklist, 187
United Nations High Commissioner for Refugees (UNHCR), 201
urban sprawl, 207
urinary incontinence, 181–82
    factors, 181
    impact of, 181

Waltzing Matilda, 290–91
welfare worker, 320
wellness clinics, 187
Westerman Aboriginal Symptom Checklist, 107
Whānau, 76
    caregiving role, 78
whanaungatanga, 76
workplace mentoring, 338
World Federation for Mental Health, 175

xeriostomia, 183

Yogyakarta principles, 228
young people
    alcohol abuse, 249
    anxiety, 257
    bullying, 250–51
    depression, 257
    developmental stages, 248–49
    drug abuse, 249
    early intervention, 252–55
    e-mental health, 252
    instilling hope, 255–56
    mental health problems, 256–57
    mental health promotion, 252–54
    non-suicidal self-injury, 256
    prevention, 252–54
    psychosis, 257
    rapport development, 246–48
    respect for, 245–46
    risk reduction, 249–50
    suicide, 256
    trauma, 249–50
    vulnerability, 249–50
    youth-focused early intervention, 245
    youth-friendly, 246
Youth Mental Health Declaration, 245

Zoloft withdrawal, 111